CHILDBIRTH IN AMERICA

DATE DUE

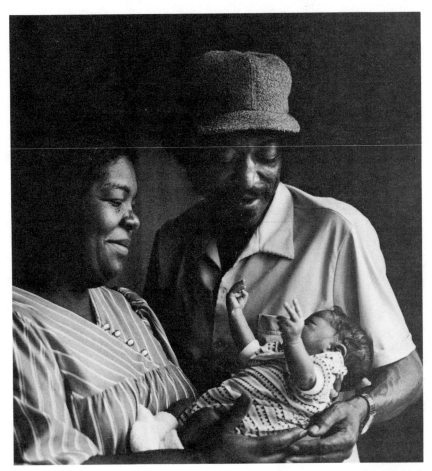

Photograph by LeRoy J. Dierker, Jr., M.D.

CHILDBIRTH IN AMERICA
Anthropological Perspectives

KAREN L. MICHAELSON
& CONTRIBUTORS

Bergin & Garvey Publishers, Inc.
MASSACHUSETTS

First published in 1988 by
Bergin & Garvey Publishers, Inc.
670 Amherst Road
South Hadley, Massachusetts 01075

890   987654321

Printed in the United States of America

Library of Congress Cataloging-in-Publication Data

Michaelson, Karen L.
     Childbirth in America: anthropological perspectives / Karen L.
  Michaelson & contributors.
     p. cm.
  Bibliography: p.
  Includes index.
     ISBN 0-89789-136-8 (alk. paper): $44.95. ISBN 0-89789-137-6 (pbk.: alk.
paper): $18.95
     1. Childbirth—Social aspects—United States. 2. Birth customs—United
States. I. Title.
RG652.M53   1988
392'.12'0973—dc19

                                                                    87-37490
                                                                       CIP

*To my mother, Sylvia Michaelson,
and my daughter, Jamaila Terrin Cohen-Michaelson*

CONTENTS

CHILDBIRTH IN AMERICA

INTRODUCTION

CHILDBIRTH IN AMERICA: A BRIEF HISTORY AND CONTEMPORARY ISSUES

Karen L. Michaelson

The time we have been waiting for has come.
A great wind sweeps through the old trees of the village,
*   bending them and shaking their fruit.*
One of the households has called the midwife....
It is the woman's time.
And now the house belongs to the women,
Busy whispering, heating water, warming oil.
The new father starts nervously as a horse at each
*   fresh sound from the house.*
And we joke with him.
Yes, life is in the balance, but we have been through
*   it all before.*

And now he is one of us.
For the mother-in-law appears and she is smiling.
And the first high cries continue like a new bird
*   chirping.*
The first lamp is lit.
There is laughing and congratulation.
Quickly announce it with music to the village.
And invite the neighbors....

—Aditi, The Living Arts of India

In every culture, the birth of a baby—the coming into being of a new member of society—is greeted with wonder and, usually, joy. Childbirth in itself is a culturally produced event (Jordan 1976; Mead and Newton 1967). "The act of giving birth to a child is never simply a physiological act but rather a performance defined by and enacted within a cultural context" (Romalis 1981). It is the culmination of the parents' cultural knowledge about self, body, gender,

1

and the meaning of social adulthood in a given society. Thus the history of childbirth in America and any discussion of contemporary issues surrounding birth must be seen in the context of the wider history of American culture.

THE TRANSITION FROM HOME TO HOSPITAL BIRTH

In British North America prior to 1760, birth at home was a "woman's affair," a social event that formed a basic part of the domestic culture in which women participated (Leavitt 1983; Smith-Rosenberg 1975; Wertz and Wertz 1977). When the time for birthing came, to help them through their travail, women gathered others who had been successful in childbirth. If necessary, even strange women would do, but a man, even if he were a skilled physician, could not be expected to understand this essentially female experience.

Equal to this desire to give birth in the company of other supportive women, however, was the fear of pain, complications and death which might accompany the birth of a child. The letters and diaries of women up through the mid-nineteenth century reflect this fear of being "down to death's door" (Leavitt 1982: 121) with each birth. Indeed, death in childbirth was not uncommon.

By the early nineteenth century, women from wealthy families began to invite male physicians into the previously female domain of the home birthing room to insure a safer birth. And as obstetric technology advanced, new techniques, such as the use of forceps and anesthesia, came under the control of these male obstetricians.

In actuality, these new techniques often caused more problems than they solved (Leavitt 1983). For example, during this period the standards of modesty prohibited male physicians from viewing the private parts of their patients, and thus the forceps were applied without benefit of sight. Countless stories testify to the severe lacerations nineteenth century women suffered in childbirth. And while the use of forceps might have provided a needed aid to the safe delivery of the infant whose progress was obstructed, their frequent overuse and misuse in normal labors resulted in an increase in perineal laceration (Leavitt 1983; Wertz and Wertz 1977).

Still, the majority of women in this period gave birth at home attended by midwives, for few could afford a physician's care. But for those who chose physicians, birth changed from an event controlled by fate to an experience where women could determine what kind of birth they would have. This perception of the ability to shape birth became more important when anesthesia was introduced in the second half of the nineteenth century. Ether and chloroform promised relief from pain during birth (Leavitt 1983: 291–92). By the late nineteenth century, the letters of middle class and wealthy women reflected a desire to turn the birth experience over to a physician in exchange for the comfort of his anesthesia and the apparent safety of his technology. As long as birth remained in the home, however, it was largely under women's control. The male physician attended the laboring woman under the careful observation of her women friends who might themselves have known as much about childbirth as he did. In the early twentieth century, however, women began to move from the home birthing room to the hospital—away from the comfort of female friends as attendants and midwives as care providers and into the hands of physicians and hospital staff. The real change in childbirth came in hospitals.

In the nineteenth century, maternity hospitals were asylums for the poor and homeless. Doctors and philanthropists believed these women needed medical treatment and moral uplift. Although less than 5 percent of women delivered in hospitals in 1900, the numbers increased dramatically in the 1920s (Wertz and Wertz 1977: 132–33). As doctors increasingly began to be looked upon as experts in the treatment of human ailments, it was not poor women who flocked to the hospital, but women of the middle and upper classes. By 1921 more than half the births in many American cities took place in hospitals. "The marked transformation in birth practice occurred because both women and doctors found hospital birth more efficient than home birth for accomplishing what they wanted" (Wertz and Wertz 1977: 133). The move to the hospital was hastened by the specialist's desire to wrest birth away from general practitioners and to systematize birth procedures within the hospital setting. (Leavitt 1983: 298). Dr. Joseph D. Lee's influential 1920 article,"The Prophylactic Forceps Operations," which reduced birth to predictable patterns by the routine use of outlet forceps and episiotomy in normal deliveries, made these procedures common in hospitals throughout the United States.

This transition to specialists and hospital birth settings was part of a larger movement toward professionalization in medicine and other fields. Increasingly, the advanced training needed to be a physician set doctors apart from lay practitioners and largely closed the profession to those who could not afford to pay for training. The training of physicians created a need for a flow of patients. This was provided by maternity hospitals for the poor, who gave up their modesty in exchange for physician-attended births. But, as physician-attended births became more and more fashionable because of the opportunity to have a painless birth through anesthesia, and as physicians increasingly desired to confine their deliveries to the structured hospital setting, women of all classes came to give birth in the hospital.

Although women sought hospital births for their safety and relief from pain, in the early part of the twentieth century hospitals were not particularly safe places to give birth. Infection spread easily in hospitals; more importantly, the misuse of drugs and the unnecessary use of innovations such as forceps kept in-hospital maternal mortality "unnecessarily high" (Leavitt 1983). By 1940, however, maternal and infant mortality had begun to decline, due to both the introduction of antibiotics and improved hospital practice (Shapiro et al. 1968). At this time, 55.8 percent of American women gave birth in hospitals (Devitt 1977). By 1955, 95 percent of American women gave birth in hospitals (Leavitt 1983: 301). Wealthy and poor alike labored "alone among strangers" in a situation over which they had little control.

While birth was safer in hospitals, women found this location a mixed blessing. For women living in a society where maids, cooks, and servants were no longer readily available, hospitals provided a quiet place to recuperate from childbirth. But these same hospitals were also sterile, frightening, and dehumanizing. When in 1957 the *Ladies Home Journal* printed a letter urging an investigation of "cruelty in maternity wards," it received hundreds of letters reporting experiences of dehumanization and lack of concern for mother and baby (Letters 1958). "Hospital delivery had become for many a time of alienation—from the body, from family and friends, from the community, and even from life itself. The safe efficiencies had become a kind of industrial production.... A woman was powerless in the experience of birth and unable to find meaning in it, for her participation in it, and even her consciousness of it were minimal" (Wertz and Wertz 1977: 173).

Although there were economic and ideological reasons for males to desire to control birth, Judith Leavitt (1982:122) points out that the perception of childbirth as a brush with death made women more willing to move to the hospital for greater safety. Women did not see this as a loss of an important part of the birth experience, but as relief from pain and a greater guarantee of life and health. In seeking apparent safety, however, they lost the strength of the company of friends.

CHILDBIRTH AND THE IDEOLOGY OF MOTHERHOOD

The transition from home to hospital and, more recently, from hospital to more homelike settings, does not merely reflect changes in medical technology or women's interaction with the medical profession. The single, most profound fact linking a woman's social role to the physiological act of childbirth is that in bearing a child, she becomes a mother. "Pregnancy and birth... herald enormous changes in the life of any mother. Even a woman who gives up her child for adoption at birth has undergone irreversible physiological and psychological changes in the process of carrying it to term and bearing it. And the woman who continues to mother will find the rhythms and priorities of her life changed in the most profound and also the most trivial ways" (Rich 1976:162). Motherhood is, after all, an institution with certain expectations for action which change over time (Badinter 1981; deBeauvoir 1953), and those expectations have changed with the evolution of women's roles in society.

The notion of full-time exclusive motherhood is fairly recent, a product of the last century and a half. Prior to that, women's work was a source of productive labor, not simply reproduction and nurturing. The home was the center of a family's livelihood, and women contributed to that by their work. Both parents contributed to the upbringing of their children, who in turn became productive members of the household. With industrialization, the home became less the center of family livelihood, and women's work became more a part of the private domain (Zaretsky 1973; Rich 1976).

Between 1900 and 1940, women's primary work became the upbringing of children. They were responsible for their children's physical and moral development from the moment of birth onward. But, women were not thought fit by virtue of their womanhood alone to be good mothers—they had to study the "science of mothering" (Margolis 1984:40–44). While women were transferring responsibility for childbirth to the medical profession, they were also transferring responsibility for childrearing to the advice of experts. Just as the rigidly controlled hospital birth experience stressed scheduling and the scientific management of birth women, were admonished to follow a rigid behaviorist pattern of control in raising their children. They were not to love and coddle their children, but to emphasize regularity, punctuality, discipline and cleanliness (Margolis 1984).

The 1940s and 1950s saw changes in the concept of motherhood. For one, mothers were urged to be more permissive with their children. But more significantly, women began to enter the workforce in increasing numbers. By 1950, 29.6 percent of the workforce were women; by 1960, 33.4 percent; by 1970, 38.1 percent; and by 1981, it had grown to 43 percent. What is more important is that these were not single women working until marriage or women working after their children had grown; they were women in their prime childbearing years and, increasingly, mothers of children under six years old.

Yet, even though more women entered the workforce in the 1940s and 1950s, a woman's primary responsibility was to her family, and especially to her children. Prior to 1960, "not only did women spend most of their adult energies raising a family rather than pursuing employment; this pattern was thought to be congruent with and supportive of a set of intrinsically female skills and preferences" (Luker 1984: 113). Even for those who worked, a paying job was merely an adjunct to women's primary role of mother. During this period the types of jobs largely open to women—low paying and low skilled—also made work less gratifying than motherhood as a primary role. Of course, for many women in American society, participation in the labor force was not new or optional. "Poor women and women of color have rarely had the luxury of being able to devote their energies full time to family care, whatever the cultural expectations" (Luker 1984: 113).

While the increased ability to limit family size made for fewer children in the home by the end of the 1950s, fewer children in the household did not imply less work for mothers, for their responsibility for creating "perfect children" grew proportionately. Indeed, in the 1950s mother and home were synonymous. Good mothers cared for and sacrificed for their children. Adrienne Rich (1976: 25) describes her becoming a mother "in the family-centered, consumer-oriented, Freudian-American world of the 1950s. My husband spoke eagerly of the children we would have; my parents-in-law awaited the birth of their grandchild. I had no idea of what I wanted...I only knew that to have a child was to assume adult womanhood." In that context, to father meant to beget; to mother meant to nurture as well as to bear a child. Childbirth had become a part of the view of motherhood as a total way of life. Nothing since Victorian literature equalled the reverence with which women's magazines of the 1940s and 1950s extolled home and maternity.

It was in this period that Grantly Dick-Read's ideas about "natural childbirth" became popular among the middle class, for he believed that birth was the exultation of motherhood. He believed that the moment of birth was a moment of ecstatic fulfillment that the doctor should not take away from a woman. His and Ferdinand LaMaze's "psychoprophylactic method" gave women the option of being conscious throughout the birth, even if they were not actually in control of the experience. His notion of the father sharing in the birth supported middle class notions of togetherness in marriage. Although the parents were to participate more actively in the birth experience, Dick-Read cautioned that the doctor ultimately knew best how to manage the laboring woman. Still, his notions were not widely accepted by American physicians of the time who thought that the natural process would take too long and disrupt carefully timed hospital routines.

THE MOVEMENT TOWARD CHANGES AND CHOICES

The 1960s, and particularly the 1970s, saw the publication of a number of books seeking the "demedicalization of childbirth" (Haire 1972; Arms 1975; among others). Many of these more polemical writings became part of the basis of the movement to regain what women began to feel had been taken from the birth experience. The rise of feminist ideologies in this period reemphasized the parturient woman's need of support from other women and her increasing desire to control the circumstances of her birthing.

Demands for greater personal control of birth came about precisely as women began to take for granted the safety of birth. The nineteenth-century women who saw birth as taking them down to death's door are a far cry from the contemporary women who perceive birth as being a far less risky business than obstetricians would have it seem (McClain 1981a,b). The notion that women have a "right" to control their own bodies and their medical treatment is a fairly recent phenomenon (Mundy 1983) and parallels broader changes in the concept of women's role in society.

The decade after the 1950s saw a growing conflict between the actuality of women's increasing participation in the workforce and the ideology of the mother at home. The opportunity for women to have status outside the home and family implied a devaluation of the idealized role of mother and wife. The media began to portray working mothers and even single mothers as optional role models. But the nurturing role remained, and the ideal mother became "superwoman," who had to balance job, children, and intimate relationships with ease. If before the 1970s working women were castigated, then since that time it is the woman who stays home who often feels the object of scorn (Goodman 1979). Luker (1984) notes that two very different notions of motherhood have developed, based on perceptions about the place women should occupy in society and about what proper family structure should be. The first, and older, conceptualization of motherhood assumes parenthood to be a natural state and values children over material things. Family influence and the presence of children often limit the options that a woman has in making life choices. The second conceptualization sees parenthood as a planned state and parenting as not simply a natural activity but one that provides the child with the best set of emotional, psychological, economic, and social resources that one can arrange (Luker 1984: 181). Motherhood is one option among many to consider in making life choices, and it does not preclude other options. For these women, motherhood has been demoted from a sacred calling to a job (Luker 1984: 205).

These two views of motherhood coexist in the present generation of women giving birth to their children and affect their planning for and experience of birth. Nelson (1983) reports that working-class women tend to focus on the outcome of the birth experience—the baby and motherhood—while middle-class women tend to see the birth itself as a separate and significant experience. Yet for most mothers today, some changes are common. In line with current notions of health and physical fitness, both pre- and postnatal exercise classes have become commonplace. Most middle-class women are concerned to some extent with the management of their birth experience and prepare for it by reading books that range from treatises on legal rights and spiritual midwifery to manuals on baby and child care. Paternal roles have also begun to change (Gral et al. 1981; Margolis 1984). A majority of husbands, particularly middle-class husbands, expect to accompany their spouses into labor and to witness the birth of their child. This reflects broader changes in mainstream American society where the intense bond of support between husband and wife has become primary over extended family ties. Even language has reflected this shift in roles: instead of using the terms "to mother" or "to father" with their weight of traditional meaning, the term "to parent" has become current as an indicator of active participation in childrearing by either gender.

THE CONTEXT OF CHOICE, CHANGE, AND CONTROL IN CHILDBIRTH

The late 1970s and early 1980s have seen an outpouring of books that offer women and men "choices in childbirth" (Feldman 1980, among others) and instruct parents how to negotiate a satisfactory birthing experience. Yet despite the increasing number of options, until quite recently most women have preferred to trust a medicated, hospitalized birth. Childbirth education, nearly universal in some communities, has made women more positive about birth, but for the most part it is still an anxiety-laden time. Moreover, the issue of the availability of technology inappropriately stimulating its use (which plagued the introduction of forceps) continues with the routine use of procedures such as fetal monitoring (Adams 1983). While doctors may now view their patients' bodies in labor and delivery, their training frequently includes a paternalistic view of women and a pathological view of the birth process (Scully and Bart 1973). The hospital staff's interactions with the woman in labor and her spouse or other companion tend to encourage a norm of "manageable patient behavior" which is advantageous to the work routine of birth attendants, rather than to the parents' access to and selection of birth options (Danziger 1979: 899).

The difficulty of effecting change is indicative of the place of the childbirth experience in the broader context of American culture. It is only recently that the experience has come to include not only freedom from undue pain and attention to the health and safety of mother and child, but also options such as the presence of significant others (husbands, friends, grandmothers, and even siblings) at the side of the laboring woman. Home birth, homelike birthing rooms in hospitals and free standing "maternity centers," the LaLeche League's support of breastfeeding, and the "natural childbirth" movement all reflect many parents' desire to be in control of the birth situation. However, the various books and articles that celebrate home birth, the presence of the father at birth, and other changes in the birthing process still presume a high standard of living. Prepared or natural childbirth in the United States has been a middle-class phenomenon. "The conditions which affect the majority of women in labor—

poverty, malnutrition, desertion by the father of the child, inadequate prenatal care—are ignored by these books" (Rich 1976: 169).

SOME CONTEMPORARY ISSUES

With the advance of technology and changes in the ideologies that support women's and men's roles in American society, a number of issues have become the focus of discussion on the quality and meaning of childbirth in America. Many of these issues are new. In the 1950s, for example, discussion of postpartum malaise was restricted for most women to a few days of the "baby blues" after birth. Prevailing ideology supported the mother remaining in the home; conflicts between family and career or between a woman's self-development and her family's well-being were, if not unknown, rarely reported. Child abuse, while it certainly existed, was rarely acknowledged as a problem. Certainly these issues are very important in examining childbirth and family formation in the 1980s and 1990s. This section, then, outlines the shape of these issues, examines their implications for the policies that shape the American birth experience, and raises a number of somewhat difficult questions that are still to be answered.

Universality and Variation in the Birthing Experience

With regard to physiology, women's birth experience crosses time and culture. The shape of the pelvis, the position of the birth canal, the occurrence of uterine contractions—all of these are part of the human species' anatomy and physiology. In every society, the human infant is born with a large brain and with a long period of helplessness during which he or she must depend upon others for support.

Yet, women's experience of birth itself varies greatly from one culture to another. In every society there are rules that govern birth and modify the universality of the physiological "facts." Rules specify the proper location for a birth to take place: in a separate birthing hut, in the mother's ancestral home, in a hospital; they specify the kinds of attendants the birthing woman may have: whether the woman labors with a single helper or in the company of the women and/or men of the community; and they specify the behavior that is deemed acceptable during labor. Even the mother's behavior towards her infant when they see each other for the first time is governed by culture. Despite the variation, there are some fairly widespread themes: "First, reproduction is a central event in the life of a woman: the bridge from childhood to adulthood. Second, childbearing is enveloped in rituals that ensure the well-being of the fetus. Third, women are almost always provided with social and emotional support during labor and birth" (Romalis 1981: 10). Jordan (1985:1) makes an apt distinction between parturition (the physiological act of birthing which is, at a gross level, universal) and childbirth: "the ways in which the process is experienced, endowed with meaning, and behaviorally managed in different societies."

One of the hallmarks of the anthropological study of childbirth has been the realization that childbirth is a culturally defined act set within the universals of a common human evolutionary heritage. That anthropological, or holistic, perspective is woven through the articles in this book. Anthropologists have studied the variations in childbirth across cultures (Ford 1964; Newton 1972; Montagu 1937; Konner 1976, among others). Before the 1950s, however, the male bias in ethnography resulted in less interest in the reproductive cycle (with some notable exceptions); male ethnographers were excluded from the predominantly women's world of birth practice and ritual (McLain 1982). Anthropological accounts focused more on descriptions of the place of birth, "taboos observed by pregnant women, and postpartum behavior of mother and father than on the actual dynamics among participants in the birth or the nature of the experience for women....The result is a record of ideal forms of behavior and a host of exotic customs, with rather more known about male participation [couvade] than the female experience" (Romalis 1981). Today, however, there is a great deal of interest in reproductive processes and practices both here and abroad. (See Kay 1982 for an excellent series of articles on cross-cultural birthing.)

The availability of more detailed knowledge of birth processes in other societies has greatly reduced the romanticization of primitive birth management as a natural, intervention-free process. The mythology of the primitive woman leaving work for an hour to give birth in a field has been replaced by the realization that women in low-technology societies often suffer long and painful labors that result in infant or maternal death (Romalis 1981). They are subjected to all manner of interventions into the birth process, and, though such interventions may not require the use of advanced technology, they are part of the ritual management that shapes a woman's birth experience. Reproduction is, after all, too important to be left to the whims of nature (Romalis 1981). There are, however, a number of differences between the model of childbirth accepted by the majority of American women and those held by their sisters in other cultures. In most non-Western societies, childbirth is viewed as a function of health, rather than of illness. The birth rituals that welcome the new member of society signify not only a change in parental status—from woman and man to mother and father—but also celebrate a successful birth (Oakley 1977). Most Americans, in contrast, accept a biomedical model of birth, that is, birth is defined as a risk to be managed by the application of science and technology, and sociocultural factors are either neutral or an impediment to proper care (McClain 1982). As Davis-Floyd notes in chapter 10 of this volume, American rituals of birth incorporate the woman and child into a technology-dominated system and celebrate the triumph of science over nature. Yet, just as different regions of the United States have differing traditions of food and custom, so they have different traditions in the medical management of birth. Some areas have been quick to accept innovation, others have been slow. Some have long traditions of lay midwifery and home birth. Still other areas of the country have childbirth traditions tied to the presence of a major medical school. And there are differences in the birth experiences of urban and rural women.

These differing medical traditions combine with cultural differences found in various parts of the United States. Ethnic cultural forms and diverse local values such as the "pioneer spirit" or the "counterculture," shape both the birth options available to a woman and the meanings she gives childbirth and motherhood. Eating or avoiding particular foods during pregnancy, ritual bathing or nonbathing after birth—such customs affect a woman's relationship to the dominant biomedical model, and affect the level of comfort various ethnic groups have with the health care system during pregnancy and birth. Moreover, the experience of childbirth in America is influenced by a woman's socioeconomic position. How many of the "choices in childbirth" recommended by contemporary birthing manuals are unavailable to women isolated not only by cultural difference and minority status but by poverty? Does the maintenance of strong lay-midwife traditions in some black and hispanic minority communities (long after white middle-class women had moved to hospitals) significantly affect the experience of birth? Certainly changes in the cost of medical care have an impact on those who have not had an opportunity to participate fully in the economy.

Many of the contributors to this book address these cultural questions along with a larger question: to what degree is the biomedical model, so widely accepted in American society, simply one culture's construct of the appropriate childbirth experience? This model is rapidly spreading: many societies are changing their childbirth practices in response to the larger forces that are redefining the birth experience in medical terms. What then happens to the diversity of birth experience by ethnic group, to the cultural definitions and meanings given to childbirth? Such practices are not often integrated into contemporary medical tradition. Even in the United States, "increasing attempts to remove childbirth from the illness model compete with continuing advances in obstetric technology" (McLain 1982).

Appropriate Technology and the Concept of Risk

The application of technology to the birthing process is the hallmark of the American biomedical model of birth. As Rapp and others point out in this book, even the language with which most Americans discuss birth events is predominantly medical rather than familial, religious, or otherwise couched in intimate terms. This is particularly true for those areas of birthing, such as prenatal diagnosis or neonatal intensive care, which have been defined by the technologies that gave rise to them. The biomedical model by and large defines the very way Americans think about birth; thus most women assume that some technology—whether it is an episiotomy, ultrasound, or some other technological intervention—will play a part in their birth experience. To take an opposing view that the biomedical model may not provide the best and safest birth experience, as do those who support out-of-hospital birth, is to oppose a widely held cultural norm and often to risk criticism not only from medical personnel, but from friends and family who accept the dominant model.

There is little cultural imagery in America that celebrates birth as a significant life experience, rather than as a medical event. There are no fecund earth goddesses nor sculptures of birthing women to refer to. Childbirth is a subject rarely talked about outside of its medical framework—what anesthesia a woman had or whether the doctor arrived on time. Judy Chicago, searching for images for *The Birth Project*, a series of art works exploring the experience of birth, discovered

> that the birth process, so central to human existence, is
> virtually a "taboo" area for open human expression. Little

attests to or explains or symbolizes or honors or renders this
primary experience.... Art usually grows from art, but this
time art is going to have to grow directly from experience. I
am making myself into a creative vehicle for the expression of
one of the most fundamental and important life experiences of
the human race (Chicago 1985:19).

In gathering the experiences of women who had given birth, she found that for
many of them this was the first time they had ever really talked about that which
had been a major event in their lives. For many American women, the folklore
and traditions surrounding pregnancy and birth, which gave childbirth meaning as
a social event involving women and babies, have been replaced by the medical
discourse of ultrasound, fetal monitoring, and other aspects of contemporary
perinatal care. Instead of joking with friends about whether a baby's lusty kicks
mean the impending birth of a football player or a ballerina, today's expectant
mother passes around the ultrasound image of the fetus, scarcely discernible to
the uninitiated, a technological confirmation outside of her own intrabody awareness that a pregnancy does, indeed, exist.

The accelerated use of technology in American obstetric practice reflects a
philosophical orientation toward childbirth as an inherently "risky business."

The various forms of obstetric technology have become the
tools of safety as the fetus is monitored for risk and guarded
against danger. Attitudes and actions are focused on pregnancy
outcome which has led to the philosophical orientation and
practical articulation of risk categories. Patients are classified
as high risk or low risk, and a number of risk-screening tools
have been developed for use in determining into which risk
category a patient should be classified (Burst 1983:47).

The concept of risk is, in actuality, a statement of statistical probability.
"Epidemiological studies isolate prevalent 'risk factors' that then become defining
characteristics of a population who are then perceived as 'at risk'" (Newman
1984:1). In and of itself, risk is a cultural artifact that has different meanings to
the medical personnel who may use it to categorize patients for specific treatments and the women who use the concept to choose how they wish to give
birth. McClain (1981a), for example, notes that women found birth far less risky
than did medical personnel, and that those who chose home births, in particular,
felt that the medical risks were greatly overstated.

The medical definitions of risk in pregnancy are often flawed. They are
derived as much from a philosophical stance that treats every pregnancy as high
risk until it is over, as from real conditions that might require intervention to
prevent a tragic outcome. Such a stance has been termed the "maximin approach"
to childbirth: "choosing the alternative that makes the best of the worst possible
outcome, regardless of the probability that that outcome will occur" (Brody and
Thompson 1981:977). This worst-case analysis is in part stimulated by a
professional reward system that gives little reward to those who treat hundreds of
patients appropriately, but severely castigates those who fail to catch the woman

with a rare and unexpected complication (Brody and Thompson 1981). Because of this and with an increased fear of malpractice charges, physicians and hospitals err on the side of caution. The effects of this reward system are also exacerbated by the tendency throughout contemporary American medicine to honor those who find dramatic cures. Women who do not receive adequate prenatal care, for example, have low birthweight/high-risk infants who are treated with the full battery of technology available in neonatal intensive care. The neonatologist who saves a very tiny infant receives more attention than does the family doctor who labors daily to guide women through a healthy, uneventful pregnancy and birth.

Another factor that contributes to the accelerated use of technology is the very way in which doctors determine risk. Obstetric risk-scoring systems are oriented toward prediction of the most severe risks—those that will result in neonatal or maternal mortality or severe morbidity. They are thus geared toward predicting the worst. They offer little reassurance to those who are low risk and do not provide information that allows a judgment to be made for lesser intervention, or no intervention at all. Risk-scoring systems also tend to lump innate risks such as congenital anomalies (which cannot usually be helped by intervention), with acquired risks, such as toxemia, for which some intervention may be appropriate (Brody and Thompson 1981). Thus, a woman whose pregnancy has gone smoothly, but who is carrying an infant with some anomaly, is treated as if she herself is high risk and is subjected to the panoply of technological interventions that accompany high-risk births. Risk scoring for the worst cases makes the maximin strategy seem necessary. The worst, after all, always has some statistical probability of happening.

Regionalization also has accelerated the use of technology in childbirth. Begun in the early 1970s, regionalization concentrates expensive technology and personnel in Level III urban hospitals, which are intended to be accessible to all patients within a given region (Burst 1983). Level I and Level II hospitals, which are likely to be in the woman's home community, treat low-risk women and infants and refer the high-risk patients to Level III hospitals. The intent of regionalization was both to insure cost effectiveness by avoiding the duplication of expensive equipment and highly trained personnel within a given geographic area and to provide better care for mother and baby. Indeed, some real benefits have come from regionalization. The Robert Wood Johnson Foundation's evaluation (1985) of eight regionalized perinatal services indicates that lives were saved and that there was less disability in infants at one year of age.

But with these positive results have come troubling questions and new risks to the woman and the family (Burst 1983). If women are transferred to a regional perinatal center, they are removed from the support of friends and family. If the infant is transferred, the parents may have difficulty visiting the distant neonatal intensive care unit. And increasingly, babies are being born in Level III hospitals. The maximin strategy in obstetric management, focused on the worst case, classes many women as "at risk" and thus candidates for birth in a regional perinatal center. Women themselves, accepting the model, are often reluctant to give birth elsewhere. There is, however, evidence that the use of interventions increases with the available level of technology and medical specialization (Adams 1983). Thus, low-risk women giving birth in a setting also geared for the management of high risk births may find themselves being subjected to unnecessary interventions in the birth process.

None of the above is intended to indicate that technological intervention is *never* appropriate. Certainly, if an infant shows classical signs of distress—passage of meconium in the amniotic fluid, extreme alterations of the rhythm and rate of heartbeat—then closer monitoring and perhaps even more extreme intervention may be indicated. But many hospitals routinely require electronic fetal monitors for all obstetric patients regardless of risk; some doctors feel it is malpractice not to use the available technology. When technology is used routinely for all obstetric cases, there is a real danger that it will become iatrogenic in and of itself. "Many obstetrical interventions form an interconnected system, with one intervention leading to additional risk factors...which in turn require new interventions" (Brody and Thompson 1981:978). Thus, the development of the all too familiar pattern of internal fetal monitoring and cesarean section (Burst 1983) or the use of anesthesia and forceps. Even the transfer to a regional center or the unfamiliar environment of the hospital itself can have an iatrogenic effect. Anxious, fearful mothers often have slowed labors, perhaps the result of the stimulation of catecholomines, which can have a profound negative effect on uterine contractions.

There is little solid proof of the efficacy of routine use of oxytocin to stimulate labor, premature rupture of the amniotic sac, anesthesia, fetal monitoring, episiotomy, or low forceps delivery (Brody and Thompson 1981). Current research focuses on whether or not these procedures are safe, not whether they are necessary. Many interventions do not result in a real decrease in infant mortality, and they do result in increased maternal morbidity and discomfort. There have, for example,

> been unwarranted claims by the proponents of fetal monitoring that the combination of fetal monitoring and the resulting increase in cesarean sections is responsible for the decreased infant mortality rates of the past several years. Such claims ignore the impact on pregnancy outcome and infant mortality resulting from improved nutrition (including the effects of the Women, Infants and Children Nutritional Program), prenatal care, the use of certified nurse-midwives, increased birth weights, decreased prematurity rates, and the availability of abortion (Burst 1983: 47)

The increased use of technology may blind both patient and practitioner to the possibility of nontechnological interventions into the childbirth process. Better prenatal care, increased childbirth education, and the presence of a support person during labor and delivery are nontechnological interventions which can have dramatic results in fostering a positive birth outcome. "Many perinatologists believe that continued reductions in infant mortality and morbidity will not occur through further improvement in high technology medicine. Instead, they look for progress at the 'low tech' end of the spectrum, through prevention of high risk births" (Robert Wood Johnson Foundation 1985: 9). Even in more difficult births, a nonbiotechnical approach may be indicated. For example, there is evidence that "walking the patient" can effectively stimulate uterine contractions in many cases, thus lessening or eliminating the need for oxytocins (Notelovitz n.d.). Flynn et al. (1978) note that the duration of labor was significantly shorter for an ambulant group as compared to a group of women who were kept in a reclining position during labor. The shortened duration of labor appears also to have resulted in less use of analgesia and fewer fetal heart abnormalities.

Many of those who advocate a nontechnological approach to pregnancy and childbirth feel that the biomedical model of birth is a construct of Western medical culture and that other models may serve as well in the safe management of birth. In this volume, the contrast has been drawn between medical models and midwife models by Trevathan and Lichtman, who see a profound difference in the ways in which midwives and doctors treat the birthing woman. While Trevathan describes a lay midwife clinic and Lichtman a nurse-midwife-staffed birthing context with real differences in the relative acceptance of the predominant medical management of birth, there are essential commonalities to the approaches they describe. They are concerned with the humanization of maternity care, the nonseparation of mother and infant from one another and from their families, a respect for the dignity of individuals and for their emotional as well as their physiological needs, and a commitment to little or no technological intervention into the natural birthing process. These are not merely cosmetic differences with the biomedical approach to childbirth; they represent fundamental philosophical differences.

The concern with relative levels of risk and the appropriate use and nonuse of technology appears in almost all of the articles in this book. Whether it is prenatal access to quality care reducing risk or the routinization of prenatal diagnosis; whether it is a question of aggressive intervention in labor and delivery or after the infant is born; or whether it is an issue of the best procedures to foster family formation and optimum infant and child development, risk factors and technological choices color the discourse. In fact, within the ranks of those who deliver babies and those who use their services, there is a great deal of debate about what constitutes a safe and humane birth. While nearly all participants in the debate would agree that "every fetus has the right to be well-born" (Notelovitz n.d.:6), the parameters of what that means are drawn at sharply different points. Phrased in terms of home versus hospital birth, of prenatal diagnosis or electronic fetal monitoring or not, the debate centers on an essential question: Just because we have the technology, must we always use it? The moral and ethical issues involved in the debate over the appropriate use and nonuse of technology are complicated by other trends in American society: the growing concern with the cost of health care, equity in access to care, the changing position of women in society, and even the meaning of children themselves within the family.

The Perfect Child

Certainly one issue that has complicated the decision to use technology in the birthing process has been the growing desire on the part of many health care consumers to have what has been called the "perfect child" (Luker 1984). Zelizer

(1985) notes that a profound change has occurred in the value of children to the American family since the 1870s. Once essential productive elements in the household economy, children in America today are economically "worthless," but emotionally "priceless." With the advent of relatively effective methods of birth control, childbirth, at least in most middle-class families, has become voluntary. Yet despite the economic costs of children, most Americans choose parenthood. They choose it in spite of, not because of, the utility of having a child: for love, emotional fulfillment, and to "feel like a family."

As women increasingly entered the labor force and had fewer children, the value of each child increased. The costs of the mother's absence from the work-place or years lost in the cycle of her career are now counted against the raising of each child. Becoming a parent is not simply a natural act, but a choice made in the context of other available options (Luker 1984). With this greater invest-ment and emotional valuation, each new baby must be "worth it" in terms of its potential for a full and emotionally gratifying life.

This presents a paradox. The middle-class woman who limits the size of her family and must balance career and motherhood is also the woman who desires the "perfect child." She also is the woman who may want more control over childbirth. Despite the desire for more women-centered alternatives in childbirth, the possibility that technology might be needed to insure the infant's safety makes many women unwilling to stray too far from the comforting confines of doctor and hospital, which promise that extraordinary measures will be taken to insure the child's maximum potential. The current emphasis on child perfectibility has made women more anxious about fetal and neonatal damage than they were earlier in the century. This, in turn, feeds the attending physi-cian's desire to use the full battery of technology available, lest he or she be sued for the wrongful birth/life of a less-than-perfect child. The chapters by Rapp, Rothman, Levin, and Guillemin clearly express the parents' quandary over the relative merits and long-term impact of the use of technological interventions versus the desire for the best possible life for any infant to be born.

Information and Choice

Much of the debate about choice and control in childbirth can be phrased in terms of information, for in order to make choices an individual must know what the alternatives are. Information itself has become a valued item in contemporary American society. The possession of adequate information gives one control over a situation, and control over one's own life is clearly a contemporary value. Americans speak of "freedom of information" and of the "right to know" as if these were inalienable rights of citizenship. The individual has the "right" to know as much as it is possible to know.

Contemporary obstetric technology makes it possible to know a great deal about the physiological condition of mother and fetus. As the contributors to this book note, prenatal diagnosis, electronic monitoring in labor, and careful monitoring of the infant's postpartum state introduce "new conceptions of what counts as relevant information and new judgments concerning who is competent to interpret information, to communicate it, and to make decisions regarding the management of birth" (Jordan 1986).

Information may, in fact, be of great benefit in childbirth. Zax et al. (1975) found that women who had received childbirth education prior to their labor and delivery had a more positive attitude toward birth and required less analgesia and anesthesia than did other women. Information about the relative risks and benefits of various procedures can help a woman decide as to their appropriateness for her birth experience.

But the value of information as a source of control is a two-edged sword. Rapp, Roth, Guillemin, and Levin suggest that knowledge itself may force choices upon people. There is really no right "not to know." Those who do not want the information that technology can give them are often cast as irresponsible. But informed consent—the notion that once an individual knows, he or she is competent to decide—is a terrible burden, despite its high value and legal standing in American society. It presumes a rationality of decision making where knowledge is often incomplete. Because information about pregnancy, childbirth and infant development is primarily medical or technical, rather than social or ethical, it does not provide the full basis for decision making in this singularly important aspect of human life.

Moreover, in American society information about childbirth is not owned universally. It is, by and large, specialist knowledge, the domain of the medical professional. "[R]egardless of what women and their attendants know about childbirth, there is in any birthing system an agreement about what constitutes relevant knowledge, important knowledge, consequential knowledge in the sense that it matters for the conduct of birth, and what constitutes irrelevant knowledge, old wives' tales, and the like" (Jordan 1983:2). In low-technology contexts, this "authoritative knowledge" is likely to be shared by the woman, other birth participants, and the birth attendant. The woman is the authority on what her body is doing; the midwife is the assistant, drawing from both her own past experience and her technical training. Because specialized tools are not used to gather information about the laboring woman, all parties have fairly equal access to whatever data are available within the system (Jordan 1986). Decisions about what to do when trouble arises thus tend to be joint decisions.

In high-technology obstetrics, in contrast, specialized instruments provide information, which is generally privileged, not shared, information. "Decisions made about birth management are made on the basis of specialist knowledge derived from technical instruments and procedures, knowledge which is *in principle* inaccessible to the woman and to other birth participants" (Jordan 1983). A woman who is told that "the monitor" indicates she needs a cesarean has no other information with which to form a decision. Her knowledge of her own bodily state is not relevant in the medical context. Likewise, parents, faced with highly technical explanations of risk factors and medical probabilities in prenatal diagnosis or for a critically ill newborn, tend to relinquish decision-making authority to the specialists who own the information.

Yet several of the authors in this book raise the serious issue of who should make decisions about pregnancy, birth, and infancy. It is the parents, after all, who must live with the results of their decisions. When information is couched only in medical terms, the right to know becomes a travesty for those who do not have a specialist education. Minimally, information for perinatal decision making must include not only the risks and benefits of various courses of treatment, but also knowledge about what it means to assume those risks.

For many women in American society, however, the issue of the right to know is moot. Information about childbirth is unequally distributed; inevitably the poor have less! Misinformation and the lack of information about basic reproductive functions may have led to the pregnancy in the first place (Johnson and Snow 1982). Poor prenatal care and other factors that often accompany poverty (poor nutrition, drug use, etc.) mean the woman is "risked out" of birthing alternatives established for low-risk women, and even those not at risk rarely have the necessary information about options that might be available. The low birthweight/high-risk infants all too frequently born to poor women are resident in the neonatal intensive care unit (NICU), a highly specialized medical context where information is carefully guarded and disseminated by the staff. Thus the poor, who often use obstetric and neonatal technology the most, are the very ones who have the least information.

Access

In some sense, all the other issues discussed in this book come to a head in the question of access to adequate care for all pregnant and birthing women. Meaningful information, appropriate technology, choices of birth place and style, and the quality of the birth are all largely foreign to the majority of poor women. Although, as Lazarus points out, all women, even poor and minority women, have the same goals and desires for a good birth and a healthy child, the poor have more high-risk babies, more babies who are sick, and a higher infant mortality rate than do women who are not poor. The reasons are complex.

To begin, low birthweight is a major determinant of infant mortality in the United States, and infants born at low birthweights are at greater risk of illness and developmental disability (Institute of Medicine 1985; Folkenberg 1984). There is a constellation of factors closely associated with the birth of low birthweight infants that are also closely correlated with women living at or below the poverty level. These include demographic factors such as low level of education, nonwhite race (particularly black), childbearing at the extremes of the reproductive age span, and being unmarried; medical factors, such as poor obstetric history, poor nutritional status, or a short time between pregnancies; and behavioral/environmental factors, such as the use of tobacco, alcohol, or other drugs and inadequate or absent prenatal care (Institute of Medicine 1985).

There are more subtle factors which also effect the course of pregnancy and childbirth for the poor. In a study of the stressfulness of life events in pregnancy, Helper et al. (1968) found that seven out of the top eleven events women rated as making it more difficult to adapt to pregnancy were events common to the lives of many poor women. These included being pregnant while unmarried, the baby's father not wanting the child, having to take care of present children without the assistance of a spouse or others, and having too little money to live on. High levels of stress in pregnancy can have an impact on the woman's overall health and, as Margaret Boone points out in chapter 3, may also be a factor in her not seeking prenatal care.

By far the most effective means of improving the health of poor infants is to reduce the chance of their being born at a low birthweight. And, according to the Institute of Medicine, there is overwhelming evidence that the most effective means of reducing the birth of low birthweight infants is early and high quality prenatal care. But as several contributors point out, poor women do not receive adequate prenatal care, and some receive no prenatal care at all. One reason for this is financial—the lack of private insurance coverage or the lack of adequate funds for prenatal care in public health care programs. Additionally, providers are often reluctant to care for poor women, whose high-risk pregnancies often result in poor outcomes (and thus the potential risk of malpractice suits). They also may feel that reimbursement rates for this specialized care are too low (Institute of Medicine 1985). Moreover, there are often insufficient prenatal care services at sites that have concentrations of poor patients. As several contributors to this book note, poor women may also perceive the available prenatal care to be less than useful, nonsupportive, and often aggravating. Combined with difficulties in arranging transportation and child care, these disincentives may cause a woman to put off prenatal care until quite late in her pregnancy.

Even when women seek out prenatal care, they may not receive high quality care, particularly if the concept of "quality" goes beyond the availability of technology. The emphasis on acute care, on curing a problem once it happens rather than preventing it, is of particular significance in the management of the pregnancies of poor women. While many poor women do have health problems that indicate caution in the management of their care, the risk-scoring system and maximin orientation mean that many poor women are routinely subjected to a series of technological interventions into the birth process. And, because most of them receive care in a clinic situation, they do not have a relationship with a personal physician with whom they could negotiate a particular birth style if the option were available. It is ironic that the poor, because of their high rates of low birthweight infants, make more use of technological interventions at birth and of sophisticated intensive care nursery equipment, yet they are the least equipped to evaluate the use of such advanced technology. Indeed, many poor women associate high-technology birthing with quality care, with the notion that everything is being done for them that can possibly be done. Because their prior experiences of birth and/or of the births of their friends may have been as high-risk patients, the information available to them about birth options is limited to a rather impersonal, highly technologized model. It is what they expect, and, because many of them do have significant medical problems and also do not question the model, it is what they receive.

There are a number of programs instituted around the United States that have addressed the issue of quality prenatal care for those who might otherwise not receive it. Characteristic of such programs are improvements in risk scoring, education of patients to recognize the signs of preterm labor, and a variety of programs aimed at the modification of behavior that might endanger the fetus, such as the reduction or cessation of smoking, the reduction of substance abuse, and the improvement of nutritional status. Some programs include linking the woman to more effective support systems in her community.

Despite the development of prevention programs in selected areas, it is clear that not only do poor women not have "choices in childbirth," but they often do not even have access to adequate care. When a woman comes into a hospital emergency room threatening to deliver prematurely, there is often little time for record keeping, much less self-conscious choice making. Middle-class concerns over power and control in birthing have little impact upon the overall powerlessness of poor women to control the circumstances of their lives.

Birth, Bonding, and Families

Because the human infant is born unable to care for its needs and remains quite helpless for a long period of time, it is necessary for a baby to have caretakers to provide for it. The content of that care goes beyond meeting the physiological requirements for growth (food and shelter) and includes affection, stimulation, and protection from abuse. Because the quality of care early in life appears to effect social and emotional development, a great deal of interest has developed in the concept of "bonding," the process by which parents and their infants develop a warm, loving relationship. Initial discussions of a "critical period" immediately after birth, during which bonding between mother (and father) and infant takes place, have been criticized on a number of grounds. For one, the bonding studies examined poor and often socially isolated mother-infant dyads. "To give a mother immediate and active contact with her newborn baby in the hospital involves more active positive contact with hospital staff than for a mother isolated from her infant. It may be that, for socially and economically deprived groups, it is this relationship with hospital personnel, accompanied by expressions of interest, encouragement and reassurance, rather than the contact with the infant, that is important and helpful to the mother" (Chess and Thomas 1982:219). In assessing the importance of early contact after birth for poor women, who may be separated from their infants because the infants are low birthweight and must be in the NICU, there is the danger of ignoring underlying problems of poverty, such as poor social support, substance abuse, and other forms of stress, which lead to a stressful mother-infant relationship.

Most researchers have backed away from the notion of a critical few minutes or hours after birth and moved toward the notion of a gradual development of affection between parent and child which begins before birth and continues long afterward. Cranley (1981), noting that a mother has had active interaction with the fetus from the time of quickening, reports that mothers talked to, played with, and otherwise had a relationship with the child developing inside of them. Such prenatal interaction occurs in other cultures as well. For example, the Eastern Ojibwa Indians believed that "a child required the tenderest care even before it saw the light of day. Both before and after it was born the mother talked to it, teaching its soul and shadow such information as the habits of animals it would encounter as it grew up" (Jenness 1935). Klaus and Kennell, whose names are closely associated with the notion of need for early mother-infant contact, have themselves said that the period after birth is not a period of imprinting, as in some animal species, but a sensitive period during which contact with the baby might enhance a mother's relationship with her baby (Kennell and Klaus 1984). That period is not the sole factor in the development of mother-infant attachment, for certainly many mothers have grown attached to babies although separated after birth or adopted well after the first hours and days of infancy. Such an important, life-sustaining relationship is unlikely to be dependent upon a single short period of time. (Klaus and Kennell 1982).

Yet there is evidence that infants who spend time in the NICU, and thus are separated from their mothers after birth, are more subject to child abuse and neglect. O'Conner et al. (1980) found that mothers separated from their infants had more serious parenting problems (physical abuse, nonorganic failure to thrive) than mothers given an extra twelve hours with their infant in the first two days of life. Newman (1984) notes that in a study of 600 victims of certified child abuse in Rhode Island, 23.6 percent had been premature, though the incidence of prematurity in the state population was only 6.1 percent. Prematurity or low birthweight should not be taken as the single precipitating factor in such abuse, however, for there is a configuration of problems that surround the raising of a vulnerable child. It is unclear, for example, whether the higher incidence of abuse among children who were low birthweight infants is because of early separation or because such children themselves are difficult and often unrewarding to care for (Egland and Vaughn 1981). "Preterm, low birthweight and sick infants are not likely to be either physiologically or socially 'competent' at birth, or even at the time of hospital discharge.... They are usually less responsive and more difficult to care for, i.e., to soothe when crying and to feed, and to have more erratic sleep patterns than most full term, healthy babies" (Bromwich 1985:7). There are subtle differences in the ways that preterm and full-term mother-infant dyads interact. Preterm infants may be less available as a social partner than their term peers, be awake for shorter times, and spend a greater percentage of their waking hours fussing and crying (Parmalee et al. 1983). Moreover, even at eight months, premature infants may be less soothable. Newman's description of the social environment of the infant in neonatal intensive care (see chapter 13), gives some indication of the possible etiology of the social unresponsiveness of such infants. It is also possible, as Cranley (1981) suggests, that the interruption of pregnancy before term interrupts the normal course of development of maternal attachment, resulting in a "preterm mother" as well as a preterm infant.

Not unexpectedly, there is a close correlation between the continuance of problems throughout childhood for low birthweight children and their low socioeconomic status (Bee et al. 1982; Cohen et al. 1982). For parents who live in multiple-stress situations, "the biologically vulnerable infant may be viewed as just one more source of stress" (Bromwich 1985:8). Parmalee et al. (1983) note that such children continue to perform less competently at ages two to five when they come from families of lower socioeconomic status. A mother who is subject to stress because of poverty and/or other small children requiring her care has difficulty maintaining the infant as high priority.

The birth of a biologically vulnerable infant creates stress even in the most integrated families. Not only can the special needs of such an infant create financial stress, but its presence in the family has an impact on family closeness, familial celebrations, and even on a couple's sexual life (White and Dawson 1981). This impact is greatest on mothers who are young, of low socioeconomic status, and who have little help or support for infant care. Early contact between mother and infant, although not essential for the growth of attachment, may enhance their relationship, particularly when combined with prenatal education and the provision of other forms of postpartum support. Some birth environments may be more conducive to early and prolonged infant contact and the creation of a positive social environment for mother and baby. Here again, the poor, who may be most in need of additional support for positive family formation, are most often excluded from such alternative nurturant birth environments. While it is important not to seek single causes when parent-child bonds break down, a positive birth environment may be advantageous to poor, as well as to middle-class women.

Support Systems

Cranley's research (1981) indicates that pregnant women with strong social support systems were more likely to form a deep attachment to their fetuses, and that higher levels of maternal-fetal attachment were positively associated with positive views of infant behavior. Mothers with strong social support are also more likely to visit their infants frequently if they are separated from them and to interact effectively with their infant when he or she is still in the hospital (Parmalee et al. 1983; Minde et al. 1980). Increasingly, social support is being considered a critical factor in maternal adaptation to pregnancy and successful reproductive outcome.

The relationship of strong social support and positive childbirth outcomes is complex. Even defining social support is difficult: a mother may live in a household with many family members or in a crowded neighborhood where there is an everyday intensity of social interaction and still have little support. Considering the number of social contacts alone ignores actual transactional processes and situational factors that mediate the actual giving of support (Gottlieb 1981). Moreover, the contacts a woman has with family and others may be negative, creating greater stress and disruption of her life (Wellman 1981; Olds 1983).

Just as early separation of mother and infant is insufficient in and of itself to explain later child abuse, the existence or absence of social support is usually not sufficient to explain complications of birth or later poor adjustment to parenting. Nuckolls (1972) was one of the earliest to note that women who had many recent life events (such as a divorce, moving of residence, etc.) and few psychosocial resources had three times as many complications of pregnancy as women with many stressful life events and many pyschosocial resources. This interaction between life stress and a woman's support system has since been studied by other researchers (Tilden 1983; Smilkstein et al. 1984; Turner and Noh 1983). Again, it is the poor who most frequently fall victim to this association between stress and social support. Poor women are more likely to experience a stresssful pregnancy, complicated by financial distress, impersonal prenatal care, and, as Boone points out in chapter 3, often the disorder and violence that attend their everyday lives. At the same time, poor women are more likely to have weak support systems—to be unmarried or in an unstable relationship, to have friends and family who can only offer limited support because of their own stressful existences, and to be otherwise socially isolated. Because these factors can have a direct negative impact on pregnancy, labor, and delivery and on later problems in maternal-infant interaction and child development, Smilkstein (1984) and some other researchers have begun to call for an assessment of psychosocial risk, similar to biomedical risking for pregnant women. Such an assessment would allow for intervention into the expectant woman's social support system during pregnancy and perhaps help to avoid later complications that might lead to technological intervention.

A number of intervention programs have been developed that are based on the notion that health education combined with efforts to strengthen a woman's social support will result in better pregnancy outcomes and healthier, better adjusted mothers and babies. David Olds' program in upstate New York, for example, focuses on unmarried, poor pregnant teenagers, and combines nurse home visits during pregnancy and after the baby's birth with attempts to involve family and friends in the mother's care. The nurses also assist the women in making contact with community resources which might provide additional support and provide education about health and parenting behaviors that might have a direct impact on fetal and infant health and development (Olds 1983; 1980). While such programs do not do away with the devastating effects of poverty and social disorganization on parents or provide the jobs and income that might make a long-term difference in the parents' lives, they do address the larger social and economic influences on family life, and on a case by case basis they do provide specific assistance to help poor women cope more effectively with pregnancy, birth, and parenthood.

The provision of social support at birth is found cross-culturally. In societies whose birthing systems are characterized by low technology, social support during labor and delivery aids both in the management of pain in parturition and in the strengthening of the will of the laboring mother to get through a difficult birth. There is evidence that in American society, too, strong social supports help to alleviate some pain in labor and may carry a woman through the birth experience with fewer technological interventions than might otherwise occur. Gaskin (1978) reports that the strong social support system provided for women in a communal context permitted even complicated births to take place without technological interventions, and there have been numerous reports that the presence of a supportive person during labor and delivery lessens the need for analgesia and anesthesia, thus reducing the possibility of iatrogenic effects. The La Leche League provided a support network for women who wished to breastfeed during a period when bottlefeeding was the norm, and it has continued to provide support and assistance to new mothers to carry them through difficult times with their infants. As Morse and her colleagues report in this volume, the presence of support for breastfeeding is critical to a mother's comfort in continuing to nurse her baby.

Alternative Birth Contexts

The development of new technologies and the increasingly hospital-centered illness model of birth has created a discrepancy between medical values and the goals of some childbearing families (Fullerton 1982). By the mid-1970s, the New York District Branch of the American College of Obstetricians and Gynecologists (ACOG) issued a position paper which, while it extolled the virtues and safety of modern obstetrics, also acknowledged that such high technology sometimes did not meet the personal and emotional needs of consumers (Cohen 1981). Soon after the International Childbirth Education Association (ICEA) responded with a long list of issues that they claimed the professional organization had ignored, including the responsibility of the individual for her own health, its failure to acknowledge that childbirth is a natural process, and its tendency to leave the consumer out of health care planning. Those involved with these issues have become increasingly polarized, with proponents of the biomedical model of health care arguing that the only safe way to give birth is in a hospital, and a growing body of parents and caregivers who assert that the only natural way to give birth is at home.

In response to this debate, a series of options in childbirth have developed which run the gamut from a traditional labor in the labor room, with delivery in the delivery room and anesthetized birth attended by an obstetrician, to home birth attended by one's intimate friends. In between are options to deliver in the same room one has labored in (either in a regular labor room or in a more homey, single-unit delivery system), to use an in-hospital birthing room or alternative birthing center (ABC) attended by a physician or a nurse-midwife, to give birth in an out-of-hospital birthing center, which may be staffed by nurse-midwives, physicians, or lay midwives, or to give birth at home, attended by any of the above.

There are, of course, differences among these options. Alternative birthing rooms or centers (often referred to as family-centered hospital care), allow the father (and sometimes other family members) to be in attendance; provide for labor, delivery, and postpartum recovery in one bed (with transfer to a postpartum unit if the mother and baby will stay in the hospital more than a few hours after the birth); provide a homelike atmosphere with equipment out of view or disguised; and allow options for various positions and procedures for giving birth. Delivery in such units is usually combined with a program of prenatal education and preparation for childbirth and often includes home visits at 24-hours postdischarge (Cohen 1981; Barton et al. 1980). Out-of-hospital birthing centers (or free-standing birthing centers) are less formal, give patients almost total freedom to establish the ground rules for the birth, allow friends and siblings at the birth, and require childbirth preparation classes. Most have some emergency equipment available but usually lack general or regional anesthesia. Within this broad outline, there are variations by region and size of population area. Dobbs and Shy (1981) found that the options for labor, delivery, bonding, and postpartum procedure were greater for women using alternative birthing rooms in hospitals with under 1,000 deliveries per year. And some options, such as early discharge and rooming-in, were available regardless of the use of a birthing room, even in larger hospitals.

The reason these options have developed is complex. The competition, stimulated by low birth rates and growing numbers of obstetricians, has caused concern among medical professionals (deVries 1983). For some physicians who considered home birth to be the choice of "fanatics," changes in hospital routine were a means of preventing women from leaving the care of the medical profession. For hospitals, fearful of empty beds, alternative birthing centers became a part of their strategy to improve their position in the "obstetric market place" (Dobbs and Shy 1981) and to attract middle-class women to use their services. Dobbs and Shy (1981), for example, found that in areas of Washington state where hospital administrators perceived out-of-hospital births to be stable or increasing, the trend was to have alternative birthing rooms, while in areas where out-of-hospital deliveries were perceived as few, or decreasing, no alternative birthing room existed or was planned by the area hospital. Moreover, cost considerations have stimulated an interest in alternative birthing. There is evidence that single-unit delivery and other modifications of the labor-delivery-recovery routine are more cost effective per patient than the traditional way of giving birth (Notelovitz 1978; Lubic 1983). The containment of costs has become an increasing concern as third-party providers, both public and private, have restricted the amounts they will pay for various procedures.

Cost also affects the consumer's choice of childbirth method, but it is not the primary reason for choosing an alternative birth place or style. Most women choosing alternative birth places do so because they have strong feelings about medical control of childbirth and a strong desire to have a birth experience consistent with their perception of birth as a natural, not very risky process. Women choosing out-of-hospital births are consistently oriented toward individual control of their own health and the childbirth environment (Fullerton 1982). Many home-birth couples distrust the medical system and are concerned about the possibility of iatrogenic risks to both mother and child. Rather than perceive the hospital as a safe place for their infant, they see it as one that is potentially harmful. Even in the case of a damaged infant, those who choose home birth may argue for the appropriateness of a nonaggressive treatment that will allow the infant to thrive or die naturally, rather than be subjected to the rigors of neonatal intensive care. Those choosing home birth typically prefer the familiar social world of their home, surrounded by family and friends, and see the hospital as a source of "culture shock" (Bauwens and Anderson 1978), where they will be subjected to unfamiliar rules and routines not of their own choosing. They often are embedded in a network of friends who have also given birth at home and are supportive of their desires (McClain 1983b). Those who choose a traditional in-hospital birth tend to have greater trust in the medical system and view childbirth as risky. In-hospital alternative settings and freestanding birthing centers attract women with views in between these; they are often a compromise when one member of a family wants a home birth but the other seeks the apparent safety of the hospital.

The issue of safety, however, is not the primary focus of the contributors to this book who examine alternative birthing contexts. There is substantial evidence that childbirth at home (McClain 1981b) is safe for most women having "normal" births. Other birth alternatives also have an excellent record of safety (Notelovitz 1978; Barton et al. 1980). The issue is whether these different birth settings provide a real alternative to women, whether they permit a woman to have control of her own birth experience, and whether or not they provide a positive, emotionally satisfying environment to women and their infants. There is increasing evidence that some settings provide more real alternatives than others. Many hospitals have adopted the term "alternative birth center" while offering few alternatives to routine hospital birth practices. They may make no attempt to limit medical intervention or allow greater flexibility in having friends, relatives, and siblings at the birth. DeVries' (1983) study of a group of hospitals offering alternative birthing centers (ABCs) found that many of them are simply rooms furnished in a homelike way, with no fundamental change in the philosophy of birth management. Physicians attending patients in the ABCs used analgesia, electronic monitoring, and local anesthesia, among other interventions. Proponents of this type of birthing center argue that this permits even high-risk patients to deliver in a homelike atmosphere, while opponents feel that opening an attractive birthing center with no real change in philosophy is more for the benefit of the medical team and cost conscious hospital administrators than the woman herself (Burst 1983).

Women expecting to deliver in these settings are frequently transferred to the regular labor and delivery unit (Barton et al. 1980; DeVries 1983). Transfer rates average about 23 percent (DeVries, 1983), and ABC protocols set out a wide range of conditions under which women must be transferred out of the unit. Any deviation from the norm, such as a prolonged second stage, is grounds for transfer. Women who use the ABC have already undergone extensive risk screening, so that any woman who is even moderately high risk is screened out. Therefore, women accepted into the ABC are the "cream of the crop" and are expected to have trouble-free, natural births. Physicians cite the high rate of transfer as further evidence of the risk inherent in childbirth and the wisdom of choosing an alternative setting within the safe confines of a hospital. Some consumers, however, see the transfer rate as one more proof that the medical profession wishes to coopt the natural childbirth movement and remain in control. Transfer rates from home births and out-of-hospital birth centers are far lower; compared with these settings, women in ABCs have reduced capacity to resist intervention and transfer. "Theoretically, of course, a mother who disagrees with a proposed treatment has the right to leave an ABC. However, few women in labor choose this course of action. Transfers may occur more commonly in hospital ABCs because of the ambiguity that surrounds the definition of 'risk' during certain events of labor. The obstetrician has a great deal of freedom in interpretation of physical signs, and the limited knowledge of the average client prevents her from contesting medical evaluations of her progress" (DeVries 1983:7–8). Clearly, in this situation women have not substantially gained control of their birth circumstances.

A part of the reason for the continued lack of real alternatives in hospital-centered births is the growth of concern for the safety of the fetus to the near exclusion of everything else (Burst 1983). Attention during labor and delivery is focused on the condition of the fetus and the mother's physiological state (slowing of contractions, blood pressure) rather than on her emotional or psychological needs. Yet, while preventing physical harm to mother and baby is necessary, this approach all too often leads to intervention into the birth process. Few mothers will argue with their attending physician when told that a given intervention is necessary "for the sake of the baby." Although there are no substantial studies of the psychological or social benefits to the infant of being born in different, equally safe, birth settings (Institute of Medicine 1983), there do appear to be some benefits to both the mother and mother-infant interaction in alternative birth settings which allow maternal involvement in the birth process and easy postpartum interaction of mother and child.

Even prepared childbirth does not often lead to the requisite knowledge to decide whether an intervention is appropriate or not. Melzack (1984) points out that the emphasis on a "painless" childbirth in many prepared childbirth classes may keep women from facing the issues which may come up as they give birth. Many women do, in fact, have intense pain and those women whose expectations of labor do not match the reality they encounter may experience more pain (Asbury 1980). Women expecting a "natural, painless" childbirth experience anger and frustration when labor is more painful than they anticipated. "Implicit in all of this is the assumption that if labor *does* become painful, it is the fault of the mother for not having learned the training regimen properly. Not only does the prospective mother face pain, then, but the pain itself becomes a token of failure. The mother is now burdened with a sense of guilt for having betrayed her own expectations as well as those of her husband and her trainer" (Melzack 1984:322). Yet, as Morse and Park point out in chapter 7, the experience of pain is perceived differently by women of different cultural backgrounds, as is the permitted reaction to the pains of birth.

In some sense, the body of information itself is the primary "alternative" in birth, for the sharing of birth-related information by parties to the birth process implies a shift in the control of that process. Fullerton (1982) cites five procedures which many women feel are non-negotiable expectations in contemporary childbirth: (1) no prolonged separation of parent and infant following birth; (2) no routine administration of analgesics or anesthesia without regard to the wishes of the laboring woman; (3) no routine perineal shave or enema; (4) no exclusion of the father or significant other from labor and delivery; and (5) no routine episiotomy. But the most common birth option sought by women is involvement in the decision-making process (Dobbs and Shy 1981). Yet, even women who are well informed about obstetric care and have definite preferences may not get what they want (McClain 1981b), as witness the high transfer rate for in-hospital ABCs to conventional labor and delivery. It is important to note, however, that many women do not view standard obstetric care as impersonal and dehumanizing. "Some women may welcome hospitalization for childbirth as a socially legitimate release from the role obligations of housewife and mother. Women may also view their home as inappropriate for childbirth because of lack of space, or because of values emphasizing modesty or privacy for the act of childbirth" (McClain 1981b:1037). Moreover, the option to choose diverse alternatives which might humanize childbirth is largely limited to the middle class and the wealthy.

> At this time, woman-centered birth is used primarily by well-educated middle- and upper-class women who are able to prepare themselves with information and assert their right to control their own experience. In addition, a smaller population of those who have rejected many major cultural institutions use lay midwives as part of their process of developing an alternative culture. The fact remains, however, that a humanized birth process is still unavailable to most people—despite the fact that birth is a universal experience and one that is central to women's lives (Chicago 1985:196).

To what degree, then, do alternative birth settings and birth styles give women control over their birth processes? Certainly the early writers who advocated natural childbirth were not advocating women's control: natural childbirth was to take place within the dominant biomedical model of the birth process, with the doctor knowing best what was good for the laboring woman. And, while the subject of alternative delivery sites raises many issues: consumer rights, responsibilities, and power; professional rights, responsibilities and power; home birth and lay midwifery or birth attendants; economics, cost effectiveness and cost containment—the real issue is control (Burst 1983). The focus on family-centered care may not, in fact, provide that control. Not only is the meaning different in different contexts—it can mean merely that the father is present or that a whole variety of options is available—but it also focuses on the family in a rather traditional sense, rather than on the woman herself. Many aspects of family-centered care tend to coopt the woman's desire to control her birth experience. Some hospitals even offer family-centered cesarean births, complete with childbirth preparation classes and the presence of the father at the birth. While this humanization of cesarean birth is positive in some senses, it also moves toward the acceptance of surgical intervention as part of "normal birthing" (Romalis 1981). Thus, family-centered care provides only half-hearted options unless it is accompanied by a real philosophical shift that significantly removes birth from the dominant biomedical model and sees it as a natural event in a woman's life. Woman-centered childbirth, on the other hand, focuses on the woman's right to know and to choose the options she feels will be best for her and her child. Women, presumably, want a childbirth experience that is safe and that promises positive outcomes for the child's development. Women choosing alternative birth settings also want to remain in control of their birth experience so that it is a celebration both of their womanhood and the coming into being of a new person.

Feminism and the Control of Birthing

The issue of control has been the primary focus of the feminist exploration of childbirth. Control of childbirth has been seen by feminists to be only one facet of women's larger struggle to control their life circumstances. The biomedical model, which dominates American childbirth, is seen as having been derived from a male perspective—a male structuring of an event that happens to women. Men have set the norms according to their own experiences, and because men do not have babies, the normal physiological processes of pregnancy and birth are deviant (Mundy 1983). To the woman who views medical treatment as a consumer good rather than as a sacred trust, childbirth takes on a political dimension that involves the negotiation of power relationships between a woman and her care provider (Romalis 1981). These power relationships are expressed in terms of male domination of the medical profession.

Thus, the compromises proposed by contemporary medicine have not satisfied those women who wish to control their birth experiences. The issue here is the social construction of pregnancy and birth, and as long as those who adhere to the biomedical model also control the place of birth and the technology used in birthing, they control the context and meaning of the birth experience. Many childbirth preparation classes are a case in point. Often these classes are sponsored by a physician or hospital and teach LaMaze breathing techniques as well as prepare the women and their partners for the hospital routine. What is offered is not really natural childbirth but prepared birth, and that preparation conforms to the biomedical model of birth. "Natural childbirth classes socialized couples into expecting medical interventions and accepting medical definitions of reality" (Mundy 1983:5). Lamaze substitutes conscious control of pain for analgesia and anesthesia, but in reality this does not translate into control over the birthing situation (Rothman 1981). Medical personnel still define the progress of labor and the events of delivery.

For some women, home birth is the only way to challenge the medical model of childbirth, for it moves the birth experience outside of the physical context of the dominant biomedical model and removes the technologies and conceptual frameworks that define birth from the control of specialists to that of the birthing woman and her supporters. Yet the feminist interest in home birth has produced several points of tension. For one, the move toward naturalism in childbirth has attracted not only feminists, but very traditional women who want birth returned to them for reasons of family. The whole notion of family-centered birth implies much about the traditional roles of men and women in the family, and the presence of the father at birth may accentuate, rather than diminish, male control of women's experience. Feminists choosing home birth and other alternatives challenge not only the medical profession but the traditional family structure. Thus the home-birth movement is often an uneasy alliance of women who want similar birth experiences for very different reasons (Rothman 1981).

Moreover, even for those who hold less traditional views of the family, there is a quandary raised by "natural" or home birth. The feminist rejection of the notion that childbirth is primarily important as a means to motherhood, with the concomitant acceptance of the importance of childbirth as an experience in and of itself, combined with the acceptance of motherhood itself as a choice to be made rather than an inevitability, leads to contradictory desires. If a woman chooses to have fewer children so that she may also pursue other options in her life, then each child born must be "worth it" with regard to those other options. Technology is the resource that promises to produce the "perfect child," and thus when physicians describe childbirth choices in terms of infant safety and long-term child development, the decision as to what kind of birth to have becomes more complicated.

Another point of tension in the feminist critique of childbirth lies in their seeing an opposition between only two models of childbirth: the biomedical and the natural. By using this framework, feminists make the assumption that women have common desires in childbirth—that they all want or will come to want conscious control over a natural birth. Nelson (1983) points out that there are real differences in what women want in their birth experiences, and that these are highly correlated with class position and cultural background. In her study, middle-class women wanted active, involved births free from medical intervention; working-class women wanted passive birth experiences with more medical intervention. Neither group necessarily gets what it wants, although it is the middle-class, feminist model of a prepared, involved birth experience which affects most reform in birthing. Because that view is widely accepted by academic writers, it is the one used when physicians and hospitals seek, in however limited a way, to humanize birth. This model may not suit all women. It is thus somewhat ironic that "those who are most interested in women defining for themselves the nature and meaning of childbirth are, perhaps, guilty of prescribing a perfect birth for all women, regardless of individual needs or motivations" (Nelson 1983:285).

Despite these points of tension, feminism has had a significant impact on the experience of childbirth in America. The notion that women have a right to control their bodies, particularly their own reproduction, has both raised the consciousness of those planning to give birth in contemporary America and had an impact on the medical profession's approach to birth. Yet, the feminist critique has been largely pertinent to the interests of the middle class. "[D]espite considerable public discussion by feminists about the need for women to seize control of labor and delivery, the fact remains that for the overwhelming majority of pregnancies, physicians have the upper hand when it comes to decision-making" (Luker 1984:109).

The Role of Policy

The issues raised above—unequal access to prenatal care, the appropriate use of technology, control over the context of childbirth—indicate a need for intervention at the level of policy into the events surrounding childbirth. Changes in the family unit, such as the sharp rise of births to unmarried women and the high rate of school-age pregnancy, have diminished the support systems which have traditionally helped women to achieve positive infant outcomes. These social changes have been compounded by the American pattern of income distribution. "The U.S. probably has the most unequal income distribution of any western industrialized nation. Budget cuts and changes in the tax structure enacted in 1981 have made the rich richer and the poor poorer, so that today the poorest fifth of the U.S. population receives 4.2 percent of the national income, while the richest fifth receives 43 percent, or more than ten times as much" (UNICEF 1983: 28–29). Poor women get less prenatal care, have more low birthweight infants at risk of increased mortality and morbidity, and, certainly, have fewer choices in childbirth.

Although it is not within the scope of a book that focuses on childbirth to discuss the root causes of poverty and inequality in America, it is useful to look at those areas of policy that are directly related to the high number of poor birth outcomes among the poor. Chief among these is the emphasis on postnatal intervention rather than prenatal preventive care. From the Baby Doe regulations, which mandated aggressive intervention in the postnatal care of critically ill infants, to the structure of third-party payments, which stint on prenatal preventive care but will pay for the technology of postnatal intervention, there is a clear policy focus on acute rather than preventive care. Cutbacks in federal programs such as WIC (the program providing nutritional supplements to Women, Infants, and Children), plus reductions in coverage for prenatal care in many state Medicaid programs have increased the number of infants born at risk and thus also the need for postnatal intervention. Even trends in the private insurance industry, such as increasing deductibles and co-payments and defining maternity benefits as optional benefits, may discourage use of prenatal services (Robert Wood Johnson Foundation 1985).

There are serious questions about the focus on intervention rather than prevention, both in terms of ethics and of cost. The use of sophisticated technology to save the life of a catastrophically ill infant is very expensive. Prenatal prevention programs, which are primarily low technology programs of education, surveillance, and nutritional supplementation, are less expensive. Calculations at both the national and state level project substantial savings for public and private agencies if better, more comprehensive prenatal care were provided for women at risk of having a low birthweight infant. Using a target group with a current low birthweight rate of 11.5 percent, the Institute of Medicine estimates that by reducing that rate to 10.76 percent through adequate prenatal care, the cost savings in postnatal care would easily equal the expenditures for prenatal assistance. Reducing the rate to 9 percent (the 1990 goal set by the Surgeon General for maximum low birthweight rate among high-risk groups), every added dollar spent for prenatal care within the target group would save $3.38 in the total cost of caring for low birthweight infants (Institute of Medicine 1985:17). These figures represent only a 13 percent and a 22 percent reduction in the low birthweight rate, well within the changes that may be anticipated with better prenatal care.

Such cost estimates are based on the low birthweight infant's care in the hospital after birth and on rehospitalization during the first year, using conservative estimates of the use of resources. One estimate is that if comprehensive prenatal care were provided to all low-income women, the federal government would save over $360 million in costs for neonatal intensive care and rehospitalization of low birthweight infants (Blackwell et al. 1983). To these costs one may also add expenditures for long-term morbidity and rehospitalization costs and for the fiscal impact of the social and emotional costs to the families of such infants. The dissolution of some marriages under the stress of caring for a severely compromised child, the loss of income if one parent must remain at home to care for such a child, the need for special education facilities, and other long-term postnatal costs all add to the monies that would be saved by the provision of comprehensive prenatal care. Moreover, better prenatal care would also give women greater choice and control of their childbirth experience, for women who can expect positive birth outcomes can make use of a far greater range of birth alternatives. Many of the low technology alternatives, such as home birth, free-standing birth centers, and the use of midwifery services, would also be lower in cost than the birth options now available to poor women at risk of having a low birthweight infant.

These estimated cost savings are not theoretical figures. Publicly supported programs of prenatal care have made a difference in birth outcomes. The WIC program, which provides supplemental food, nutritional counseling, and strong links to other prenatal services for pregnant women, has reduced infant mortality and the rate of low birthweight infants in those areas where evaluation of the program has taken place (Institute of Medicine 1985). Sokol et al (1980) report that improved prenatal care through the Cleveland Maternal and Infant Care (MIC) program resulted in participating women experiencing 60 percent less perinatal mortality and a 25 percent lower rate of preterm deliveries than comparable women not enrolled in the project. In rural Georgia, a nurse-midwifery program that provided prenatal care to low-income women who had no private physician halved the incidence of low birthweight in that region (Reed and Morris 1979).

A review of the positive results of comprehensive prenatal care has led the Institute of Medicine to recommend that the federal government take a leadership role in enhancing the capacity of prenatal care to reduce low birthweight. This leadership role should consist of the provision of funds for comprehensive prenatal programs and a federal statement that describes model prenatal care in order to encourage a uniform understanding of such care throughout the country. However, federal leadership in providing adequate prenatal care in the mid-1980s has not been forthcoming. Poland (1984) reports that a recent World Health Organization (WHO) survey of 23 European countries found that, although they had a gross national product far below that of the United States, these countries had made a serious commitment to maternity services. These included health insurance, paid maternity leaves of at least twelve weeks, child care allowances, special privileges when traveling on public transportation, free milk, vitamins, and baby equipment, and special working hours. In the United States, however, a strong anti-interventionist perspective at the federal level has resulted in budgetary cuts for prenatal programs, ironically at the same time that the government has attempted to legislate greater intervention in the neonatal intensive care unit. Several contributors to this book document the effects of the federal role and raise serious ethical and political questions about America's national commitment to the health of its mothers, infants, and children.

Questions of policy lead back to the universals in birthing discussed above. To insure its survival, every society must make provision for the birth and care of healthy infants. If particular cultures are to carry on, and, indeed, if the human species is to survive, the health and well being of the next generation must be insured. At the same time, all societies make rules that govern pregnancy and birth, presumably to guarantee the successful birth of that society's new members. A society whose rules or policies potentially inhibit positive birth outcomes exhibits an internal pathology that may indicate a weakening of the society's will to carry on and remain viable. It is no accident that infant mortality is used as a yardstick of a nation's health and well being! The issues raised here—from the lack of access to care, to individual control of the birth experience—are part of the measure of American society today.

ABOUT THIS BOOK

The contributors to this book address the critical issues that have arisen as new technologies pose choices in previously unquestioned arenas and new ideologies provide varying options for the relationship between parent and infant, and parent and parent. The articles are organized to move through the birth experience, from pregnancy through the early postpartum. In each, the factors which structure significant decisions provide a focus for discussion: in pregnancy, whether to have amniocentesis or not; in childbirth, how to choose between alternative birth styles and locations; in the postpartum period, when to intervene in the lives of critically ill infants. Some authors analyze the cultural variations in the birth experiences of the diverse ethnic minority communities that make up the American population. Others consider the social, cultural, and economic factors that affect differential access to care throughout pregnancy and birth. Still others address the changing impact of gender roles on the birthing experience.

Each of the articles is based in field experience—research in the real-life contexts of pregnancy and childbirth in America. The authors draw on their experiences in lay-midwife run clinics, public health facilities, and neonatal intensive care units to evaluate the more abstract questions raised by practice in each of these contexts. They combine their observations with interviews with health care professionals, pregnant women, and new mothers to obtain an in-depth sense of what the issues in and experience of childbirth in America are today.

The contributors are all professional social scientists, most well past their doctoral degrees with many years of teaching and research between them; a few are just beginning their professional careers. They come to this book with varied backgrounds and experiences. Some are established scholars whose professional interest turned to these issues after the powerful experience of the birth of their own child; others are childbirth practitioners who returned to the university to obtain further degrees and the scholarly skills with which to analyze their practice; still others have been engaged in long-term research on these issues and have served as expert witnesses and givers of testimony for congressional consideration. They are joined in this volume by both their scholarly interests and their concern for making the American social and cultural context of pregnancy and childbirth, and the entry into parenthood, a positive and humane experience.

NOTE

I am indebted to the work of Dorothy and Richard Wertz and Judith Walzer Leavitt for much of the material which appears under the heading of the history of childbirth in America. The material presented in this introduction is greatly abbreviated; those who wish a more complete understanding of the historical antecedents of American birth practices should consult the works by these authors cited in the Bibliography. I would also like to thank Jo Wade, Grant Ramsey, and Nathan Maling for their assistance in producing the final manuscript, Jim Bergin and his staff for their careful editing and consultation, and, especially, each of the contributors for their patience and encouragement as we worked together to complete this book.

SECTION I

DECISIONS IN PREGNANCY

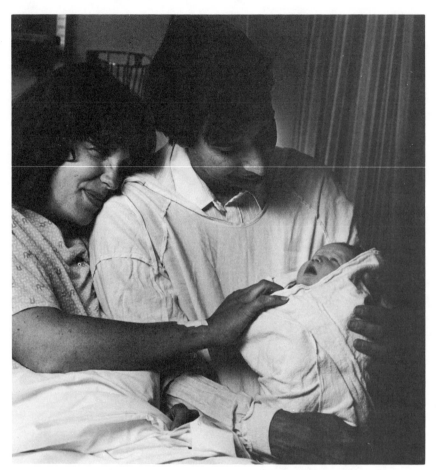

Photograph by LeRoy J. Dierker, Jr., M.D.

DECISIONS IN PREGNANCY

Having my baby,
You're a woman in love and it's love that's growin' in
*   you....*
Didn't have to have it.
Wouldn't put you through it.
You could have swept it from your life but you wouldn't
*   do it,*
And you're having my baby....
*   Paul Anka, "(You're) Having My Baby"*

...the overwhelming weight of the evidence is that
prenatal care reduces low birthweight. This finding is
strong enough to support a broad, national commitment
to ensuring that all pregnant women, especially those at
medical or socioeconomic risk, receive high-quality
care....
*   Institute of Medicine, Preventing Low Birthweight*

In most societies, pregnancy is a period of both joy and care in which appropriate behaviors are culturally defined and few decisions are necessary. There is joy in the approaching addition to the larger family unit—the birth of an heir, perhaps, or another pair of hands to labor in the fields and later to support the parents in their old age. There is care that the growing fetus will not be damaged in the womb. A woman may be given special foods to eat to encourage the growth, health, and/or particular gender of the infant. She may be instructed as to situations to avoid where such dangers as the "evil eye" of an envious neighbor or the curse of a barren woman might fall upon her and forever mark or injure her child.

A woman who becomes pregnant in contemporary America may have a body of folk belief and advice from others to guide her. But radical changes in technology, the transition in family structure, and the growth of the medical model of perinatal management make the American woman's cultural context for pregnancy far different than any known before in less industrialized societies. The pregnant woman in America faces a number of decisions that will profoundly affect the outcome of her nine months of waiting. The first signs of pregnancy— missed menstrual periods, nausea, tenderness of the breasts—may be greeted not with joy, but with dismay by women who lack the support of spouse or family to see them through pregnancy, birth, and parenthood. Certainly, the first

35

decision a contemporary American woman faces is whether or not to continue her pregnancy. For many, that decision is clearcut: the child is wanted or not wanted, termination of the pregnancy is or is not a viable option within the woman's personal moral context. And yet, as medical technology provides more information about fetal development, the language of science and the language of morality become painfully intertwined. Barbara Katz Rothman's chapter points out that in today's world, information itself has a moral quality. For many, the right–or the duty–to know if one is carrying a healthy child presupposes the necessity of acting on that information. As technology is applied to more and more women and provides earlier and safer analyses of fetal status, the juncture of decision and information become an issue that must be addressed in terms of quality of life, the relative rights of parent and child, and society's broader commitment to assisting the disabled.

All of these issues must be seen in cultural context, for it is culture which defines the differential reality of the fetus, the definition not only of handicap, but also of whether an infant is a viable member of society. Western culture places primacy on the survival of the infant through the aggressive use of technology, as seen in section 3 of this book. At the same time, cultural definitions of the perfectability of the infant through the intervention of technology create new questions related to whether fetuses should live or die. The American fascination with the newest capabilities of technology surround parents' conceptualization of their reproductive experience not only in pregnancy, but in the reasons put forward for increased intervention in childbirth and in the aggressive treatment of critically ill newborns in neonatal intensive care. In chapter 3 Rapp describes how the very language used in prenatal diagnosis structures parents perception of the appropriate course of action in medical terms, just as Davis-Floyd, in the next section, sees the language and ritual of hospital birth as molding the very way women think about birth, their infants, and their own bodies. Here, too, the ability to make decisions about the fate of a fetus or a newborn is often controlled by the medical definition of the situation. Both Rapp and Guillemin and Levin (see section 3) talk about the ways in which medical ideology and terminology structure parental decision-making by controlling the parameters of discourse.

Most women decide to continue their pregnancies. Even pregnancies that are not at first welcomed are often accepted as they progress. Indeed, attachment to the baby-to-be grows throughout pregnancy, so that the postpartum interactions described in the final section of this book have their roots in the prenatal period. Factors that create stress during the prenatal period may compromise the growth of attachment to the infant developing within.

Most women, no matter what their social, cultural, or economic circumstances, have the same desire for the successful outcome of their pregnancy: a healthy child. As Wenda Trevathan points out in chapter 14, women come to their pregnancies with a common heritage which is part of their biological make-up as human beings. Yet, if women have a common biological heritage with which they embark upon pregnancy, they come to this significant life process with very different social, cultural, and economic resources. Differential access to these resources, particularly during the prenatal period, may determine the course of the pregnancy, the birth event, and ultimately the health of the infant and its ability to be integrated into the sociocultural environment within which it is born. While ethnic differences have often been reported as determining behavior during pregnancy and the resultant successful reproductive outcome, the chapters in this section, plus Trevathan's in the final section of the book, strongly indicate that socioeconomic factors, rather than cultural norms, determine whether or not a woman receives the kind of adequate prenatal care that will result in the birth of a healthy infant. The chapters by Boone, Lazarus, Poland, and Sargent and Marcucci, cross a gamut of socioeconomic and ethnic populations and make it clear that those without access to social and economic resources receive a different level and quality of care than do those who have access to such resources. The pregnancy experiences of poor women are qualitatively different from those of middle-class women; while a middle-class woman may select the kind of care she wants to have, the poor must accept the care available at public clinics.

It is not that care at such clinics is technically bad. In fact, because public clinics are often the training sites for medical residents, the technology available at such clinics may be quite advanced. Indeed, Poland points out that many poor women associate advanced technology with quality care and actively choose to be treated at a clinic associated with a teaching hospital, where such technology is likely to be available. What makes public-clinic care of lower quality than the care available to those who can pay for their physician's services is a combination of impersonality, lack of continuity of personnel, inconvenience, and, all too often, staff attitude. Boone, Poland, and Lazarus show how long clinic waits, the inability to communicate adequately with staff, and other negative features associated with clinic care result in a reluctance on the part of pregnant women to seek the adequate prenatal care they need to insure a successful reproductive outcome.

Two chapters in this volume, however, present models which indicate that adequate care can be made available to the poor and that healthy infants result from such care. Sargent and Marcucci reveal that the Khmer, despite the fact that many are poor and that they are culturally different than their caregivers, seek and receive prenatal care with the assistance of social workers specifically assigned to assist them with their pregnancy needs. In Trevathan's research, women quite as poor as those described in some of the other chapters in this book have good reproductive outcomes in the context of a lay midwife-run clinic.

A comparison of all of the research populations represented here makes it evident that one very important factor in securing a good outcome of pregnancy is strong social support. This support may be in the form of family, as among the Mexican women giving birth in Trevathan's clinic, or it may be provided by an external source, such as the social worker and translator in Sargent and Marcucci's research. What is increasingly apparent is that those with poor support systems, such as the women Boone describes, have low birthweight infants and other complications of pregnancy and birth. Throughout this volume, the need for a support system corresponds to successful reproductive outcome, whether it is evident in the overall health of the infant, in the ability to bond with the newborn and to succeed in nourishing it, or in the ability of the parents to adjust to the newborn and care for their infant in a nonabusive manner.

The authors raise questions of policy–of whether equality of access to care and the reduction of infant morbidity and mortality are truly goals which are being pursued in American society. Poland, in particular, points out that there are structural causes within society that result in inadequate prenatal care and that government policies can and have made a difference in access to care. Lazarus, too, raises the issue of perinatal policy, bringing as well a perspective on the relationship of feminist concerns for a woman's control over her own body to the context of women who are poor, pregnant, and have control over little of what takes place in their lives.

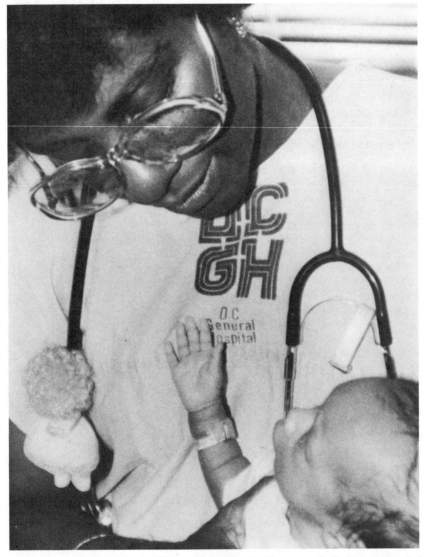

Photograph by Maurice Thompson, D.C. General Hospital

POOR WOMEN, POOR OUTCOMES: SOCIAL CLASS AND REPRODUCTIVE HEALTH

Ellen S. Lazarus

INTRODUCTION:
THE PERSISTENCE OF REPRODUCTIVE PROBLEMS

Despite the most advanced technology and facilities in the world, the United States continues to have a high rate of infant and maternal mortality relative to other industrialized nations. While the infant mortality rate has been reduced through technological advances in perinatal medicine, the establishment of perinatal health programs, and improvements in sanitation and nutrition, at least fifteen nations have lower infant mortality rates (United Nations 1980), and six have lower maternal mortality rates. The National Center for Health Statistics (1984b) reported that in 1982 the infant mortality rate was as high as twenty-seven deaths per 1,000 live births in some cities in the United States (e.g., Washington, D.C., and Detroit) and there is evidence that both maternal and infant perinatal morbidity and mortality may be both underreported and under-estimated (Smith et al. 1984; Zemach 1984). Most alarmingly, the decline in the national infant mortality rate leveled off in 1985 (*New York Times* 1985) and infant mortality is now actually increasing in some cities, such as Cleveland and Youngstown.

American women bear a high number of low-weight (less than 2,500 grams, or 5 lb. 8 oz.) babies. This condition is considered to be the most important correlate of infant mortality (Hutchins et al. 1984). Low-weight babies are twenty times as likely to die within the first year of birth as infants of normal weight (Surgeon General's Report 1979). Low birthweight is associated with the increased occurrence of mental retardation, developmental difficulties, and disorders of the central nervous system (Heckler 1983).

In addition, teenage pregnancies have increased in the United States at a higher rate than all other industrial societies, and there is a growing concern over both the increase of sexually-transmitted disease and of illegitimate births (Public Health Reports 1980). In New York City, for example, more than a third of

39

all births are to unwed mothers (*New York Times* 1984b) and in Cleveland half the births in 1984 were illegitimate (Cleveland Vital Statistics 1984).

POVERTY AND CHILDBIRTH

This chapter focuses on this national crisis in reproductive health by examining the social circumstances in which perinatal problems occur. Poor women living in inner-city ghettos, the rural South, and Appalachia overwhelmingly have high-risk pregnancies, low birthweight babies, and babies who die within the first year of life. Reproductive problems are perpetuated through the conditions of poverty. Poverty, therefore, is a most appropriate and vital issue upon which to focus in both research and in policy directions.

This viewpoint is not a new one, nor has the government been unaware of it. With the establishment of the Children's Bureau in 1912, the federal government became directly involved with the health of women and children. The following year it commissioned a study to provide information on the determinants of infant mortality. Family income, housing, employment status of the mother, and early care of mothers and infants were cited as crucial factors in determining whether babies and mothers lived or died (Davis 1978).

Since that time, and particularly during the last thirty years, a great deal of evidence has accrued to indicate that high infant mortality and low birthweight are tied to income rather than to race or ethnicity (Fogel 1981; Richardson 1967). In a review of the literature in the United States and Britain, Osofsky and Kendall (1973) found a significant relationship between socioeconomic level, pregnancy outcome, and child development. Low-income women tend to have more closely spaced pregnancies and more numerous pregnancies; they begin childbearing at an earlier age and continue later in life. It has been suggested that along with these factors, low maternal educational attainment, single marital status (Stickle and Ma 1977), lack of good perinatal care, lack of education about the course of pregnancy and birth, poor obstetric care (Erickson and Bjerkedal 1982) and high levels of stress (Oakley, Macfarland, and Chalmers 1982) may contribute to the complications of pregnancy, premature deliveries, and lower birthweights. These in turn increase the risk of perinatal mortality and morbidity.

Federal birth statistics, however, do not normally distinguish socioeconomic status but tend to focus on ethnicity and minority status. Although blacks and hispanics are proportionately poorer, there are more poor white women than any other group of poor women in the United States (U.S. Bureau of the Census 1980). Research and policy attention, however, continues to be directed to race and minority status and diverted from social class. The Department of Health and Human Services, for example, states that the rate for black infant mortality is almost double that for white infants, as it has been for the past twenty years (Heckler 1983), but no mention is made of the poverty associated with this racial group. However, comparison of the birth statistics for two hispanic groups in the United States—Puerto Rican and Cuban women—reveals the association of class with birth outcome. Puerto Ricans are at substantially higher risk for low birthweight babies than Cuban women. More of the former are unmarried and undereducated. Over twice as many Puerto Rican mothers as Cuban mothers in the United States are unmarried teenagers. Of Puerto Rican mothers:

46 percent completed high school
48 percent were unmarried
69 percent of births were to unmarried 15-19 year olds
9 percent had low birthweight babies

Of Cuban mothers:

73 percent completed high school
14 percent were unmarried
1 percent of births were to unmarried 15-19 year olds
5.8 percent had low birthweight babies (Ventura 1984).

Puerto Ricans in the United States are predominantly poor (U.S. Commission on Civil Rights 1976), while Cubans are mainly the descendants of middle-income or professional Cubans who emigrated after Castro came to power in 1959 and are generally more educated and have greater access to resources.

It is vital that certain groups (e.g., black, hispanic, native American) be targeted as at risk of having low birthweight infants, but it must be for the right reasons—not because of their culture, but because they are poor. Only then can appropriate solutions be developed and carried out.

The obstetric literature in the United States, focusing on technological innovations and pathology, has virtually ignored ethnicity and socioeconomic factors in reproduction (Snow et al. 1978). Social scientists, however, are beginning to concern themselves with how social and cultural factors contribute to biological and medical problems in pregnancy and birth (cf. Boone 1982; Kay 1982; MacCormack 1982). If we are to enlarge our understanding of how perinatal conditions arise and why they persist, we must investigate these factors. If we want to understand the causes of these problems rather than merely the extent to which they exist, ethnographic research can provide an invaluable perspective. It examines the actual circumstances in which poor women live and have babies. Surveys do not. They cannot adequately address questions of causality, for they are limited to descriptive characteristics. Moreover, most survey data (e.g., education, race, marital status) used for vital records are derived from birth and death certificates and sometimes from hospital records (e.g., data on smoking, nutrition, alcohol consumption). The accuracy of this information is questionable. During my own experiences as a researcher, I was made aware of numerous instances in which the information in hospital records was vastly different from the information I obtained firsthand.

In this chapter I examine the circumstances in which poor women manage their pregnancies and receive perinatal health care. While my conclusions are derived from my own ethnographic research in an intense study of two small groups of women, it is my contention that, in general in this country, the accoutrements of poverty—unemployment, lack of support, poor education, lack of continuity of care in public clinics with long waits and the resultant stress created—are clearly more significant factors in reproductive problems than is ethnicity. The literature cited below, communications with other social scientists who have worked in similar situations, and my familiarity with other public outpatient clinics and their clientele serve to reinforce this conclusion.

Because the condition in which poor women live and have babies and the kind of perinatal care they receive are different from those of middle-class women, their concerns and the issues they face also differ. In the latter part of this chapter, I discuss concerns and suggest directions for dealing with these problems.

THE RESEARCH PROJECT

During 1981 and 1982 I conducted a research project which was in part designed to investigate the issue of ethnicity and socioeconomic factors in reproduction. My priorities were to disentangle ethnic factors from socioeconomic factors as determinants of pregnancy management, to investigate how women who receive their care at a public clinic manage their pregnancies, and to evaluate the kind of health care they receive.

Fifty-three low income women, twenty-seven Puerto Rican and twenty-six "white" women (a category used in census tracts), were studied from early in their pregnancies up to the postpartum period. The women received their care at the public outpatient clinic of a large county teaching hospital located in a midwestern industrial city. Making a detailed case study for each woman enabled me to develop an understanding of her pregnancy and birth within the circumstances of her life and to view this experience as an evolving process rather than as a static event. Approximately 500 interviews were conducted with the women in the study throughout the antepartum, intrapartum, and postpartum periods. I visited their homes, met their families, and was present at many of their labors and births. Over 150 interactions with these women and clinicians were observed. In addition, resident physicians and nurse-midwives were interviewed at length about clinical care and their perceptions of patients.

TABLE 1. Demographic Characteristics of Informants

	Puerto Rican (N=27)	White(N=26)
Mean age at pregnancy	21.8	22.4
Age range	17–29	16–39
Primaparas (first births)	9 (.33)	15(.58)
Multiparas (second or more births)	18 (.66)	11 (.42)
Mean years of education	10.5	10.6
Mean number of living children	1.12	.88
Mean age at first birth	18.5	19.5
Age range at first birth	13–24	16–26

Except for the ethnic distinction, the women who participated in the project had very similar demographic characteristics. Both samples included teenagers: there were nineteen between the ages of sixteen and nineteen. The other women were in their twenties; the only exception was one white woman who was thirty-nine. Many were unmarried and over 60 percent had not completed high school.

Perinatal outcomes indicated that the Puerto Rican sample was slightly more at risk. Twenty-four percent of the Puerto Ricans had low birthweight infants, compared to 21 percent of the white sample.

Ethnicity and Social Factors: Life Conditions of the Women

One of the most significant findings in this study was that the Puerto Rican women did not perceive and manage their pregnancies differently from the white women. They did not have different expectations of clinical care and their behavior in the clinic did not differ from the other group. This was true even for women who did not speak English. A language barrier was an important factor that contributed to a lack of communications at the clinic, but the women did not have different beliefs about pregnancy and birth. Despite the fact that the Puerto Rican women maintained a strong cultural identity and did participate in some distinctive traditional practices (Lazarus 1984), these practices had no bearing on their perinatal management and outcome. Contrary to other findings they did not follow the "hot-cold" syndrome associated with hispanic health (cf. Harwood 1971), nor had most heard of it. Regardless of whether or not the Puerto Rican women were born or brought up in the mainland United States or in Puerto Rico, all were influenced by the biomedical model of pregnancy and birth now prevalent in both the United States and Puerto Rico.

The Puerto Rican and white women shared similar social circumstances and daily experiences. A lack of opportunity to change their lives and an underdeveloped sense of self-definition were notable. Women were dependent on government assistance in the form of food stamps, Aid for Families with Dependent Children (AFDC), public housing, the Women, Infants, and Children Program (WIC), and Medicaid.

Another prominent factor was the complicated, often unsatisfying relationships between the women and the fathers of their babies. Most of the women belonged to female-headed households. Either because of divorce, widowhood, separation, or unstable or nonexistent relationships, most were assuming sole parental responsibility for the baby. Some of the younger women were living with their parents and sometimes grandmothers took responsibility for raising the baby. Although families did not condone out-of-wedlock babies, in most cases the babies were accepted. Of the teenage women between sixteen and nineteen years old, only seven of eighteen were married, and one was engaged. Many of these marriages were fraught with difficulties.

Unemployment was prevalent, undermining relationships and contributing to stress. Many of the fathers were unemployed and seeking jobs of any kind. A few had lost federal government job training in the wake of budget curtailments of social programs; others worked at temporary jobs. Several women voiced frustration that their mates did not work because they were lazy, while others complained about drinking problems.

Conversations with my informants and with other women who used the clinic led me to believe that, with few exceptions, the absence of conjugal relationships was the rule. Other studies focusing on women of low socioeconomic status have come to similar conclusions. Auletta (1982), in his study of the "underclass," stated that in 1979, 12.8 million people in the United States—

just over half of those families classified as poor—lived in families headed by a woman or were women living alone or with nonrelatives. In this same year, 41 percent of all Puerto Rican families in the United States were headed by women.

Carol Stack (1974), writing about survival strategies, found that poor black urban couples often did not chance marriage. Welfare benefits and ties in kin networks provided greater security for women and children. I found these same patterns prevalent among the women in my study. Poor relationships with males led to dependency on "welfare." Since the men had low-paying jobs, if they were employed at all, welfare cuts affecting the "working poor" made such marital relationships even more tenuous. Some women preferred that the baby's father help out financially but not live with them. This arrangement provided more independence and greater financial security. Several women mentioned that in marriage men were in charge but women had the responsibility. Moreover, in the state where the research took place, as in half the states in the country, women are eligible for Medicaid or AFDC aid only if a father is not present in the home or if he can demonstrate a disability. Government policy in this regard, therefore, militates against two-parent households when parents are poor.

The tedium of the women's lives was another clear pattern that emerged from the study. Daily routines did not change much for women with children except for the days spent at the public prenatal clinic. The younger and single women complained that they could not go out as much and have "fun, drink, and dance at parties." Only one young woman remained in high school. For the rest, day after day was spent housekeeping and watching daytime television, particularly soap operas.

Almost all the women were able to function on a daily basis, taking care of their homes and, if they had them, their children. The women had very different personalities and needs and varied in their ability to seek assistance. Some were apathetic. Faced with decisions during their pregnancies, a few women let themselves drift, let things happen to them. Social workers at the hospital who counselled women with physical, emotional, or social problems had to teach women to take responsibility for themselves and to develop control over their lives. They described this as one of the most difficult and challenging aspects of their jobs. Conversely, a few well-motivated women sought social services; for example, one woman enrolled under a grant program at a community college, where she took a paramedic course while welfare provided daycare. But for most of the women, extra programs with long waits and without transportation or babysitters were too inconvenient or overwhelming.

Having a baby gave meaning to the lives of women who had few options in life. Women experiencing the birth of their first child tended to romanticize motherhood. A baby brought prestige and a sense of identity when little else in their lives provided opportunity for self-fulfillment. As enthusiastic and excited as they sometimes appeared, however, they were usually depressed and bored. They were becoming mothers under circumstances that offered little hope for them to change or improve their lives. Their lack of education and skills and their worries about money were compounded by an economy in which unemployment was extremely high and recent cutbacks in federal financial-assistance programs had been made. The women's lack of knowledge about labor and birth, complications in their often high-risk pregnancies, and their past experiences contributed to fears and anxieties. All of these factors led many of the women to view their pregnancies with alternating feelings of delight and depression.

Life conditions may not in themselves cause high-risk pregnancies and births, but they provide an explanation of why pregnant women who are poor experience high levels of stress. Studies in Great Britain indicate that stress is higher in lower socioeconomic groups, reflecting the quality of life. Furthermore, an association has been made between stress and anxiety in pregnancy and higher rates of toxemia, asphyxia, stillbirth, low birthweights, and the poor physical condition of infants (Oakley, McFarlane, and Chalmers 1982). In sum, I found that both white and Puerto Rican women in the clinic faced many of the same problems, problems that middle-class women do not usually experience. The common denominator was poverty.

The Management of Pregnancy

An examination of health beliefs, attitudes, and practices, including family planning and diet, provides insights into how pregnancy and birth are managed, as well as into related problems.

Over 75 percent of the pregnancies in this study were unplanned. The main reasons were a lack of knowledge of or access to birth control. Many of the women had used birth-control methods casually and sporadically. Religious beliefs, however, were not a factor in the use of birth control, although they were significant for some with regard to abortion. Teenagers, in particular, had not used birth control. Frequently cited reasons were: "I was afraid my mother would find out"; or "I was afraid to ask." Most women felt they should have used birth control before they had sex for the first time. Some reasoned that they failed to use contraception because "I didn't think I would get pregnant." Fear of health risks or unpleasant side effects were cited as major reasons for ineffective use or nonuse of contraception. Most of these comments referred to the use of birth-control pills; most women were unfamiliar with other methods of contraception.

There were a number of complaints about the IUD based either on personal experience or the stories of friends or relatives. Only one woman had used a diaphragm before her pregnancy. She and several others were planning to use this method after the birth. Several who had tried the diaphragm found it undesirable. Although a few women, who felt that they had had enough children, expressed a desire to be sterilized after the birth, only one had a tubal ligation directly after the birth.

During their pregnancies, all but one woman in the study told me that she would use birth control after the baby was born. Nurse-practitioners at the clinic family-planning services stressed teaching women to understand the variety of options for family planning. But knowledge of and access to birth control are not the only factors in the rate of subsequent pregnancies. Because of apathy, dissatisfaction with available contraceptive methods, or carelessness, a number of the women did not use birth control after giving birth. Difficulties in obtaining appointments at the family-planning clinic and the inconvenience of coming to the clinic were reasons cited. In addition, many of the women told me that the fathers of their babies did not like to use condoms. Several times I met women at the clinic who had delivered their babies, but who were returning for a pregnancy test. Before I left the clinic, one of my informants had an abortion, and another was expecting another baby. I have since learned of other similar occurrences. Middle-class women I have subsequently interviewed also informed me that they had initially had sexual activity without the use of contraception, but had financial access to abortion and the incentive to terminate an unwanted pregnancy. However, most of the middle-class women believed it was relatively easy to contact their private physician or a family-planning agency for contraception.

Women acceded to the importance of good nutrition, but when I asked them to describe a healthy diet, they could only speak in generalities. Their diets varied, but generally they were not protein deficient. Most were able to afford to eat meat, but often it was fried. Consequently diets were high in fat and calories, and complex carbohydrates, such as vegetables and whole grains, were lacking. They ate a great deal of highly sugared and salted "junk" food. Middle-class women I have interviewed also demonstrate a poor knowledge of nutrition, but, because they usually get enough protein, minerals, and carbohydrates, their ignorance makes relatively little difference. Also, reading much pregnancy literature enables middle-class women to become aware of the need for high-calcium, low-salt diets and of the association of mother's diet with fetal growth.

Physicians at the clinic did not usually talk to patients about appropriate nutrition despite the fact that the physicians all agreed that proper nutrition was essential during the perinatal period. Resident physicians admitted that they had little training in or knowledge of nutrition. The division of labor in the clinic was such that if women were defined as underweight, overweight, or diabetic they were referred to a nutritionist after the physician's examination. Some women said that this was useful, but many were anxious by then to leave the clinic and saw the conference with the nutritionist as a waste of time.

About half of the women smoked, eighteen heavily, though they were not ignorant of the hazards of smoking. Informed in the clinic of the association between smoking and low-weight babies, some cut down from two packs to one pack a day, but most found it too difficult to stop completely. Smokers also tended to drink a great deal of coffee. One woman told me she drank three or four pots of coffee a day (ten cups in each) along with her pack of cigarettes. Despite the fact that two years before, her pregnancy had ended in the premature delivery of her daughter at six months, no one at the clinic had ever asked about her eating habits.

A few women used marijuana occasionally during pregnancy, but none were using "hard" drugs. None of the women were heavy drinkers. The women did not exercise either before or during their pregnancies, and many did not think they should start during pregnancy. Several of the nurses suggested stretching exercises to women who complained about cramping muscles. One nurse attempted to set up an exercise class with a physical therapist at the hospital. Nevertheless, few clinic patients expressed an interest in participating in these classes. Middle-class women, on the other hand, talked enthusiastically about recreational walking and even jogging, and some attended private aerobic classes for pregnant women.

Most of the women, including those who already had children, had a limited knowledge of pregnancy and birth. They had accumulated bits and pieces of the dominant biomedical model from their clinic encounters, through their past experiences (i.e., being a diabetic, having a miscarriage), from friends and family, and to some extent from radio, television, magazines, and pamphlets. Few women read any of the numerous and readily available books relating to childbirth.

It was difficult for many of the women to articulate what they knew and to distinguish their rational thoughts from their feelings. They often felt uneasy and tense during their pregnancies. They were concerned about having enough money, about being alone, about unhappy relationships. They worried about pain during childbirth, of something going wrong with the pregnancy, the labor, and the delivery, or the possibility of an unhealthy baby. When I asked women if they knew what was happening to their bodies during labor and delivery, their answers varied from: "Yes, I understand it all because I've been through it before," to "I know the basics," to "I'm not sure," and "I don't know anything." Further probing indicated that even those who said they knew what to expect revealed that what they expected was "a great deal of pain, bleeding, and all that stuff."

On the other hand, middle-class women who see private doctors for their care knew much more about the changes in their bodies during pregnancy and about the mechanisms of pregnancy and birth. This knowledge, coupled with fewer financial concerns and stronger support from the father of the baby, contributed to much more relaxed pregnancies. However, when it came to actual labor and delivery, middle-class women said that they too did not know what was happening, that their doctor was in charge, and that therefore they did what they were told. Several women mentioned that their childbirth preparation course prepared them for natural childbirth, not for the cesarean sections they ultimately had.

Women in my study received advice from family and friends. Because of the general nature of the advice, it did not interfere with the information given at the clinic, nor did it provide much practical help. However, it was the source of some emotional support. They heard comments such as: "Eat right, don't drink or don't smoke," "Take care of yourself." Some of the women in both groups manifested vague beliefs in folk explanations. These beliefs generally appeared to fill a gap when other explanations were not given. Typical folk beliefs were: "If the baby kicks early, it's a boy," "Heartburn means the baby is going to be hairy," and "Chicken soup is good for you." But medical explanations from resident physicians and midwives were far more important to the women.

Women in my study depended upon the clinic for a great deal of psychological and educational help because they did not have this support outside of the clinic. Often they did not have the supportive relationships that middle class women do, the financial ability to make life more pleasant during their pregnancies (for example, automobile transportation, exercise classes, baby sitters), or their own doctor. But clinic procedures and the impersonal doctor-patient relationship left them frustrated and with unfulfilled expectations regarding care.

Care in the Public Clinic

In the United States, over 98 percent of births take place in hospitals (Public Health Reports 1980). Nationally, most low-income women do receive prenatal care (Ventura 1984) and this was the case at the county hospital where the research took place. In 1983, out of 3516 women who gave birth at the research site, fewer than forty-five had two or fewer prenatal visits.[1] Hospital officials expect "no-care" figures to rise because of deteriorating economic conditions for the poor. On the average, the women in this study first visited the clinic in the fourteenth week of pregnancy and made ten visits during the prenatal period. Usually there were several weeks between the making of the first appointment and the actual appointment date.[2]

For the small but significant percentage of the women nationally who receive no prenatal care, and for those negatively affected by the growing reduction in Medicaid services (Norris et al. 1984) and the Maternal and Infant Care Program (M&I) services, serious problems exist. Women in comprehensive prenatal care and infant followup programs have been found, in large scale studies, to experience significantly improved perinatal outcomes despite low sociodemographic characteristics and high obstetric risk (Sokol et al. 1980; Showstack et al. 1984). One study found that participation in the Special Supplemental Food Program for Women, Infants, and Children (WIC) is associated with the reduction of Medicaid newborn costs and with the increase in mean birthweight (Schramm et al. 1985). Seventeen women in my study participated in the M & I Program. They were provided with more services and support than the other women, and this helped to prevent their "slipping through the cracks" in the system, the plight of many women receiving care in a public clinic. The twenty-five women in the WIC Program said that the dairy coupons helped them plan their food budgets.

All of the women in the study wanted healthy babies and desired quality medical care. They believed this care was available at the clinic. Coming to the clinic reassured women that satisfactory progress was taking place and that any problems would be diagnosed and treated. They expected their births to be medicalized procedures controlled by the medical profession. Based on their own experiences or those of friends with high-risk pregnancies they believed that there were certain inherent biological risks in pregnancy and birth and that it was therefore important to attend the clinic.

Even with their access to quality technical medical care, women were disappointed. The impersonal atmosphere in the clinic and the indignities that they felt they suffered there left many of them frustrated and dissatisfied. Certain characteristics of the care system undermined compliance and the attitudes of residents and patients toward one another. Chief among these—and the subject of the vast majority of the complaints, were the long waits, usually two or three hours, often longer, at the clinic. The second most frequent complaint was the lack of personal continuity of care, caused in part by the rotating service in the resident-training program. The medical record, not a person, was usually the chief link in care from one visit to the next.

The lack of continuity, coupled with the long waits, led to an absence of rapport between residents and clients. Women were rushed, or at least felt rushed, and were hesitant to ask questions. Bored and frustrated from the long waits, they were often passive and vaguely hostile by the time they were seen. This demeanor tended to reinforce the doctor's stereotype of the "disinterested clinic patient." Many of the women were self-conscious about their lack of knowledge about pregnancy and birth and their ignorance of medical terms, but they were too embarrassed to ask questions. However, it was readily apparent that women desired explanations for their conditions, tests, and medical procedures. Over and over I heard: "I like it when the doctor explains. It helps you to deal with things." One women expressed the opinion of many:

> If it was my first baby I wouldn't come—too scary here—never in a million years. I feel more comfortable seeing a woman doctor because I can talk to women better at the visits. Also, the exam is embarrassing. For the delivery it doesn't matter. The doctors spends about five minutes with me [in the clinic]. That's okay if there is nothing wrong but how would they know when they spend so little time with you...? Sometimes I feel like a guinea pig. If I wasn't worried because of my last preemie I wouldn't come back. They are experimenting on me. It's nerve wracking. One doctor tells you one thing, another something else. This medical student told me I had to have a cesarean when the doctor last week said it wasn't necessary to have a repeat cesarean. Now I don't know what to do. That makes you hate to go. They didn't take my blood pressure. I had to tell them afterward. I didn't see the nurse. Even if the nurse was around I wouldn't have wanted to see her at that point. I got out at 4:30. It's hurry up and wait.

Resident physicians were usually rushed and often exhausted. In the five to ten minute communication with the patient, they sometimes did not ask women about compliance and self-care. Sometimes they assumed that noncompliance was due to patient disinterest and ignorance and therefore focused exclusively on the technical examination. The midwives, with more experience and a longer allotted appointment time (approximately 20 minutes), were able to supplement the physical exam with birth education.

The emphasis in obstetrics/gynecology resident training is on learning pathology and surgical and other technical skills. Clinical care is considered unexciting, and clinic patients are not a priority. Junior residents are pressured by more senior residents to keep on schedule and not take more than the expected time with a patient unless a serious problem arises. To aggravate the lack of rapport resulting from this attitude, the obstetric residents I observed did not give patients information about prenatal care or birth. Information was provided by a nurse after the patient's examination by the doctor. At this point, however, women were anxious to leave the clinic. The nurses, themselves harried from a backlog of patients and duties, sensed the women's feelings and often skimped on teaching or on the handling of patient problems, complaints, and anxieties. Women were also constantly subjected to other indignities. One example was the lack of privacy during interviews with nurses. Conditions such as this reinforced the women's belief that they were unimportant to the clinic personnel, while to me it emphasized their lack of control over the management of their pregnancies.

The organization of health services affects the kind of care that women receive, in particular the doctor/patient relationship. Public-clinic patients receive different care from those who obtain services for a fee in private obstetric practices. In a study analyzing discourse between doctors and patients, Todd (1984) found that obstetrician/gynecologists in private practice had more control over the interaction and thereby had more influence on female patients than did residents in clinics. My observations of clinical interactions indicate that power is indeed distributed differently in private and public medicine, but that clinic patients still have very little control over their care. Physicians practicing in public clinics share a great deal of authority with administrators and to a lesser degree with nurses. They therefore have less individual power than private physicians. As a consequence, clinic personnel, including physicians, are able to blame the system for inadequacies in the delivery of care and to assume less responsibility to patients. In public medicine, then, the physician has less control, but so does the patient. Private patients, who are usually more educated and have a higher income, can more readily choose a physician (or an alternative birthing experience) for their prenatal care and birth. This is not to denigrate the very real problems that women of higher socioeconomic classes face, but poor women have even greater difficulty acquiring satisfactory health care.

Women who use public clinics have little choice about where to receive care. They find talking to clinic professionals more difficult than do more affluent patients. Similarly, relatively inexperienced and generally middle-class residents have problems communicating in their brief interactions with women from a different socioeconomic background. Poor women find it difficult or impossible to manipulate the complicated clinic system for their own benefit. Receiving care in a public clinic is but one expression of poor women's powerless position in society.

The women in my study were aware that they had little control over their care, but that in itself was not vital to them. Much more important, they wanted a doctor who knew their case and who cared about them—a desire also expressed by women who can afford to choose private care. Over the course of their pregnancies, clinic patients were exposed to many different resident physicians, nurses, aides, clerks, and sometimes social workers, yet the clinic structure was such that few people actually knew who the women in my study were. The women felt that no one cared or would or could give them the social support they needed.

During pregnancy, most women have similar desires. These include a satisfying experience, a healthy baby, quality care, and a positive relationship with a health professional who listens and does not make them feel stupid. Medical management of childbirth is clearly the kind of care that most women receive; few poor women are aware of any alternatives, and few actually want alternatives. Even so, the feminist view that women should have control over their bodies and their decisions about birth (c.f. Boston Women's Health Book Collective 1985; Romalis 1981) has led to small but positive steps in the medical management of childbirth for poor women as these changes have been incorporated into perinatal care at public institutions and teaching hospitals. Notable among those at the study site were the teaching of Lamaze "natural childbirth" classes and encouraging patients to bring the father of the baby or a friend to labor and delivery for support. Also, women were not given enemas or shaved in preparation for birth. Breastfeeding, while not encouraged, was accepted.Women who took the Lamaze course appeared calmer during labor and birth than other women. Interestingly, those who took the course were either women who were expecting their first baby or those who were not in a relationship with a male. A possible explanation is that these women had more time and fewer household responsibilities preventing them from coming back to the hospital for the course. Although attendance at Lamaze classes was encouraged, most women could not or would not commit themselves to attend. Even when alternatives were offered, poor women did not readily avail themselves of them. The reasons were many—it was too difficult to travel to the hospital one more time; there was no one to babysit or no one to go with; or the hospital was too far away to take the bus at night.

CONCLUSIONS AND IMPLICATIONS

Many of the problems associated with pregnancy and childbirth can be linked to poverty. While epidemiological studies of childbirth are useful in showing the distribution of birth problems, they have significant limitations. Birth statistics must be interpreted with caution because they are not always accurately obtained and because the data that are obtained are limited to certain readily available information.

As a result, these statistics often ignore significant issues, in particular ethnicity and poverty. Because it is the common factor in so many perinatal problems, the poverty issue should be central in policy considerations. Although race or ethnicity should not be confused with class,[3] they often are. My study was limited to two groups of low income women at one hospital. Further studies are needed to compare the health care and health risks of specific races and ethnic groups both within the same class and across different socioeconomic levels.

Ethnographic studies that examine the forces shaping perinatal beliefs and practices, the relationships between a pregnant woman and those who assist her, and the patterns of care she receives are a necessary supplement to epidemiological studies of childbirth. Knowledge of the social situation of birth provides an understanding of how life circumstances may contribute to perinatal problems. For example, not having enough money affects nutrition, not having social support creates anxiety, unemployment leads to friction and stressful relationships.

Even women who are not poor face some of these problems. Ethnic beliefs, in themselves, can play a role in poor compliance and communication between doctors and patients. My findings, however, indicate that women from different backgrounds all want the same things: to receive quality care and to be treated with dignity and kindness. Racial prejudice in health care certainly exists and should be addressed. However, regardless of ethnic background, unmarried teenage mothers are predominantly poor, not well educated, and are dependent upon government programs for assistance and public clinics for medical care. These are the women who have low birthweight babies. The causes are complex, but the association with poverty is obvious. Perinatal problems must be seen in relation to the position these women occupy in the social structure. It is clear from this study, in which both poor white and Puerto Rican women had similar patterns of problems, that poverty rather than ethnicity is the critical element in reproductive health.

Most of the pregnancies observed during this study were unintended. Prevention of pregnancy must not focus on access to family planning alone. A well-designed study of family-planning clinics, staffs, and teenage clients found that compliance was significantly greater when family-planning nurses provided strong support and reinforcement (Nathanson et al. 1985). Programs must address the larger issues of these women's lives and be initiated for both young women and young men. Employment opportunities can contribute to a sense of self-worth and dignity, and job training as well as jobs and day care should therefore be a national priority. Many of the women in my study dropped out of high school *before* they became pregnant; they believed that school was uninteresting and irrelevant to their lives. Emphasis should be placed on getting people to finish high school so that they are more employable. However, worthwhile programs have to be developed for them to want to do this. People must see that they have choices, and so the choices must really exist. Supportive programs in schools and health institutions are needed to teach teenagers to deal with social relationships; in particular these programs must help develop an understanding of the consequences of one's actions, including sexual relationships, pregnancy, birth, and the consequences of raising a child. Controversial high-school health clinics in St. Paul and inner-city Chicago which provide family-planning information and contraception are considered very successful by participants. The National Urban League has begun an anti-pregnancy campaign which is aimed at young men. Support groups for unwed teenage fathers have been started in New York City by neighborhood groups and Planned Parenthood. These programs do not reach everyone, but they provide emotional support, encouragement for involvement, and techniques of coping with child rearing, all of which ultimately significantly reduce child abuse. There must also be meaningful sex-education programs and counselling with followups.

Perinatal education and prenatal care are other areas that clearly need improvement. Prenatal care and relationships with clinicians in the public clinic control the perinatal process and influence how women think about pregnancy and birth, and as a consequence they can contribute to stress in pregnancy and childbirth (Oakley et al. 1982). What is needed are programs that effectively educate women to manage their pregnancies, that prepare them for labor and delivery, and that teach them how to deal with pain. Such programs, along with educational programs that provide school children with information about reproduction, responsible planned parenthood (including options for birth control), and the importance of prenatal care are found in Sweden. When combined with obstetric standards, wherein obstetricians' attitudes are seen as a major factor contributing to the success of the system and where peer review of obstetric care is common, these programs have led to a unified approach to quality obstetrics and have been cited as the cornerstone of Sweden's low infant mortality and morbidity rates (Hein 1982). If instituted in this country, these programs might make it difficult to blame the patient or her socioeconomic status for poor birth outcomes. Clearly, technological expertise is not enough.

While it is not possible to quantify quality care and its effect on pregnancy outcome, the findings of this research as well as that of others suggest that care significantly affects well-being. One example is the satisfaction women felt with experienced midwives at the clinic who were able to provide continuity of care, emotional support, and education. "The effects of warmth and kindness on measurable outcomes of pregnancy may be difficult to demonstrate, but these qualities are simply good in themselves. Many things that really count cannot be counted" (Enkin and Chalmers 1982, 285).

The overall solution for providing optimal care for all pregnant women may lie in the total reorganization of health care throughout this country. Until and unless that happens, specific clinic functions must be examined closely to see where certain problems can be eased. In the hospital clinic where my research took place, a Health Maintenance Organization program is going to be developed in several primary care areas, including obstetrics. To attract Medicaid patients, for whom they will now have to compete, staff secretaries and clerks are receiving instruction on how to be more attentive to patients. Although the reasons for change are financial, women will benefit as a result. Long waits, depersonalized service, and lack of continuity of care are difficult to eliminate in a busy teaching hospital, but these are not merely minor inconveniences; they seriously affect health care, and in particular, communication between doctors and patients.

The contradictions between the priorities established by the medical system in training obstetricians in teaching hospitals and in the provision of care to clinic patients also affect communication and raise basic questions about resident education. Nonclinic patients are also affected, though perhaps less directly, for it is in such public clinics that obstetricians develop the values and professional attitudes towards patients that they will take with them to their future private practices (cf. Carver 1981; Scully 1980).

The Department of Health and Human Services has listed priority objectives to be reached by 1990 for reducing infant mortality and high-risk birth: administering block grants, supporting high-risk screening programs, providing assistance to states to develop and implement perinatal care, and conducting research on growth retardation (Koontz 1984). But no mention is made about the quality of health care or of preventing perinatal problems in the first place. And, there is current evidence that the goals for the reduction of low birthweights for black infants are considered unfeasible (Koontz 1984). Furthermore, studies on the environmental causes of low birth weight have not been initiated (*Public Health Reports* 1983). Federal, state, and local agencies, and community and private organizations should pool resources; however, this cannot be done without leadership and funding from the federal government. Meanwhile, the current administration has reduced desperately needed services in the M&I Programs and in the WIC program through cutbacks in spending, and has restricted eligibility for Medicaid and AFDC. Funds for community health centers and migrant programs have been cut. Thus, instead of increasing services and providing more preventive care, the existing situation calls into question the degree to which reducing infant mortality is truly a priority in this country. Finally, because poverty is central to the problem of poor reproductive outcome, it too must be addressed.

NOTES

I would like to thank Gregory Pappas for comments on an earlier draft of this chapter. This research was supported in part by the Perinatal Research Center, US PHS grant # MO1-RR00210.

1. The obstetric/gynecology department did not keep records of how many women were actually asked for this information.

2. By way of comparison, in a twenty-two state survey in 1981, Puerto Rican mothers had a median of 9.3 prenatal visits (Ventura 1984).

3. Even when both racial and socioeconomic factors are differentiated, race is still used as "a proxy measure of social phenomena" (Wise et al. 1985).

2

ADEQUATE PRENATAL CARE AND REPRODUCTIVE OUTCOME

Marilyn Poland

Reproductive outcome is one criterion often used to reflect the overall health of a population. In the United States, the infant-mortality rate (the number of live-born infants who die in the first year of life per 1,000 live-born infants) has long been considered a barometer of the nation's general health and a reflection of the effectiveness of its health care system. The fact that the United States has ranked no better than seventeenth among highly industrialized nations in its infant-mortality rates has been a concern to health providers (Chase 1977: 662). While the overall infant-mortality rate has been falling in recent years to a new low of 10.9 per 1,000 in 1983, there are large differences in group-specific mortality rates. In Michigan, for example, the infant-mortality rate among blacks has been higher than that of whites for many years. Recently, this disparity has become more apparent. In 1982 the rate for black infants was 24.6, more than twice that for whites (9.7 per 1,000) (MDPH 1984).

The strongest predictor of infant mortality in industrialized countries is the birth of very low birthweight infants, or infants weighing less than 1,500 grams at birth (Lee et al. 1980: 759). Factors associated with the birth of small infants include poverty, race, age, high parity, inadequate social supports, previous birth of a small infant, inadequate weight gain, substance abuse, and poor health habits such as lack of medical care (Gortmaker 1979: 653; Earhardt et al. 1970: 743; McCormick 1985: 82; Boone 1982: 233). One study reports an increase in infant-mortality rates accompanying economic swings and attendant stress (Brenner 1973: 145). Several other studies report a significant improvement in pregnancy outcome with utilization of prenatal care, especially by poor women (David and Siegel 1983: 531; Greenberg 1983: 797). Women who attend more than six prenatal visits have infants with higher birthweights than those with less care (Taylor 1984: 9). Furthermore, comprehensive high-risk antenatal clinics are particularly effective in reducing the likelihood of a poor outcome (Sokol et al. 1980: 150).

Following these themes, the two studies presented here examine the socio-demographic, attitudinal, structural, and maternal correlates of prenatal care-seeking and low birthweight infants born to predominantly black mothers in Detroit, Michigan. Two research questions were posed: (1) What demographic, structural and attitudinal differences are associated with amount of prenatal care? and (2) What effects, if any, do maternal characteristics and prenatal care have on pregnancy outcome?

Between 1980 and 1984, an average of 19,000 live births occurred each year in Detroit. Over one third, or 7,000 infants per year, were born at the major obstetric facility of Wayne State University, Hutzel Hospital. Changes in health-seeking behavior and patient outcomes in large university-affiliated perinatal centers often reflect health-related social changes in the populations they serve. The two studies undertaken in this hospital were (1) a study of medical records during a period of economic recession to examine sociodemographic and maternal factors associated with lack of prenatal care and pregnancy outcome, and (2) lengthy interviews with postpartum mothers who received varying amounts of prenatal care to determine attitudes and beliefs underlying care seeking. Together these studies provide both qualitative and quantitative evidence of both the correlates and effects of prenatal care in a low-income, primarily black popula-tion at high risk of pregnancy complications.

THE FIRST STUDY: THE HOSPITAL RECORD

Methods. The records evaluated consisted of half of all the charts of walk-ins (N=244) and a comparison group (N=260), both drawn at random from the hospital's delivery records for 1980 and 1982. Walk-ins were women who came to the hospital in labor and did not receive prenatal care by a physician associated with the hospital. The comparison group was drawn from those who had attended the hospital's prenatal clinic. Information from the medical records, including sociodemographic, maternal, and pregnancy-outcome variables, were coded for analysis. Additionally, written comments that the staff attributed to patients were recorded. Sociodemographic variables included marital status, zip code, race, and insurance. Maternal-health factors included maternal age, gravity, parity, number of abortions, hypertension, diabetes, number of prenatal appointments, and illicit drug use. Additionally, a "risk score" was determined based on an empirically documented list of maternal criteria associated with poor pregnancy outcome (Hobel et al. 1973: 1). One or more of the following variables denoted a woman as being "at risk" for complications of pregnancy: para 5+, diabetes, heart dis-ease, age less than 17 or greater than 34, hypertension, previous low birthweight infant, greater than 42 weeks gestation, use of illicit drugs or alcohol, breech presentation, multiple birth, cephalopelvic disproportion, and acute uterine bleed-ing. Pregnancy outcome variables were: length of gestation (measured by Dubo-witz Score reflecting the infant's gestational age), birth weight, one and five minute Apgar scores, and length of hospitalization for mother and infant (Dubowitz, Dubowitz and Goldberg 1970: 1).

Results. Analysis of hospital statistics revealed that the number of walk-ins doubled from 145 deliveries during the early economic recession in 1980, to 344 deliveries at the peak of recession in 1982. For the total walk-in group in this study (that is, half of the total number of walk-ins in both 1980 and 1982), 88 percent were black, and 71 percent were single. When they registered in labor, 24 percent had no insurance, 60 percent had Medicaid, and 16 percent had private insurance. Although hospital statistics reported the 244 women in this study as walk-ins, an analysis of their medical records indicated that while 41% had no prenatal care, 38 percent had been seen by a doctor and were either referred to the university service due to a pregnancy complication (referrals), or they had lost their insurance and were sent to the hospital to deliver. Hospital staff refer to the latter patients as "dumps" and the practice as the "dumping syndrome." Finally, 21 percent had no clearly identified care-seeking patterns. This latter group was not included in the comparison analysis.

Sociodemographic, maternal, and pregnancy-outcome factors of the remaining 193 walk-ins were compared for 1980 and 1982. Results indicated no differences in maternal-health (risk) factors or pregnancy outcomes over the study years. Although more women had no insurance in 1982 (27.5 percent versus 19.8 percent) and fewer had private insurance, these differences were not significant. However, when walk-ins who were at risk for complications (N=108) were compared across years, there was a significant drop in those with private insurance and an increase in those without insurance (P<.05). Further, it was anticipated that no care walk-ins would have a poorer pregnancy outcome than the referrals. When these two groups were compared, no care walk-ins were significantly more likely to have no insurance, to be drug addicts, to have smaller babies (mean of 2,610 grams versus 2,890 grams) and to have longer infant hospitalization (mean of 5.5 days versus 4.0 days, p <.01).

TABLE 1. Comparisons Between Referrals, Walk-Ins, and Clinic Patients

Variable	Walk-ins (N=100)	Clinic (N=260)	Referrals (N=93)
No Insurance	32%***	10%	16%
Substance Abuse	38%**	6%	8%
Low Birth Weight	40%**	19%	30%"
"AtRisk"	63.3%*	41.1%	51.4%
	Means	*Means*	*Means*
Parity	2.1***	1.0	2.0***
Gravidae	3.5***	2.	3.2***
Abortions	4**	.79	.28*
Weeks Gestation	37.4***	39.23	6.9**
Birth Weight (grams)	2610***	3210	2890***
Apgar (one minute)	7.1**	7.7	7.3**
Infant Days in Hospital	15.5**	4.0	4.8

Significance levels: * p <.05; ** p <.01; *** p <.001
Note: Levels of significance indicate comparisons of means of adjacent columns.

Comparisons between walk-ins (referrals and no care groups) and the hospital clinic patients over both years are seen in Table 1. Walk-ins were more likely to have been at risk for health problems during pregnancy, they had shorter pregnancies, produced smaller babies with lower Apgar scores, and came from zip codes located more often in east Detroit where fewer prenatal clinics were located.

Since the walk-in group differed from the general clinic population due to a large percentage of drug addicts, the no-care walk-ins who were not drug addicts were compared with nonaddicted clinic patients. Table 2 presents these differences. Although maternal risk scores were similar for women in both drug-free groups, walk-ins were younger and had higher parity, fewer abortions, and outcomes marked by shorter gestation and smaller infants who spent more time in the hospital. A two-way Analysis of Variance (ANOVA) which included group, birthweight, and length of gestation revealed significant ($p < .05$) differences between groups for birthweight when length of gestation was controlled. In other words, infants born to women without care were smaller than babies born to mothers who received care and who had pregnancies of the same gestational length. Stepwise multiple regression analysis, using birthweight as the criterion variable and maternal age, parity, prenatal care, and previous low birthweight baby as predictor variables, found that two factors—having had a previous low birthweight infant and amount of prenatal care—predicted 21 percent of the variance. The other factors did not contribute significantly to the birthweight.

Some medical charts contained statements that reflected patient and physician attitudes along with reasons for referrals. For example, charts of many drug addicts contained references to patient hostility and refusal to follow some medical procedures. Two of these women left the hospital against medical advice. Two referrals who went into premature labor were told to go to Hutzel Hospital by their physicians because their Medicaid insurance would not cover the cost of lengthy hospitalization. Another woman reported being sent to the hospital when she lost her insurance and was told Hutzel was a "charity" hospital, despite the fact that it is a private institution.

TABLE 2. No-Care Walk-Ins Who Were Not Drug Addicts Compared with Nonaddicted Clinic Patients

Variable	Means	
	Walk-ins (N=72)	Clinic (N=236)
Age	22.3	24.0*
Parity	2.12	1.09***
Gravidae	3.45	2.89
Abortions	.4	.8**
Hct	34.4	35.9**
Weeks pregnant	37.4	39.2***
Birth weight (grams)	2671.5	3210.3***
Infant days in hospital	5.5	4.0

Significance levels: * $p < .05$;   ** $p < .01$;   *** $p < .001$

THE SECOND STUDY: INTERVIEWS WITH THE WOMEN

Methods. This study focused on women who delivered at Hutzel Hospital over the summer of 1984 and who were identified by hospital statistics as "walk-ins" (women who delivered without receiving care by a physician associated with the hospital). A comparison group was selected as the next "clinic patient" to deliver. The forty-two women who agreed to be interviewed were asked about the amount of care they received, their experiences with prenatal care (both traditional and folk health activities), and their attitudes toward medical care during this and previous pregnancies. These questions were asked in an open-ended interview format. The women also completed a questionnaire containing Likert-type scaled questions that reflected the amount of help and support they received over their pregnancy from family, friends and others. Examples of these questions are: "How much can you count on your family for help if you should need it?" "Compared to other families you know, how would you rate your own family for closeness?" How much does your mother help you?" "How much does your father help you?" "How happy are you with your relationship with the father of your baby?" "How much can you count on his family for help?" and "How many friends do you have that you can talk to about problems?" The scores from each question were totaled so as to represent amount of support, and information from the medical chart was collected as in the first study. One new variable was obtained: adjusted weight gain during pregnancy, computed as weight on admission in labor minus nonpregnant weight (by history) divided by the average expected weight by month of gestation (Niswander 1981: 30).

Results. Forty-two women participated in the study; forty were black, and two were white. Table 3 describes their demographic characteristics. Walk-ins and clinic patients were combined and subdivided into three levels of traditional medical care by a formula that takes into account the month of pregnancy they registered for care, the number of visits they had, and the length of pregnancy (Schwartz and Poppen 1982). Of the forty-two women, seven were classed as having adequate care, thirteen as having intermediate care, and twenty-two as receiving inadequate care.

TABLE 3. Demographic Characteristics of the Sample (N=42)

Characteristic	Mean	Range
Maternal age	23.8	17–41
Parity	2.3	1–8
Number of prenatal visits	5.3	0–14*
Length of gestation (weeks)	36.6	22–41
Weight gain	20.3	0–49
Birth weight (grams)	2,807	720–5,940

* 12 women received no care

Analysis of Variance (ANOVA) by level of care followed by a Student Neumen Kuels procedure was performed for demographic and pregnancy outcome variables. Women in the inadequate-care group had higher parity (mean 1.3 children *versus* 0.8, p <.05) and shorter gestations (mean 34.7 weeks *versus* 38.6 weeks, p <.05) than women in the other two groups. There was a positive linear relationship between amount of prenatal care (by group) and weight gain adjusted for length of gestation (p <.05). Women receiving inadequate care gained an average of eight pounds under average weight gain, while those in the intermediate- and adequate-care groups gained an average of one pound and five pounds, respectively, over average expected weights.

The interviews themselves focused on early symptoms of pregnancy, advice women received from family and friends, decisions about where, when, and why to seek care, experiences with antenatal care, and suggestions to improve access and quality of prenatal care.

How did the women know they were pregnant? Most women pointed to a missed menstrual period as their first indication of pregnancy. Three had irregular periods and were three to four months pregnant before they became suspicious. Other indications included throwing up, "feeling evil," eating more, and "having a fish dream." Nine saw a doctor in the first trimester to confirm the pregnancy, while two bought pregnancy kits at a drug store and confirmed the pregnancy themselves.

Where and why did the women go for prenatal care? Of the forty-two women interviewed, thirty received some prenatal care, while twelve did not. The thirty women used a variety of health facilities, including health department and hospital clinics, private doctors, and an HMO, and ten women used emergency drop-in centers. Eighteen women used two or more of these facilities, depending on convenience, cost, and nature of the services.

The women who preferred the drop-in centers liked the convenience of not having to make an appointment or wait for long periods to be "checked." The centers were also located close to home, charged the women no more than $10, and supplied vitamins "cheaper than in the drugstore." Two of the three women who saw private physicians enjoyed a continuous relationship with one doctor and expressed dismay when their physicians referred them to "clinic doctors" at the university for pregnancy complications. Another woman attended the prenatal clinic of a hospital close to her home, but elected to deliver at Hutzel because "it's a better hospital for mothers and babies." Seven women registered at the university's high-risk clinic. They valued the technical expertise of the physicians and missed few appointments after they registered. Most women receiving care in clinics complained about long waiting periods and seeing different doctors at each visit. "You have to see so many doctors and they tell you different things." Despite the impersonal nature of the care, most felt that university doctors were "the best" and "they have all the tests in one place." Two women went to Hutzel Hospital specifically because they anticipated benefiting from the new technology. "I wanted to go to Hutzel because they do a lot of ultrasounds," and "They can tell you the sex of your baby."

What advice from others and self-help measures were available? All women mentioned special things they did to care for themselves, such as eating good food, taking vitamins, and avoiding strenuous activities. Many received advice about pregnancy from family and friends, including warnings about the danger of raising their arms and choking the fetus with the umbilical cord and things to avoid doing "so the baby won't be marked." Some women registered for care only after a relative (usually the mother) or a friend gave them money or provided transportation. The twelve women who received no prenatal care had all been urged to see a doctor by friends or relatives. Interestingly, all twelve bought vitamin pills or used pills left over from a previous pregnancy "to keep your strength up."

Why did women receive different amounts of care? Comments made by the women are summarized by level of care. The seven mothers who received adequate care were either primiparae (N=4) or had had complicated pregnancies in the past (N=3). One woman saw a doctor regularly at an emergency walk-in clinic until she came to the university to deliver, and two were referred to the clinic at the university by private physicians because they were "high risk." The rest were followed at hospital-based clinics. All had insurance, and they felt that prenatal care was very important because "you could be having complications and may be able to find out before it's too late." "It's important to get checked cause anything could happen to the baby or to yourself." One added that although she felt that prenatal care was very important, "after a while all they do is weigh you, check your urine, and measure your stomach." Another added that in retrospect she did not feel that "it is necessary to go that often. Prenatal care is hard to get across like the fact that smoking is bad for you. But once you start going, you tend to keep it up. If I get pregnant again, I probably won't start so early."

The thirteen women who received intermediate care were primarily multiparae, and at the time they realized they were pregnant all but one had either private insurance or Medicaid. The one mother without insurance delayed registering for care because "I hate to go through all the hassle of getting on Medicaid and then making an appointment." All but one felt that prenatal care was important, yet all either registered in the second trimester or missed several prenatal appointments. One woman avoided some appointments because "I didn't want to get bothered or poked," while another avoided care in the last two months because "I was too big to be walking all that far to catch the bus." Four women described "hassles" with health personnel. "They ask you a lot of questions and send you to a lot of people." Another described being turned away from the clinic because she was one hour late. "The bus was late. When they turned me away I said forget it and I wouldn't come no more." One mother went to an emergency drop-in clinic to be "checked" because "prenatal care is not that important. As long as the baby moves and the mother feels okay, you don't need to see the doctor. Poor people can't afford to see the doctor all the time." One woman thought prenatal care was "boring." Others missed appointments due to moving or lack of transportation. One registered in the second trimester because of not knowing where to go for care.

The twenty-two women who received inadequate care were generally multiparae, all were critical of the medical system, and many felt that prenatal care was not very important. Three had no insurance and were not eligible for Medicaid. "I went to the social worker to see if I could get on Medicaid. She told me I wasn't eligible, and to go to Hutzel Hospital when the baby came." Another paid $40 for prenatal vitamins and to be "checked" once by a doctor. "I couldn't afford to go back." Seven other women were Medicaid-eligible but failed to seek insurance or medical care. These women had a more laissez-faire attitude toward prenatal care. All multiparae but one had received prenatal care with previous pregnancies. This one woman was a heroin addict and had a seven-year-old son with cerebral palsy. "I know that if I had gotten some care my son might not have been born that way. I meant to get some with this baby, but I went into labor early." Several women indicated that they thought care was only important with the first pregnancy. "I knew what to expect from my first pregnancy. You only need care the first time you're pregnant. After that, you know what to do for yourself." Some mothers felt that a few prenatal visits were necessary, but frequent "checks" were not needed. "I went to a drop-in clinic to be checked a few times. I didn't need no special care because I took my vitamins, and I was doing okay." The following statements represent the various opinions of the women:

"I didn't go for care because I felt fine and the baby was moving."
"My mom had eight kids, and she taught me everything about pregnancy and kids. I didn't need no classes or prematernity care."
"I didn't feel like seeing a doctor. I guess I was lazy."
"As long as you deliver at a good hospital like Hutzel, you don't need all that prenatal care."

Several women described problems with health personnel. "Some social workers have nasty attitudes." One teenager complained about a nurse at the teen clinic "who said I was too young to be pregnant again. She upset me and I left." Other women "hated" or "feared" doctors. Two women reported that the clinics they attended during a past pregnancy had closed, and they were reluctant to register at a new facility.

Twenty-one of the twenty-two women who were not registered to deliver at a hospital called the Emergency Medical Service (EMS) when they went into labor. One woman was driving to jury duty when she stopped at the Emergency Room at the university to be "checked" for cramps. Many described feeling "scared" in the EMS van. Five women were first taken to hospitals close to their homes but were quickly transferred to the university service because they had no insurance or were in premature labor. One woman who knew she was at term told the EMS driver she was in premature labor because "I wanted to deliver at a good hospital. I knew they would take me to Hutzel." Another added, "As soon as I heard they were taking me to Hutzel, I could relax."

DISCUSSION

Gaps in reproductive and infant health care in the United States are thought to contribute to the nation's high infant-mortality rate. In addition, factors such as maternal age, parity, socioeconomic status, chronic illness, and poor health habits are associated with low birthweight infants, who are at greater risk of dying (Manniello and Farrell 1977: 667; Gortmaker 1979: 653; Brooks 1980: 2). Prenatal care has been shown to ameliorate the effects of these factors on reproductive outcome in high-risk women from low-income families.

The statistical analysis of Hutzel Hospital medical records taken during the recession supports the findings of others—women who have no insurance, higher parity, previous complications of pregnancy, and poor health habits and do not receive prenatal care have smaller babies (Eisner et al. 1979: 887; McCormick 1985: 82). The information is best understood when placed within the context of an examination of community-wide changes during the recession that resulted from cutbacks in medical services on care-seeking and health delivery patterns.

The medical-records study was done during a time of economic turmoil. At that time, there were federal, state, and local cutbacks in services to the poor. The Michigan State Department of Public Health lost $24.2 million for its programs from September 1981 to January 1983 (Walker 1983: 4). Maternal and Child Health programs lost $6.7 million at a time when demands for services increased (Walker 1983:5). Three major health centers closed in Detroit (two in east Detroit) and Wayne County, affecting 600 women and 11,000 children (Poland 1984: 5). Local family planning projects were cut by 25 percent, reducing service to 21,500 patients. Utilization of free Detroit Health Department clinics increased by 23.5 percent from 1978 through 1982 at a time when city health jobs were being cut (Walker 1983: 5). Hospitals also felt the economic pinch. During the recession, Medicaid reduced its funding for a prenatal visit by almost 75 percent, and payments to hospitals were delayed by as much as six months (Poland 1984: 7). All hospitals in Detroit were forced to make cuts. At Hutzel Hospital, health-education personnel, social workers, nurses, and nutritionists were laid off. Community hospitals and private physicians turned away some Medicaid patients.

The results from the review of medical charts reflect some of these community conditions. First, while the increase in high-risk walk-in patients with Medicaid delivering at Hutzel between 1980 and 1982 does not prove that hospitals and physicians were selectively referring, comments made by referred walk-ins describing sudden transfers to the hospital, late in the third trimester, for chronic health conditions or for no apparent reason at all support the impression of the hospital staff that patients were being "dumped." The phenomenon of selectively referring the poor has been documented by others (Himmelstein et al. 1984: 494). The care of high-risk pregnant women and infants is costly, and reimbursement by Medicaid is modest. Some hospital clinics in Detroit limited numbers of Medicaid patients they would accept (Walker 1983: 11). One large hospital refused all adult pregnant women on Medicaid until the sharp reduction in total numbers of deliveries at that hospital threatened recertification of its obstetrics residency program.

Second, while services were reduced over the entire metropolitan area, the east side of Detroit was affected more than other areas. The high number of walk-ins from that area may have reflected the reductions in prenatal services. The recession produced a dramatic increase in the number of people without work and without insurance, and those receiving welfare saw a reduction in benefits. It would seem that during this economic downturn, pregnant women experienced a withdrawal of services at a time when they were most needed.

Third, some of the women who might have benefited most from prenatal health care—the poor, the drug addicted and/or those with previous low birthweight infants—did not receive care. The study of medical records is limited to sociodemographic and pregnancy-outcome information. It does not describe the process of seeking and receiving care. Interviews with women about their attitudes and experiences with prenatal care offer some insight into their different care seeking patterns.

SEEKING PRENATAL CARE

Despite a proliferation of programs to provide prenatal care to the poor, women who are at risk of having small infants may not benefit from these programs. Women varied considerably in their perceptions of the value of prenatal care and in their experiences seeking and receiving that care. These variations were associated with patterns of prenatal care.

There was a general belief that prenatal care was most important for women who were pregnant for the first time and for those who had health problems or had a significant chance of developing complications. Although care was seen as important for first pregnancies, its importance related to information obtained by the woman and her experience of pregnancy. It is during this vulnerable first time that women learn what to expect, how to detect problems early, and what to do for themselves. The monitoring of fetal movements and general feelings of maternal well being are also part of a system of signs and symptoms which indicate health status during pregnancy. Some of this information can be learned from health personnel, though much is imparted by friends and female relatives, especially the woman's mother. Folk beliefs pertaining to special foods and activities were seen as important in preventing harm. The use of prenatal vitamins by almost all of the women demonstrates the widely held belief that vitamins contribute to a good pregnancy outcome.

Another attitude which was fairly common was the devaluing of the "preventive" aspects of prenatal care in favor of "high tech" procedures such as sonograms. Some women viewed routine aspects of prenatal care such as checking urine and weight gain, as not worth the time and effort necessary in seeking them, especially early in pregnancy. As the pregnancy proceeded, women felt that being "checked" assumed greater importance. Some also believed that strenuous activities, such as taking the bus, were unhealthy late in pregnancy, and this belief interfered with weekly appointments. The time of labor and delivery is a period of greatest vulnerability. The women who were interviewed wanted to have their babies in a good hospital. There was an underlying theme from women who received intermediate or inadequate care that prenatal care was not all that necessary as long as they delivered in a good hospital.

The frequent use of emergency drop-in centers instead of specially designed high-risk antenatal clinics for poor women is a new phenomenon. The need to catch problems early, before subjective signs become apparent, provides incentive for some women to see physicians to be "checked." The precise timing or reasons for periodic checks is unknown and would be interesting to assess. According to the women, periodic checks in drop-in centers represented medical confirmation that the pregnancy was proceeding normally, without the hassles of making appointments or traveling long distances. These centers also gave the women a feeling of control over the timing of the "checks." The women were aware that the care at these centers was inferior to that offered at hospitals, but the relief from hassles and staff with "bad attitudes" was sufficient incentive for their use.

Many of the women who sought care at clinics described long waits, transportation problems, and discourteous staff. Confusion resulting from sudden changes in location, cost, and type of available services frustrated some of the women and prevented them from seeking care. Women who were at greatest risk for complications—those with poor health habits such as drug abuse, multiparous adolescents, and infrequent clinic attenders—reported punitive attitudes and actions by health professionals. These problems undoubtedly are worsened when clinics are closed and staffing is cut because of funding cutbacks.

There is evidence that pregnancy outcomes are better when high-risk women attend special antenatal clinics (Sokol et al. 1980: 150). The analysis of hospital records from Hutzel Hospital indicates that women receiving prenatal care had a better pregnancy outcome, even when length of gestation was controlled. It is unfortunate that high-risk antenatal centers established for the poor often discourage these women from receiving care. Large antenatal clinics are often staffed by physicians-in-training on a rotating schedule. Many women may be scheduled for the same time and have to wait for long periods, seeing an array of different physicians during the course of a pregnancy. According to the women, and to other studies, this method does not encourage the use of "preventive" services by the poor (Poland 1976: 45). The poor tend to use fewer preventive-health services than other income groups, preferring to use acute emergency services. Boone (1982: 235) has suggested that physicians should develop a broader approach to the problems underlying poor pregnancy outcomes among the disadvantaged. If prenatal care, a preventive service, is deemed important by the medical community, it will have to be seen as necessary by women, and procedures will have to be offered at low cost and scheduled at the women's convenience. Reduction in funding for such services makes such an approach to the delivery of prenatal care difficult and ultimately perpetuates the pattern of poor prenatal care and low birthweight infants.

3

SOCIAL SUPPORT FOR PREGNANCY AND CHILDBEARING AMONG DISADVANTAGED BLACKS IN AN AMERICAN INNER CITY

Margaret S. Boone

The anthropological study of pregnancy and childbearing in cultures around the world suggests the universal importance of several social factors that ensure a successful reproductive experience for mother, infant, and society. Structural factors include a network of kin to impart knowledge and family name to a new infant, and economic and political institutions to support the mother and infant until the dependency of both lessens. There are also religious and moral orders to legitimize support roles, which developed during the evolution of the hominids to serve the survival needs of mothers and infants. While the flexibility of support roles increased during these millenia—that is, while it became *less* important who gave "maternal" support to an infant or "family" support to a pregnant woman—it became *more* important that support be given. The growing complexity of social structure, language, and the economy meant that a child needed a long, intensive period of socialization which, in turn, depended on the participation of a primary caretaker, usually the mother, and on social systems which sanctioned roles that served her needs. Even where survival is most precarious, where "scientific" medical care is most rudimentary, or where sex-role inequality is most exaggerated, all societies stress the importance of pregnancy and childbearing by providing some type of special care for mother and infant.

Epidemiological patterns in modern industrial societies clearly demonstrate that the health of mothers and infants varies by social class (for example, by education and occupation) and by race. Failure to provide care for mothers and infants in most societies can elicit gossip, scorn, or open hostility. In American society, failure to provide support for minority women and children is implied by their patterns of poor health. Although the "fault" for poor health is not easy to assign, maternal and infant health statistics for individual cities can embarrass the politicians and bureaucrats who are responsible for the distribution of health resources. Their task is difficult because the responsibility for poor health among

TABLE 1. Selected Vital Statistics for American Females, Mothers, and Infants, by Race, 1982[a]

	White	*Black*
Life expectancy for females	78.8 years	73.5 years
Maternal mortality rate[b]	5.8	18.2
Low birthweight rate[c]	5.6%	12.4%
Infant mortality rate[d]	10.1	9.6

[a]Data Sources: *Advance Report of Final Natality Statistics, 1982,* DHHS Publication No. 84–1120; *Advance Report of Final Mortality Statistics, 1982,* DHHS Publication No. 85–1120. Washington D.C.: U.S. Government Printing Office. National Center for Health Statistics, U.S. Public Health Service.

[b]Maternal mortality is the number of maternal deaths per 100,000 live births.

[c]Low birthweight cutoff is 2,500g, approximately 5 lb., 5 1/2 oz.

[d]Infant mortality rate is the number of infant deaths within one year of birth per 1,000 live births.

minority women and children is diffuse. It is even more difficult when the causes for poor health and poor pregnancy outcome among minority women are unclear.

Although infant birthweight is one of the most sensitive indicators of population and health quality, it is also known to respond to a variety of exogenous and endogenous factors, and to different factors in different environments. Epidemiologists identify four factors that best help to identify American women at high risk of poor pregnancy outcome: race, education, marital status, and previous poor pregnancy outcome (Brooks 1980; Reed and Stanley 1977; Wallace 1978). However, these variables do not unambiguously distinguish women with good and poor pregnancy outcomes *within* a disadvantaged, inner-city black population:

> Where illegitimacy rates are very high, marital status fails to separate high- and lower-risk women. Where reproductive age is young and fertility levels high, young age also ceases to distinguish them. If the delivering group is young, unmarried, and poorly educated relative to the population of the United States, then greater age, married status, and more education may not imply differential keys to security for the pregnant woman. To be older (or younger), legally married, and a high-school graduate in a disadvantaged population may not mean that a woman is healthier, better supported, under less stress, or has better access to medical services.... These factors do not confer a reproductive advantage, as in the general population, and their lack of significance sets apart as qualitatively different the context of pregnancy in the ghetto (Boone 1982:233).

If standard indicators fail to identify minority women at high risk, further research could clarify the reasons for low birthweight and high infant mortality among women in this, and possibly other, lower socioeconomic strata. This chapter explores the factor of social support—an important variable in pregnancy outcome which has received increasing attention in the literature in recent years (Barnard 1980).

THE IMPORTANCE OF SOCIAL SUPPORT

Because anthropological research shows that support for mothers and infants is critically important in all cultures, social support has become an important research topic in attempts to explain poor pregnancy outcome in the United States—one of the most medically advanced yet socially stratified societies. This discussion explores social support for poor black women in a northeastern American city and suggests mechanisms through which inadequate social support causes or exacerbates more commonly and easily measured conditions associated with poor pregnancy outcome, such as chronic maternal health problems, lack of prenatal care, and substance abuse.

While health statistics suggest the gross effects of poverty on reproductive health, the more qualitative components of lower-class life-styles remain elusive and difficult to measure in relation to health conditions. Subjective self-reports, ethnographic reports, systematic case studies, and surveys of "positive well-being" have become increasingly sophisticated and useful in illustrating the relative degree of psychological distress and social alienation during pregnancy and its aftermath. However, few studies have quantified any of the social or cultural dimensions of disadvantaged life-styles for the purpose of analyzing their effect on pregnancy outcome. Standard correlative measures, such as years of education and rate of marriage, fail to distinguish poor from successful pregnancy outcome among poor black women in the study population examined here. Therefore, new measures have been devised to test the importance of social support in relation to poor pregnancy outcome. Qualitative findings are then used to further explore the meaning of social support for inner-city black women at the time of pregnancy and birth.

Findings come from two related studies: one in 1980 and the other in 1984. The analyses focus on samples of disadvantaged black women who live in a city that consistently maintains one of the highest rates of low birthweight delivery in the United States. The reasons for this pattern are not well understood, although previous research suggests one basic explanation: Poor pregnancy outcome is somehow related to the high rate of black births and the high black rate of low birthweight deliveries. Infant mortality and low infant birthweight among the disadvantaged present a major challenge to policy makers who have limited dollars to solve complex health problems. If social support can be demonstrated as an important factor in pregnancy outcome for these women, then services that address their unmet needs for social support can be more realistically considered by those who design and administer inner-city health programs. To date, while innovation has not been dismissed as an inappropriate response, the social-support factor has been relatively ignored.

METHODOLOGIES FOR THE TWO STUDIES

Study One: The Epidemiological Study. The original project on which this chapter is based was conducted as a combined quantitative/qualitative study of low birthweight and infant mortality among black women who delivered at a public, inner-city hospital. The city's black population is characterized by a number of poor health indicators, including the highest U.S. rates of some types of cancer and high rates of alcohol-related deaths. In 1977–78, women at the public hospital gave birth to infants under 2,500 grams (the low birthweight standard of approximately 5 1/2 lbs.) at a rate of 15 percent, which was twice the national average. In addition to samples of women having low birthweight infants, random samples of women with normal-weight infants were also drawn from the obstetric records. A statistical analysis compared samples of women (N=105 each) giving birth to either *very* low (454g to 1,500g) or normal weight (2,501g and over) infants. Because birthweight was the selection criterion, the infant outcomes varied dramatically. In the *very* low birthweight sample, 20 percent of the infants lived, 53 percent died, and 27 percent were stillborn; in the normal-weight sample, 99 percent lived, 1 percent were stillborn, and there were no infant deaths.

A comparative case-control study using these two samples statistically tested and isolated a number of social and health factors that distinguished women with normal and *very* low birthweight infants: alcoholism, smoking, a history of hypertension, lack of prenatal care, and migrant status from the South. A medical-record review also implicated overall poor health and a variety of chronic diseases, inability to contracept effectively, very rapidly paced childbearing, relatively poor social relationships and psychological adjustments, and violence (Boone 1982:232–33). Eight in-depth interviews provided rich detail on the cultural beliefs and attitudes of some of the women who had suffered infant deaths, and suggested hypotheses to explain the relationships between social factors and poor pregnancy outcome.

Study Two: Operationalization of the Social Support Factor. Because all factors isolated in the first study could be implicated—either directly or indirectly—in the mother's receipt of inadequate support, the social support factor was operationalized and analyzed with data from a second study. Two additional samples were drawn from the original inner-city black delivering population: one more sample of women having normal-weight infants and a sample of women having low birthweight infants who were not *very* low (infants in the range of 1,501–2,500g). There were 120 women in each of the two new samples; thus there was a total of 450 women who were coded for "stability of social support." Together, the samples represented all ranges of infant birthweight except births under 454g, which were termed "incomplete abortions" and not figured into mortality statistics.

Social support was operationalized by making two assumptions. It was assumed that women who had a stable level of social support would (a) tend to list *someone* as the "responsible person" (the person to be contacted in case of an emergency) on each admission to the hospital; and (b) this would be the *same* person over time. The second study also examined residential locations of all women over a period of from five to seven years, with residences taken from a series of three hospital admissions. The first address was from the original delivery in 1977–78; the second address was the one closest to April 1980; and the last address was the one closest to the followup date in 1984. The result was a series of addresses for each woman, along with the identities of the individuals listed as "responsible persons" for all admissions. A scale (Figure 1) combined the two dimensions: Dimension A (the notation of someone, anyone) and Dimension B (the sameness of that person in a series of three admissions).

FIGURE 1. Matrix of Scores for Stability of Social Support

		Matrix of Scores						
				DIMENSION B				
		a	b	c	d	e	f	g
Best	D							
3 of 3 admissions	I	15	x	x	12	x	x	9
2 of 2	M	x	13	x	x	x	9	x
1 of 1	E	x	x	11	x	x	x	x
2 of 3	N	x	11	x	x	x	7	x
1 of 2	S	x	x	9	x	x	x	x
1 of 3	I	x	x	8	x	x	x	x
0 of 1	O	x	x	x	x	5	x	x
0 of 2	N	x	x	x	x	4	x	x
0 of 3		x	x	x	x	3	x	x
Worst	A							

Dimension A: Whether someone is listed at all as a responsible person

Dimension B: The sameness of that person over time: (*Best*) a=3 persons, all same; b=2 persons, both same; c=1 person listed; d=3 persons, 2 of 3 same; e=0 persons listed; f=2 persons, different; g=3 persons, all different (*Worst*)

Resulting scores for social support ranked from highest to lowest: 15, 13, 12, 11, 9, 8, 7, 5, 4, 3.

While most women had three recorded admissions, the scale could also be applied to women who had only one or two admissions by ranking the presence and sameness of responsible persons for those admissions only. When notations were missing, assumptions about these responsible persons were consistently made in a "conservative" direction, i.e., by making assumptions that would imply greater stability of social support for the pregnant woman. With this scale, social-support scores were assigned to all 450 women and examined by sample and by other variables. The scores are in ranked numerical order relative to one another and they are not analyzed as interval level data in this chapter.

TABLE 2. Identities of Responsible Persons in the First Study, by Sample

Responsible Person	Very Low Birthweight 454g–1,500g	Normal Birthweight Over 2,500g
Mother	59	61
Other female relative	20	15
Husband	15	18
Woman's father	1	3
Other relationship	9	8
No responsible person listed	1	0
Total in Sample	105	105

The operationalization of social support in this fashion follows logically from findings on supportive individuals in the first study. Seventy-five percent of the women in all samples were unmarried at delivery, and 75–80 percent of.all women listed female relatives as responsible persons on admission to the hospital in 1977–78. Table 2 shows the frequencies with which types of responsible persons are listed by women in the first study. The rates did not differ significantly between samples of women with normal and *very* low birthweight deliveries. In 65 percent of all cases, the responsible person lived at the same address as the woman.

Few of the women in the original samples or in the samples drawn for the second study had married between the 1977–78 delivery and follow-up in 1984, so few had made a change from a parent to a spouse in the notations made for responsible persons. Mothers remained the most frequently mentioned individuals. However, results from in-depth interviews with eight women who had had infant deaths suggested that the individuals listed were not always the most supportive. Interview data from women with *very* low birthweight infants who died revealed that mothers and other female relatives were *not*—at least for these severely disadvantaged women—the sure source of social support pictured in the literature on inner-city family structure. Instead, young women were more likely to rely on girlfriends, especially as a source of emotional support following the delivery (Boone 1985a:1004–5).

QUANTITATIVE RESULTS ON THE SOCIAL SUPPORT FACTOR

Distribution of Socioeconomic Indices. Social support was one of three indices that were assumed to be related to socioeconomic position in the United States. These measures were developed especially for the population under study and took into account the nature and quality of the data available. It was hypothesized that: the worse the socioeconomic indicator, the more likely the woman was to have a low birthweight infant. In general, this contention was supported, but distributions also suggested relationships among the indices and other variables which further explained the meaning of social support for the inner-city black woman.

First, a "disadvantaged index" scored each woman in the original two samples on the basis of the six dichotomous variables found to be statistically significant in the first epidemiological study. This index combined demographic factors (migrancy from the South, or not; residence in the first study's "high-risk area," or not), and medical factors (prenatal care, or not; hypertension history, or not), with substance abuse factors (smoker or not, alcoholic or not). Together these factors indicated an especially disadvantaged status in this particular population of women. Figure 2 shows the distribution of the disadvantaged index scores by sample from the first study (the only samples for which data on all variables were available).

FIGURE 2. Percent Distribution of Disadvantaged Index Scores among Inner-City Black Women with Normal and Very Low Birthweight Infants

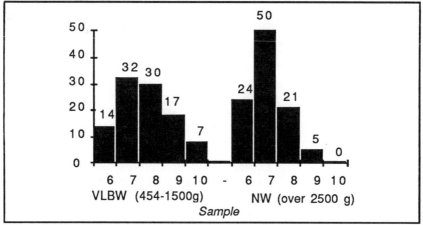

Best = 6, Worst=10

Second, a residential-stability index was developed by simply assuming that the greater the number of residential moves in a specific time period, (a) the greater the residential instability, (b) the more unstable the lifestyle, and (c) the greater the likelihood of having a low birthweight infant. Each of the 450 women was scored on the basis of the number of moves between the 1977–78 delivery (which were randomly distributed throughout the two years with respect to infant birthweight) and the followup date in 1984. Third, the stability of social support was examined as the third index. Figure 3 shows the distribution of these scores by sample from the second study.

Social Support and Infant Birthweight. Low social-support scores in the sample of women with *very* low birthweight infants are especially obvious in comparison to social-support scores in the other samples. The mode is only 9 in the *very* low birthweight sample, while it is 11 in the other two. Like many other results in both studies, these findings point to the existence of a small but particularly disadvantaged subgroup of women, i.e., those with low scores.

However, the proportion of women with the highest score in social support is greatest in the worst sample, those with *very* low birthweight infants. Twenty-two percent of women with the smallest infants have social support scores of 15, compared to 11 percent and 15 percent in the other samples. This points to another subgroup of very young women whose notations for responsible persons remain very stable because they are living at home with their parents throughout the time period.

FIGURE 3. Percent Distribution of Social Support Scores among Inner-City Black Women, by Infant Birthweight

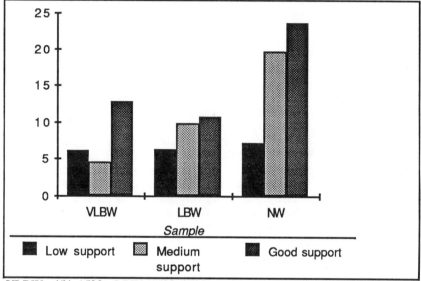

VLBW= 454–1500g, LBW=1500–2500g, NW=over 2500g

Social Support and Residential Stability. In comparing the number of residential moves with social support, there is a proportional *decrease* in the number of residential moves with *increase* in social support score. Half of the women with low support moved two or more times in the five to seven years spanning this analysis. Not surprisingly, this suggests that residential stability and stability of social support are related, and that both are negatively related to pregnancy outcome as measured by infant birthweight. In this disadvantaged in-ner-city black population, frequent residential moves do not signify upward mo-bility, as they may in more middle class and suburban groups.

Social Support and Abortion. Previous poor pregnancy outcome is perhaps the most useful medical history variable in the prediction of infant death or low birthweight delivery among all American women, and more specifically among the women in this study. Both previous miscarriage and previous infant death were used to assess the relationship between previous poor pregnancy outcome and the infant's birthweight for the 1977–78 delivery. The difference in rate in the original *very* low birthweight and normal weight samples was statistically significant ($\alpha=.05$ for both tests). Furthermore, whereas previous abortion has proved *less* useful as a predictor among women in general, it was *equally* useful in this particular population. Rates for previous abortion differed significantly ($\alpha=.01$), and the *very* low birthweight sample had a much larger proportion of women with two or more previous abortions.

The distributions of social-support scores by previous abortion among women in the original samples (the only ones for whom abortion data were available) suggest that women who receive less social support also tend to be those with more previous abortions. The analysis suggests that (1) there are proportionately more women in the *very* low birthweight sample who have had two or more abortions; (2) there are substantial numbers of women in both birthweight samples who have both good support *and* two or more abortions; and (3) the largest proportion of women with two or more abortions occurs in the *very* low birthweight sample among women with low social support. The last finding supports the notion of an especially disadvantaged segment of the reproductive population (those with low support and high abortion rates) in which high rate of abortion combines with other factors to produce a poor pregnancy outcome. However, the second finding shows that high abortion rate need not necessarily be associated with low support, as for example, among very young women who were living at home with their families at the time of the 1977–78 delivery and continued to live at home and list their mothers as responsible persons. In other words, lifestyle can be quite stable and the abortion rate still be high, especially among the very young. Also, for some women, abortion is apparently not as detrimental to a future successful pregnancy as among those with low or only moderate levels of support and whose life circumstances are not as stable.

QUALITATIVE RESULTS ON SOCIAL SUPPORT

Investigation of the social support factor in qualitative terms involves both "negative" findings on the lack of social support and "positive" findings on the presence of violence toward pregnant women. Negative and positive findings range from those in the immediate household environment to those in a larger social context. It is not simply that the disadvantaged black woman receives support from her immediate family and none from medical or political institutions, or support from welfare institutions and none from her family. Uncertainty concerning support characterizes her interactions at *all* levels of society and in many reciprocal relationships and other situations. Negative evidence for poor social support is found throughout the data on women with *very* low birthweight deliveries and is of several types:

(a) *Lack of housing support from nation and city* . Some women were among the homeless, a population which remains ill defined and poorly counted in the United States. One woman had no permanent home, although she did have relatives in the city. The fact that many homeless persons have nearby kin is a fact recently recognized in studies from New York City (Main 1983). The reasons for their lack of reliance on these relatives are still poorly understood, although findings here suggest the failure to support does indeed extend to those circumstances surrounding pregnancy and childbirth for disadvantaged black women.

(b) *Lack of employment and health insurance.* Because of the absence of full-time steady employment, most women did not have health insurance. Many women came to the public hospital because of this fact, and some were transferred, even during labor, from private hospitals to the public hospital for this reason.

(c) *Inadequate support from household and family.* Women in their twenties were often referred to family-planning services with notations in their medical record that they "wanted no more children," "can't take care of any more children," and "It [having more children] is unfair to my mother [with whom the woman and her other children lived]." A similar realistic assessment of their lack of resources is often apparent among women with low birthweight infants. The inaccessibility of family members for needed support at childbirth and for child-rearing can be due to an absence of supportive individuals in the entire kin network. For example, one woman was married and in her late teens when she had her third pregnancy and first infant death. Two years later she and her one child (the second pregnancy was ended by abortion) had moved back home with her parents. Her father was an alcoholic and her mother was nonsupportive—noted simply as "no good" in the record. While the absence of social support is spoken of in harsh terms in both medical records and personal interviews, these words cannot fail to convey a clear picture of the inadequate support for mothers and infants.

(d) *Poor social support and substance abuse.* Alcohol and drug abuse are important contributing factors in the failure of support networks for disadvantaged black women because they impede both the giving and receiving of social support. At followup, one alcoholic woman was noted by her boyfriend to be "staying drunk and not doing anything...She is driving me out of my mind and is wrecking not only her life but my life and the kids'. Looking at her makes me sick!" With the overriding factor of substance abuse, it becomes obvious why legal marriage fails to distinguish women with normal and *very* low birthweight infants. Married women with drinking problems had disrupted relationships with their families just as unmarried women with similar problems did. Neither were capable of relying on the social support which was potentially available. Furthermore, the medical complications brought on by chronic alcohol abuse increased the overall level of need evident in the case histories. The concept of "a need for social support" in many ways overlooks the "multiple-abuse complex," which would, even under the best circumstances, call for a lengthy and varied regimen of home and institutional support. This is illustrated in the following case description:[1]

> A. was divorced and 35 years old when she delivered a one pound infant who died after a week in the premature intensive care nursery. At the time of delivery she was suffering from both gonorrhea and anemia. It was her tenth pregnancy, pre-

ceded by four normal-weight deliveries, three abortions, and two miscarriages. A. also had a history of anxiety, was an alcoholic, and chain-smoked two packs of cigarettes per day. However, she did receive public assistance [which a number of unemployed women did not] and had received prenatal care during pregnancy.

No matter how severe the consequences, alcohol abuse does not engender the same guilt feelings as those expressed by pregnant heroin addicts in this study—although both drugs prevent adequate social support of mother and infant. Heroin abusers in the *very* low birthweight sample show sadness, dismay, and acquiescence to the fact that they are at fault in "causing" their infants' deaths. Although their social lives are disrupted, in general heroin users appear to be more socially active and involved with friends and kin than female alcohol abusers.

(e)*Self-induced abortion and homicide*. Perhaps the ultimate expression of the pregnant woman's inability to obtain or offer social support in this black American subculture is a woman's own effort to curtail a pregnancy, or, once it has resulted in a liveborn child, her attempt to end the child's life by her own actions. These cases do occur, despite the fact that legal abortion services are readily available in this northeastern city. (In fact, the rate of abortion for the years of this study exceeded the rate of live births.) In spite of the availability of abortion, two of the cases of prior abortion were openly recorded as self-induced. One woman threatened to abort herself on admission two months before delivery. She had two children and said she could not care for any more. Another woman, who was in her mid-teens, had requested an abortion, but it was denied because her pregnancy was too far advanced. Her infant was delivered at approximately seven months in the admitting office and lived one day.

Despite these cases and the many complaints and hesitations voiced about having more children, purposeful infanticide appears to be relatively rare in the population studied. In all the samples studied for the years in question, the coroner's office had only one case of infant death due to child abuse. Most interesting about this one case was the very young age of the mother, her overall poor health, and the high degree of involvement of the woman's own mother. As noted before, there are indications that severely disadvantaged black women may not receive the unconditional support from their own mothers and female kin that one is led to expect from the literature on black female networks. While peers—girlfriends—are supportive and nonjudgemental about early and out-of-wedlock pregnancies (the mean age for first pregnancy among *all* women was 18 years), the women in older generations—both relatives and health-care personnel—could be quite harsh. Mothers sometimes rejected their pregnant daughters and the newborn infants.

Positive evidence for poor social support is also found in the numerous references to violent events that actively work to mitigate against physical and psychological well-being for the pregnant woman. Notations about events such as these are more common in the medical records of women who delivered low birthweight infants. Violent events developed in a wide variety of contexts and at various points in time:

(1) *Direct attacks during pregnancy.* Four of the 105 women with *very* low birthweight infants were subject to direct physical attacks during pregnancy: one recorded having been hit with a baseball bat at two months of pregnancy; one was hit in the face with a bottle at four months; one was struck with a hand and required sutures at six months; and one "had a fight and was pushed in the abdomen" nine days prior to delivery. Two of the infants lived, two died.

(2) *Evidence for previous attacks.* Scars are recorded as the main evidence for previous attacks among other women. Two women had stab wounds, and a third had a gunshot wound. Two other alcoholic women had histories of assaults: one was kicked and the other struck.

(3) *Accidents and street assaults.* Violent events do not occur only in domestic circumstances, but also as more random events that reflect an inhospitable environment. One woman was accosted on the street during her pregnancy. Another had her pocketbook stolen, which prevented her from taking her high blood pressure medicine and thereby complicated delivery. One of the alcoholic women mentioned above had a history of falling as well as being struck. Yet another woman was hospitalized following an automobile accident in which her abdomen hit the dashboard.

In summary, evidence for violent events is of various types and can be traced to a number of domestic and urban problems. However, these events all constitute an important part of the life circumstances, if not the lifestyle, of severely disadvantaged inner-city black women. Their victimization has both direct and indirect effects on pregnancy and childbearing.

HEALTH POLICY CHANGE

For the health policy makers of major United States cities, childbirth among the poor presents an array of challenges and problems, including the provision of services to pregnant women which, in less disadvantaged populations, are provided more commonly by a woman's kin and friends. It is far simpler among inner-city women to fault absent or abusive boyfriends and husbands, absent or ineffective support structures such as churches, or to blame the woman's own inability to plan her family. Fault-finding avoids the basic need to improve the health of mothers and children by altering mainstream medical models along more realistic lines which must include the improvement of social support for the disadvantaged—a factor that is a "given" in most other American childbirth contexts.

This chapter suggests the importance of the social-support factor in childbirth, from both a theoretical perspective and from detailed research findings on samples of inner-city black women. When social support is operationalized in even so crude a fashion as the listing of responsible persons on hospital admission, findings clearly show that infant birthweight relates to the degree of support obtained by the mother around the time of childbirth. Social support also relates to other factors such as substance abuse and abortion which can act in an additive manner to cause poor pregnancy outcome among an especially disadvantaged population of inner-city women.

Demonstration of the importance of the social-support factor presents a clear dimension for the development of new options by health policy makers. Combinations of health program goals—prenatal care, abuse withdrawal, health style changes—should be supplemented with firm, institutionalized social-support aids if these are not provided by a woman's cultural support networks. Without a supportive environment, the expensive acute-care treatment programs for mothers and infants will not produce long-term beneficial effects, seen principally in the reduction of low birthweight rates.

NOTES

Special thanks are extended to the former patients and staff of the District of Columbia General Hospital and in particular to its former executive director, Robert Johnson, and its medical director, Lawrence Johnson, M.D. Thanks also to research assistants Wanda Dianne Glover and Helen Campitelli. The research/action project described here as the first study was funded as a Public Service Science Residency from the National Science Foundation, Grant No. OSS-7917826. The second study—"The Inner City Hospital Feasibility Study"—was designed and implemented in 1983-84 at the U.S. Census Bureau as a census-coverage evaluation project. Socioeconomic variables used in that study were useful in the present analysis. Preliminary results from the second study were presented in "Analysis of Inner City Census Coverage Using Local Hospital Administrative Records (with David C. Whitford) at the American Statistical Association meeting, Philadelphia, Pa., August 1984. The views expressed in this chapter are those of the author and do not necessarily reflect those of NSF or the Census Bureau.

1. Details are modified and rearranged to ensure the anonymity of the women. No case describes any single, real individual. Letters bear no relation to the names of the women.

4

KHMER PRENATAL HEALTH PRACTICES AND THE AMERICAN CLINICAL EXPERIENCE

Carolyn Sargent and John Marcucci

An understanding of the cultural transformations resulting from refugee adaptation to American society requires sensitivity to individual variations within the context of general cultural traits and features. Because the beliefs, attitudes and practices of pregnant Khmer women differ from those of the clinic staff who provide them with prenatal care, it is necessary to "appreciate, explore, and document the cultural meanings and social relationships that shape health care systems" (Anderson et al. 1982: 326). A broad understanding of Khmer principles of health and wellness is thus necessary in order to explain the divergent cultural and social constructions of pregnancy and to facilitate communication between Khmer clients and American providers (cf. Kleinman 1975).

KHMER PERCEPTIONS OF HUMORAL EQUILIBRIUM

The analysis of concepts and behaviors associated with pregnancy necessitates a consideration of humoral principles in Khmer medicine. The principle of maintaining the relationship between mind and body in moderated equilibrium is common to the great cultural traditions of both East and West.

> The great traditions of medicine were formulated from generic and cosmological concepts. All of them were humoural theories; four humours in the Mediterranean tradition...three humours in the South Asian tradition.... The equilibrium of these qualities maintained health, and their disequilibrium caused illness, whatever the number of humours. Equilibrium was regulated by an individual's age, sex, and temperment in dynamic relationship to climate, season, food consumption, and other activities....Therapy utilized physical manipulations,

79

modification of the patient's diet and surroundings and numerous medications. (Leslie 1976: 4)

Unlike the metaphysical shift to Cartesian reductionism in the West and the corresponding concern in medicine with germs and individual organ systems, the cultural traditions of Asia continued their holistic cosmological beliefs concerning the importance of maintaining life forces in equilibrium. The Khmer principally derive their understanding of body humors from the Sanskrit tradition of Ayurvedic medicine, which is prevalent in South Asia (Obeyesekere 1977; Nichter 1980; Manderson 1981; Amarasingham 1980). Early Khmer indigenous medicine was based on animistic beliefs of spirit intrusion and the natural effects of pharmaceutical products derived from the forest; but by the thirteenth century Theraveda Buddhism began to assert a notable influence on indigenous Khmer culture (Hall 1968:22). With characteristic syncretism, the Khmer incorporated Buddhist humoral concepts into their medical tradition.

For the Khmer, Theraveda Buddhist monks were the teachers of healing and thus responsible for the cultural transmission of the concepts of physical and spiritual harmony. However, through time, the adaptation of these Buddhist teachings to indigenous beliefs and other cultural influences, particularly the Chinese belief in the equilibrium of opposing qualities of "yin" and "yang," modified the conceptual significance of life forces expressed in the body's humors. While all of the traditional Ayurvedic humours of "wind," "bile," and "phlegm" are found in indigenous Khmer medical beliefs, the humor of wind, due to its intrinsic characteristic of movement, receives special attention in the Khmer belief system. The Khmer are particularly sensitive to the equilibrium of wind in their bodies because this humor controls the movement of blood and its corresponding effects which "heat" or "cool" the body. Although phlegm and bile are important to health, their effects are specific as compared to the more general and holistic attributes of wind in its effect on health and illness. A variety of symptoms are attributable to a disequilibrium of wind, such as fever, headache, fatigue, diarrhea, vomiting, stomach cramps, and localized aches and pains. The Khmer follow the medical practices of dermabrasion and cupping, the use of mentholated medicines, and dietary modifications to restore the equilibrium of wind and thus insure the proper movement of blood which will heal the affliction.

DESCRIPTION OF THE RESEARCH POPULATION

The twenty-two pregnant women interviewed in this research reside in an east Dallas neighborhood. Approximately half of the 5,000 Khmer refugees residing in the Dallas-Fort Worth metropolitan area live in this neighborhood. This population experiences frequent new arrivals from refugee camps as well as secondary migration from other cities in the United States. The length of residence in Dallas among women interviewed ranged from five months to three years. The neighborhood in which the majority of the refugees reside has a decided ethnic cohesiveness evident in mutual-assistance associations and the presence of a variety of ethnic general stores, which cater to the needs of these refugees by providing imported foodstuffs, medicines, and other household goods.

The Khmer women were selected as a convenience sample, primarily identified through contacts with refugee agencies in Dallas. Structured interviews were designed for an open discussion of the questions. All interviews were conducted in the Khmer language and at women's homes. The women ranged in age from eighteen to forty; 32 percent were pregnant for the first time; one woman had nine previous pregnancies. While this group averaged three previous pregnancies, 55 percent had no previous hospital delivery. Of those who had delivered in hospitals, 14 percent reported their most recent hospital delivery as being in a hospital in Cambodia, Thailand or Indonesia, and 4 percent had delivered in hospitals in the United States. Fifty-four percent of the women were in the second trimester of pregnancy when interviewed, 23 percent were in the last trimester, and 23 percent were in the first trimester.

THE FIRST PERCEPTION OF PREGNANCY

The women relied on a variety of signs to first detect their pregnancies (see Table 1). Most Khmer women clearly indicated that cessation of menstruation signals pregnancy. However, 64 percent of the women confirmed that they were pregnant based on alterations in normal body functioning. Four women consulted physicians and confirmed pregnancy via laboratory testing. In one case, a woman experienced the first evidence of pregnancy as an imbalance in body humors, expressed as a "hot" body with secondary characteristics of heart palpitations. Women complaining of humoral imbalance often comment on such heart conditions; palpitations are believed to result from a disequilibrium of the hot/cold relationship as well as the humor of wind, held to be responsible for proper blood circulation. Khmer women regarded vomiting and lack of appetite as normal symptoms of early pregnancy. The first three months of pregnancy are referred to as *chang koun* ("the baby is stronger than the mother"), a term indicating that the fetus is developing into an independent being. This process, like any body change, requires a readjustment in body humors. It is therefore to be expected that an initial period of disturbance such as vomiting, fatigue, and lack of appetite would accompany fetal development.

TABLE 1. Determination of Pregnancy

Means of Determination	Percent
Ceased menstruation	32
Vomiting, no appetite	19
Lab test	19
Just knew	14
No menses, just knew	4
Tired and hungry	4
"Hot" body, palpitations	4
No response	4

HEALTH STATUS

Most (59 percent) of the women interviewed claimed that they had no particular health complaints and considered themselves to be in generally good health. Regardless of this initial response, the women reported a variety of common complaints, especially those conditions that are perceived as problematic by Khmer women: vomiting, fatigue, dizziness, swelling, phlegm, palpitations, abdominal pain, bodily aches and pains, disequilibrium of wind and other nonspecific complaints (see Table 2).

For those who experienced vomiting, the duration of the complaint averaged three months. Approximately one-third of the women did not attempt to treat the vomiting, considering the problem to be a self-limiting condition. However, 33 percent did treat the vomiting by practicing dermabrasion, that is, by rubbing the limbs, chest, and back with a coin and mentholated lubricant. The purpose of this treatment is to restore the body humors to equilibrium; dermabrasion is considered particularly effective in treating disequilibriums of wind (for more detailed discussion of Khmer medical practices, see Sargent et al. 1983: 69–70).

One woman employed *choup*, or cupping on the forehead, to alleviate nausea and vomiting. *Choup*, like dermabrasion, restores the humoral balance, and is also especially useful in treating headaches, flushing, nausea and similar complaints. Customarily, cupping is practiced with a small bottle or cup in which fire from alcohol or a candle creates a vacuum as it is placed on the forehead. The effect is to break the capillaries on the forehead and thus allow excessive wind to leave the body.

Although most women practiced both dermabrasion and cupping, they did so for bodily complaints not associated with pregnancy per se. Interestingly, one woman substituted mentholated plasters on her forehead rather than employing the usual cupping procedure. One woman combined dermabrasion with the use of Western medications to control vomiting, while another practiced both dermabrasion and cupping. One woman modified her diet by eating some sugar to restore humoral balance and hence relieve vomiting and nausea.

Approximately 55 percent of the respondents complained of excessive fatigue. The duration of the fatigue ranged from one to eight months; 30 percent suffered only one month in early pregnancy, while 20 percent complained of fatigue throughout their pregnancy. Most women did nothing to treat the fatigue, considering it an inevitable aspect of pregnancy, although two women observed

TABLE 2. Complaints of Pregnancy

Complaint	Percent
Vomiting	55
Fatigue	45
Aches	41
"Wind"	41
Dizziness	36
Phlegm	27
Swelling	3
Other	36

that they slept more. Thirty-six percent of the women experienced dizziness during the first trimester. Forty-three percent of those complaining of dizziness used either dermabrasion or cupping to alleviate the problem.

Many women (41 percent) complained of bodily aches and pains, particularly in the back and legs, lasting for as long as four months. As would be expected, those complaining of back and leg pain were primarily women in the later months of pregnancy. With regard to treating aches and pains, 75 percent of the women thought that one was obliged to put up with such discomfort, but 25 percent took some remedial action, such as massage, extra rest, and relaxation. Swelling (edema) was not a major complaint of these women. Only 5 percent noted swollen limbs or other edema, despite the fact that 23 percent of the group were in the last trimester of pregnancy, when such edema often occurs.

One-third of the women experienced excessive phlegm, complaining of the need to expectorate frequently. The condition appeared to last for as long as two months and is considered to occur at any phase of pregnancy. The most common remedy for this problem was lemon or lime juice, which is believed to cut the thickness of the phlegm. One woman consulted a physician and received medication to alleviate the problem. Additionally, abdominal discomfort was a problem to 27 percent of those interviewed. Most considered this normal and did nothing about the problem, although one woman in her last trimester consulted a *chmoop* (indigenous midwife) for therapeutic massage.

The affliction of wind, a disturbance in humoral balance, affected 41 percent of the sample. The duration of this complaint ranged from one to eight months, so that it is difficult to generalize regarding the phase of pregnancy during which a woman is most likely to suffer from this problem. In their attempts to restore humoral harmony, most (56 percent) women practiced dermabrasion or cupping. One woman said that dietary changes helped to restore the equilibrium of her body.

Palpitations affected 50 percent of the women intermittently during their pregnancy, but no one suffered for more than two months. Khmer women consider palpitations to be a serious condition, one that is difficult to treat. Correspondingly, 73 percent did not consult anyone regarding treatment, nor did they practice any type of self-treatment. Of those who did seek treatment, 27 percent performed dermabrasion, and one consulted a Vietnamese physician as well.

Women also reported other pregnancy related problems. Of the 36 percent having other problems, 75 percent reported having chills. This finding is particularly interesting given that pregnancy represents a "heated" state for the pregnant woman. However, this does not mean that a pregnant woman cannot experience an imbalance of hot and cold humors. Accordingly, a woman may judiciously treat herself with hot or heating foods.

DIETARY REGULATIONS

According to the general theory of humoral pathology, the regulation of the metaphysical hot and cold attributes of food is necessary to the maintenance of good health (Leslie 1976: 4, 181; Foster and Anderson 1978: 60). Studies of the relationship between food preferences and health maintenance in Asia have demonstrated significant variation in classification of foods and adherence to recommended dietary regimens throughout the region (Manderson 1981; Laderman 1983). In an effort to investigate this variation further, the Khmer women were interviewed about their diets during pregnancy. The women were questioned particularly regarding foods believed to enhance health during pregnancy, knowledge of vitamins, and on foods which are thought to be detrimental to health.

Hot and spicy foods comprised the largest category of foods believed to be harmful to the pregnant woman. Specifically, red pepper was noted by 64 percent of the women, and one woman suggested that fermented fish sauce also had excessive "heating effects." Since pregnancy is already considered to be a hot state, additional hot foods might dangerously imbalance the body, causing the mother ill health and possibly harming the infant. However, 18 percent of the women did not consider any particular foods to be generally harmful to pregnant women, and three women observed that they never eat red pepper due to the risk of overheating their bodies.

With regard to beneficial foods, all women mentioned an array of meats, including pork, beef. chicken, and fish. Beef ranked highest among nutritious meats, followed by pork, chicken, and fish. A variety of vegetables and fruits were also considered to induce strength and were recommended for pregnant women. Among fruits and vegetables, most women mentioned lettuce, cabbage, tomato, and a wide variety of fruits. Cabbage was considered a particularly nutritious vegetable by 64 percent of the women. Five women thought that sweets were nutritious. Overall, it is worthwhile to note that the foods advised during pregnancy correspond closely to what might be considered a healthy adult diet.

It is also worth noting that the adult Khmer population in general does not routinely consume dairy products. None of the women in this sample suggested that milk, cheese, or other dairy products were either nutritious or preferred foods. Nonetheless, clinic personnel recommend consumption of dairy products for pregnant women, a recommendation which is consistently ignored by Khmer clients. Alternative sources of calcium, such as cabbage, are quite palatable to Khmer women.

The majority of the respondents were familiar with the term *vitamin*. Most of these women believed that vitamins increased one's strength. One woman mentioned that vitamins keep a person from being tired and help blood circulation, while another suggested that vitamins prevent illness and maintain a healthy body. Several women had only a vague understanding of vitamins; one knew that vitamins were good for the body but did not know what kinds of foods contained vitamins; another had heard the word from Americans but did not know what it meant; and a third knew that vitamins were available in pill form but did not know the purpose of the pill.

Only 14 percent of those interviewed took the vitamin pills that were given at prenatal clinic visits. Most women received a supply of vitamins at the clinics but decided not to take them, usually due to the nausea resulting from the pills. Thirty-two percent of the women said that they had received iron pills from the clinic and claimed to take them routinely. Still, most women were confused about the distinction between prenatal vitamins and iron supplements. Significantly, almost all of the women observed that it is unwise for a pregnant woman to ingest oral medications while pregnant—the introduction of a novel substance into the body at this time may be harmful. In addition, the heating effects of any medication considered to be strengthening may be injurious to the health of the pregnant woman, given that pregnancy is an intrinsically hot condition.

In her discussion of humoral balance and diet in a Malay population, Laderman concluded that the "richness of ambiguity and variability of interpretation of Malay systems of food avoidance, at the practical level, do not allow us the liberty of formulating a simple cause and effect relationship between traditional food beliefs and nutritional health" (Laderman 1983: 186). Correspondingly, Khmer women do not seem to adhere to a strict dietary regimen based on humoral principles. Among the women interviewed, diets varied according to the individual woman's sense of her own humoral balance and her interpretation of the consequences of eating certain foods. For example, most women adhered to the traditional restriction on eating red pepper during pregnancy—red pepper is believed to cause excessive heat in the mother and child and to provoke un-natural growth of hair on the infant. However, 18 percent of the women did eat some red pepper, claiming that their health would not be adversely affected and that they were not concerned about excess hair on the baby. In addition, they claimed it was more important for them to consume foods that they found deli-cious during their pregnancy. In general, most women observed that it is impor-tant for each woman to know her own body and its needs, and that food choices are based on this premise.

PRENATAL CARE

Routine prenatal care in the first trimester is not a traditional feature of Khmer obstetrics. However, 82 percent of these women sought prenatal care, the majority (41 percent) in the third month of pregnancy, although first visits ranged from the first to the eighth month of pregnancy. It is important to note that these women were strongly encouraged to seek prenatal care by caseworkers from local refugee agencies. In most cases, the women were driven to clinic appointments by a caseworker or community volunteers—thus transportation did not pose an insurmountable problem for the pregnant women. Correspondingly, 75 percent of the women commented that they had no difficulty keeping clinic appointments as long as someone fluent in English was available to accompany them.

Cost also did not appear to be a factor constraining clinic use: 33 percent of the women did not pay at all due to caseworker intervention; 39 percent paid the minimum fee of $5; 11 percent paid between $5 and $30; 5 percent paid more than $30; and 11 percent had medical insurance which covered a portion of the cost. At the county hospital and satellite clinic which these women attended, fees are based on a sliding scale according to income level. In the opinion of most Khmer women, the cost of this service is very economical compared to the cost of private physicians. However, in spite of the cost—$20 per office visit—22 percent of the women consulted Vietnamese physicians in private practice in the neighborhood for diagnostic and treatment purposes during pregnancy.

Women had a variety of reasons for seeking prenatal care. Twenty-eight percent went to the clinic in order to deliver at the hospital, and equal percentage went to the clinic because the caseworker said that they should go, and 20 percent wanted to monitor their health during pregnancy. An additional 6 percent stated that their husbands insisted that they go to the clinic, 6 percent were advised to go by their mothers, 6 percent said that prenatal care is an American custom, and 6 percent said somewhat obscurely that it was easier.

Because only one of the women speaks English, it is important to consider the availability of translators in the clinic setting to facilitate communication between patients and practitioners. Of the sixteen women who discussed this issue, 88 percent said that a translator was available during their appointment. In most cases, the translation was provided by the Khmer caseworker who accompanied the women to the clinic. Considering those women who said they had access to a translator, 63 percent reported that the doctor said that they were in good health. However, 25 percent said that the doctor did not report the status of their condition, and two of these women expressed great dissatisfaction with the lack of information.

All women who attended prenatal consultation noted that the doctor told them to return for a subsequent visit, and most appear to have consulted a physician at least twice. It is evident that the intervention of refugee agencies encourages reliability of followup care.

In assessing clinic care, women commented on the gender of the practitioner. Of the 77 percent who remarked on this point, 29 percent were examined by a man, 47 percent were examined by a woman, and 24 percent had been examined by both a man and a woman. The majority of these women (61 percent) preferred a female practitioner, while only one woman said she would prefer a man. The remainder expressed no preference. The fact that women preferred a female practitioner is indicative of the modesty which prevails between the sexes in Khmer culture. In general, it is considered inappropriate for a man to view a woman's body below the waist, even in the context of a conjugal relationship. The women interviewed did feel comfortable with a woman practitioner, however, and 83 percent remarked that they would not feel afraid if examined by a woman.

THE SHIFT FROM MIDWIVES TO HOSPITAL DELIVERIES

Among the alternatives available to Khmer women seeking prenatal care is the indigenous midwife, or *chmoop*. Although the researchers are aware of several midwives practicing in the Khmer community, 55 percent of the women interviewed stated that they did not know any *chmoop*. However, in one instance a *chmoop* arrived at the household shortly after the informant stated that she was unfamiliar with any midwives in the area. Thirteen percent of the women consulted a midwife for advice and treatment during pregnancy. A primary reason for consulting a midwife was to obtain a massage, which is said to alleviate various aches and pains and to ensure proper positioning of the fetus. However, 32 percent said they would not consult a *chmoop* regardless of availability.

Given the relative availability of midwives, it is interesting that all of those interviewed intended to deliver their babies at the hospital, though three of the women said they would prefer a home birth nonetheless. Half of the women explained their plans in terms of increased safety of a hospital delivery. One woman specified that she had delivered a stillborn child at a midwife-assisted home birth, and she was convinced that hospital personnel would be more competent. Further, 19 percent of the women claimed that hospital delivery is easier than home delivery due to the availability of effective medications. An additional 14 percent said that American law necessitated hospital delivery, that those who delivered at home would be imprisoned.

Informal discussion with members of the refugee community suggests that the opinion that home birth is illegal is widespread and includes the concern that the midwife who assists such a delivery will be arrested. For this reason, midwives who assist at home deliveries are reluctant to cut the umbilical cord. Indigenous midwives, therefore, often advise pregnant women to deliver at the hospital, and even those women who might prefer a home birth feel constrained to bear their children in a hospital setting.

Analysis of the reproductive histories of the women indicates that 36 percent had previously delivered in a hospital in refugee camps in Thailand, Indonesia, or the Philippines. One woman had delivered her most recent child in the county hospital in Dallas. Five other women had delivered their most recent child at home, either in Cambodia or in a refugee camp. It appears, then, that a decided move away from home births is emerging in the Khmer refugee population in Dallas, given that no respondent said that she planned to deliver at home. This shift results from the influence of refugee agencies, Cambodian leaders, and indigenous practitioners themselves who fear the consequences of assisting at deliveries without certification.

THE VIEW FROM THE CLINIC

In examining concepts and practices associated with pregnancy among the Khmer population, it is necessary not only to consider the perceptions of Khmer women, but also those of clinic personnel. Ten staff members at a satellite prenatal clinic used by Khmer women were interviewed concerning their experiences with this group of women. Staff included the director, assistant director, a nurse-practitioner, one physician's assistant, two registered nurses, one lab technician, three clerks and a Cambodian interpreter.

In general, staff observed that Khmer women tended to keep appointments and seemed to comply with instructions. Khmer clients did not seem to be constrained by modesty when the examining practitioner was female; however, they appeared extremely uncomfortable if any male, even a spouse, were present in the examining room. The interpreter noted that one older woman objected to the presence of a young (18 year old) woman —the interpreter—in the room during her examination. Staff described Khmer women as quiet, reserved, shy, and subservient, asking few questions and limiting replies to yes or no.

The Khmer response to pain drew the attention of some practitioners who observed that the women tended to be stoical and expressionless even during experiences which they themselves defined as painful. Interestingly, the clinic staff perceived that Khmer women fear blood tests, though the women themselves did not indicate this to be the case. According to the Cambodian interpreter, women did fear iron pills, which they thought might harm their bodies.

The primary problem involved in treating Khmer women was perceived to be the lack of communication, although since the arrival of the interpreter, communication had been greatly enhanced. Prior to this time, husbands or other men accompanying the woman were asked to translate; however, because certain subjects are not considered appropriate conversation between the sexes, men did not serve as effective translators. Similarly, children who were used as translators had difficulty discussing reproductive matters. The current interpreter has assisted not only in conveying information between staff and clients, but in explaining dimensions of Khmer culture to puzzled personnel. One nurse-practitioner, for example, commented that she was astonished the first time she saw marks of dermabrasion on a patient and was further surprised to learn that the woman's husband did it *for* her, not *to* her. Clinic personnel are now better informed regarding indigenous treatments, such as moxibustion (a procedure in which a mixture of kapok, herbs, and roots is ignited on the skin in order to restore internal harmony), dermabrasion, and cupping, due to the translator's interpretation of these practices. This awareness has facilitated staff ability to distinguish between signs of abuse and treatment markings.

In giving an overall assessment of the Khmer clientele, several staff members observed that the involvement of agency caseworkers in recruiting pregnant women to attend the clinics has greatly increased the number of women attending the prenatal clinic. Prior to this involvement, those Khmer clients who came to the clinic were seeking birth control or were making postpartum visits. Regardless of the purpose of a clinic visit, Khmer women were observed to need the accompaniment of a friend, relative, or caseworker not only to translate, but to provide a sense of security.

CONCLUSION

This study suggests that for the Khmer, humoral theory continues to form the basis of the beliefs and practices of health care during pregnancy. Humoral principles affect the interpretation of discomfort during pregnancy as well as the corresponding choices of treatment. Health care during pregnancy does not represent a radical departure from that which is considered effective for the typical adult. However, for the pregnant Khmer woman, additional concerns arise, such as the risks of oral medication, of overheating the body, and of the introduction of unfamiliar substances into the body. Significantly, though humoral equilibrium is a consideration in diet during pregnancy, women emphasized the importance of individual variability in dietary requirements.

With regard to prenatal care and delivery preferences, the intervention of voluntary agencies has clearly affected patterns of prenatal care and choice of delivery assistance. The majority of women were receiving clinic prenatal care and intended to deliver at the county hospital. Although several indigenous midwives reside in this community, only a few women stated that they preferred to consult a midwife either for prenatal care or delivery. The reluctance of women even to avow their knowledge of local midwives appears to result from agency and community pressure to rely on hospital care.

From the perspective of clinic personnel, Khmer women are reliable clients who present problems primarily when appropriate translation services are not available. Staff members, in general, have a limited understanding of the Khmer cultural context. However, even in a six-month period, the presence of a Khmer translator on staff has expanded the understanding of relevant Khmer medical practices and from the point of view of the staff, has facilitated communication and rapport with clients.

5

THE DECISION TO HAVE OR NOT TO HAVE AMNIOCENTISIS FOR PRENATAL DIAGNOSIS

Barbara Katz Rothman

Women who are medically defined as "at risk" for genetic problems in fetal development are expected to choose to have, or choose not to have, amniocentesis for prenatal diagnosis of possible problems. Amniocentesis involves the removal, via the abdomen, of a small amount of the amniotic fluid which surrounds the fetus at approximately the sixteenth to eigtheenth week of pregnancy. Results are available at about the twentieth week, the midpoint of pregnancy. Amniocentesis for prenatal diagnosis is most commonly done to test for Down's syndrome, a cause of mental retardation and physical problems. There is no treatment available at present for fetuses so affected. Thus, if the diagnosis is positive for Down's syndrome, the woman has the choice of continuing or terminating the pregnancy.

The risk of Down's syndrome increases with maternal and paternal age. Current medical practice treats pregnancies as appropriate candidates for amniocentesis when the pregnant woman is thirty-five years of age or older. The age limit has moved down from forty and continues to move downward at the present time, with women in their early thirties often considered "amnio-eligible."

The research reported in this chapter is based on interviews with sixty-two women who had amniocentesis for prenatal diagnosis and sixty-four women who chose to refuse amniocentesis. The women, who responded to advertisements in magazines, come from all across the United States and range widely in education, occupation, and parity. All women were interviewed either late in their pregnancy or, more commonly, after the birth of their baby.

DECIDING TO HAVE AMNIOCENTESIS

Why do women choose to have amniocentesis? Framing the issue—the very act of asking that question—begins to distort women's experiences, for the decision to have or not to have amniocentesis may be more or less consciously experienced as a decision, an opportunity for choice. A woman can simply show up for all scheduled doctor's appointments and have amniocentesis scheduled and performed as part of her regular prenatal care without any more of an experience of decision making than attends the routine blood tests and urinalysis of pregnancy management. Or, a woman could just "do nothing," including seeking no prenatal medical care, and thus not have amniocentesis without ever having made a deliberate decision. For none of the women interviewed was the decision that fully routinized, but it was clearly more of a conscious decision for some than it was for others.

Almost all respondents who were over thirty-five gave their age as the reason they chose to have amniocentesis. That is, asked why, they answered, "because of my age." People do not often need well thought out reasons for why they do the expected, accepted thing. It is rather like asking someone why they wash their hands. The only necessary answer is "because they get dirty." It is self-evident and does not warrant a discussion of the meaning of dirt or the value of cleanliness. Hands get washed when they are dirty; amnio gets done when you are over thirty-five. It has become routine.

SOCIAL SUPPORT AND THE DECISION TO HAVE AMNIOCENTESIS

When pressed to think more about why they chose amniocentesis, women often mentioned medical encouragement. Among the women interviewed who chose to have amniocentesis, almost all were encouraged to have the procedure by their medical advisors, and in the few cases where there was not active encouragement, the medical providers were neutral. No woman who chose amniocentesis felt that she received *any* discouragement from *any* medical representative, though in many cases one medical provider remained neutral while another encouraged the amniocentesis. Sometimes it was an obstetrician who encouraged the amnio while a genetic counselor, to whom most women over thirty-five are referred if they are considered amnio-eligible, remained neutral, and sometimes it was the other way around. Some women saw a certified nurse midwife in addition to or instead of an obstetrician; two of the midwives encouraged amniocentesis and the rest remained neutral.

Medical encouragement was not the only encouragement for women who chose to have amniocentesis. Almost all were also encouraged by their husbands. A few husbands were, in the wife's opinion, neutral or "wanted it only if I wanted it"; several women felt that the husband "insisted on it." No woman felt that she was discouraged by her husband from having an amniocentesis she wanted.

Most women also discussed the decision with at least some of their intimate friends, and most of them were encouraged to have the amniocentesis. Some felt that their intimate friends tried to remain neutral, but only two women felt any discouragement from any intimate friends. The woman's parents followed a somewhat similar pattern. About half of the women who had amniocentesis discussed the decision with one or both parents; approximately one-third of them encouraged the amnio, and, according to the women's perceptions, the rest remained neutral. The sole exception was a woman who said that she discussed it with both her parents and her priest: "They tried to appear neutral, but I felt they discouraged it."

Siblings were less commonly consulted, but among women who did, most felt encouraged to have amnio. No sibling discouraged the amniocentesis, though two remained neutral. Most women did not discuss the amniocentesis decision with casual friends or co-workers. Only one woman reported any discouragement from this source. In sum, only four women among the sixty-two who had amniocentesis experienced any discouragement from any source at all. Amniocentesis, for most women, was acceptable within their social worlds.

All of this encouragement, this pervasive atmosphere which assumes that the amniocentesis will be done as a matter of routine, may carry the woman straight through without second thoughts. But the procedure may come to be questioned as the woman learns more about amniocentesis:

> I honestly didn't think about it too much; it was understood, assumed by my OB that I would do it; I didn't feel I had an option....When I got to the medical center for the test and had all the risks spelled out is when I almost backed out.

What was first experienced as support, even welcome support, may begin to feel like pressure as the pregnancy progresses. Another woman explained:

> Before pregnancy, before I understood fully all that was involved in amnio, I thought it was a good idea and my husband agreed and we didn't discuss it further. I ignorantly assumed that you could find out results before three months, before it really felt like carrying a baby. But the more steps I took in the direction of the amnio, the more of a "bad dream" it became. This is primarily because I felt trapped by an earlier agreement with my husband to have an abortion if the baby was defective. As the pregnancy progressed, I was less and less sure I could "terminate"—which seemed like a euphemistic term for killing the baby and then delivering it. I was afraid that it would be devastating to learn the baby had an abnormality and even more afraid my husband and the doctor would put pressure on me to abort. Instead of being able to lean on my husband for support, I felt myself drawing away in anger and feeling alone and isolated.

Thus the decision to have amniocentesis occurs in a social context in which the support is more or less overt, more or less welcome, but consistently there.

WHAT AMNIOCENTESIS CAN OFFER

Although some people never really articulate their reasons for having amniocentesis and simply go through the procedure because it is expected, others choose to have the test aware of what it offers them: "Since my husband and I both have full-time careers, we felt we couldn't do justice to a baby with 'special needs.'" "I live in a rural area with no medical, social, or developmental help for birth defects...[also] this is my husband's second family and he did not want any problems with the child."

Even if women start out expecting to abort for Down's syndrome, very clear on what they want from the test, the very act of going through the amniocentesis procedure itself may make considering the need to abort more difficult. The way the technology makes knowledge available makes acting on that knowledge more difficult.

> It was easy to say at the beginning of the pregnancy that I would have an abortion. However, as part of the procedure, an ultrasound is done. We could see the baby, and she became real to us. After that it was extremely difficult to think of aborting....The procedure is performed so late and the pregnancy is advanced enough that abortion is not a simple matter. It seems much more like murder.

Other women who choose amniocentesis are fully convinced they are doing the right thing. They do not speak of murder but of being free of guilt, of doing the responsible, appropriate thing. One woman interviewed in another study (Burke and Kolker 1982), based her moral argument on her commitment to the community and on the scarce resources available to the children of the world. A trained technician, she valued the contribution technology could make:

> It's a feeling that I have a responsibility and I have fulfilled it. I have done all I can do that is medically feasible and advisable, at my age, to ensure that any baby I have will be fine. There still may be defects beyond amniocentesis—indeterminable ones. But as I said, I have done what I can and I can't blame myself for what I couldn't have done.... I am a technician. I wanted the information technology could give me because I did not wish to add another burden to society in this world.... I felt at least we'd *tried* to assure that our issue to the world would be a benefit, not a burden. If the test were wrong, we'd feel no guilt.

Another woman addressed the quality of life owed to the unborn child:

> I think that questions about the civil rights of the most severely handicapped and of the unborn are important to ask. Even so, I *personally* do not believe in life at any cost. I would prefer not to abort an unborn fetus, but I would do it and not feel guilty if we had concluded that it was best for us and for the unborn child. The quality of life counts for a lot— and decisions about it differ for different individuals.

DECIDING AGAINST AMNIOCENTESIS:
SOCIAL SUPPORT—OR ITS LACK

Although women who have amniocentesis are typically doing the expected thing, women who are over thirty-five or otherwise "at risk" and who choose not to have amniocentesis more often have to justify their decision, for they are going against behavior expected of the at-risk woman. Women who choose not to have amniocentesis are often placing themselves in conflict with the expectations of their own medical providers. Some deal with the potential for conflict by never discussing the issue. For example, few of the women who wanted *not* to have amniocentesis sought genetic counseling, for many of them believed that counselors pressure clients toward having amnio. Some women actively closed off the opportunity for discussion, noting that there was "nothing to discuss" with their doctors.

The medical personnel who were consulted by the sixty-four women who decided not to have amniocentesis did indeed encourage them to have the test, with just a few exceptions. One obstetrician discouraged amniocentesis for a woman who had a late miscarriage just a few months before this pregnancy. A history of miscarriage or of infertility are two of the few medically recognized reasons for refusing amniocentesis in high-risk pregnancies. Still, most of those who refused amniocentesis went against medical advice, and for them outside sources of social support became even more important.

Although all of the married women who had amniocentesis discussed the decision with their husbands, about one-fifth of those who did not have amniocentesis never discussed their decision with their husbands. Of those who did, almost half of the husbands were neutral. The rest, agreeing with the wife, did not want her to have the amnio. There was only one husband who wanted his wife to have amniocentesis among those who refused: they flipped a coin, and she won.

With the husband often neutral or not consulted and medical people only rarely discouraging the woman from having the amnio, where did the social support come from for those who refused? Slightly more than half of the women discussed their decision with their intimate friends. Some of these friends encouraged them to have the test, more of them were neutral, and the remainder discouraged it. This last group, accounting for about one-fourth of all the women who refused, provided support for the decision not to have the procedure.

Few women mentioned any other sources of social support for the decision not to have amniocentesis—few friends, co-workers, siblings, or other family members actively supported the woman. On the contrary, more women received some encouragement to have the amniocentesis—from co-workers, casual friends, parents, in one case a mother-in-law, and in another a "a high school friend seen at a reunion who'd had it done." Making an unpopular decision can thus be an isolating experience:

> I want to mention that within my reference group—friends
> who are professional women in their 30s and pregnant or with
> young children, mine was the unusual decision. I kept trying

to see things the way the others did, but for me their reasoning just didn't work. Once I had made my decision not to have amnio, I tried to avoid the subject, and I felt lonely with my decision.

Unlike the self-evident reasons for doing the expected, doing the *un*expected requires people to be ready to account for themselves, to defend and explain the reasons for their actions. When women who are at risk refuse to have amniocentesis and are asked why, they more often have thought-out answers.

THE ABORTION QUESTION AND THE DECISION NOT TO HAVE AMNIOCENTESIS

It is generally understood that women will refuse amniocentesis if they see it entirely as a prelude to a potential abortion and if they see abortion as totally unacceptable. This is commonly seen as the "right-to-life" position. Some women who refused amniocentesis clearly espoused that position, but even more women disassociated themselves from it, stating that "I'm not a right-to-lifer, but..." The "but" usually reflected the distinction between other people's *right* to abort and one's own *personal willingness* to do so, at least under these conditions.

The right-to-life basis for refusing amniocentesis is by now a familiar argument: "Because *in utero* treatment is in its infancy, prenatal diagnosis today is used to seek out and destroy 'defective' infants. I believe this is morally wrong." But discomfort with or unwillingness to have an abortion are by no means limited to those who lay claim to a right-to-life argument. One woman, herself a paraplegic, reported knowing several victims of spina bifida, one of the conditions diagnosable through amniocentesis: "The idea of killing a baby so afflicted broke my heart. As with other defects, there are so many degrees of impairment."

Often the lateness of these abortions distresses women who might be more tolerant and accepting of earlier abortions: "Amnio results come back so late, around 20 weeks; the fetus is no longer a clump of cells but a baby. Even if I would consider abortion in the first few weeks, I never could at 20 to 21 weeks."

It is not simply the issue of lateness as measured in weeks of gestation, ounces of fetus, or even "viabilty" that causes women to question amniocentesis. The problem is expressed in the tangled language of *fetus* and *baby*: At what point does the fetus become a baby, *my* baby, my child no matter what.

> At some point I began to feel more and more strongly that this fetus *was my baby,* and as this emerged as a strong reality, it no longer depended on the baby's health, normality, or perfection. Just as my older child is my child "in sickness or in health," so was this one. I was then commited to caring for the baby no matter what.

One woman expressed this sense of commitment as the responsibility a mother has, even before birth, to the newly incarnate being.

Some women placed this sense of commitment in a religious or spiritual context. Religion and spirituality can offer an alternative to the value of control over nature espoused by modern society in general and medicine in particular. This alternative belief system says that things happen for a reason, and value lies in rising to meet the challenge of accepting what the world offers. It can be expressed simply, as in one woman's proclaimation: "I was ready to accept whatever God had planned for me." Another expressed this world view as a "trust in the universal flow of life and death. I do not feel there are any mistakes." This kind of thinking, this acceptance of a universal plan, of lessons to be learned, runs deeply contrary to the world view offered by medicine and by a technological society which stresses the value of taking charge, making decisions, and controlling one's destiny.

> I also believe, and this is my main reason, that this babe, already conceived, with his own soul and being, was and is right for us, in our spiritual path, and feel he's God given and needs to be accepted as is. I find it hard to talk about this main reason. It's easier for me to rattle off as I did [about the risks] because I know it's more socially acceptable. Y'know?

FEELING SAFE

Not all people who decide against amniocentesis do so out of a solid philosophical grounding. Some just feel safe, are confident that there is no problem with the baby. Just as some women draw an irrational feeling of complete safety from having had amniocentesis and having done everything medicine has to offer and now feel that nothing will go wrong, other women make their bargains with different gods. Eating right and living right, having a "healthy life-style" makes some women feel secure:

> I did not feel the need [to have amniocentesis]. I eat a very natural diet and get plenty of fresh air. I do not feel that my body is "slowing down"... as rapidly as city-dwelling women. I feel very young. Also I trust my intuition. I felt everything was okay.

One of the most common and readily accepted ways to feel safe is to play the numbers game. Thirty-five is the arbitrary cutoff point, but a woman between thirty and forty can consider herself borderline. Some of the women who had amnio said they would not have had it if they were "a year younger," "under 35" (she's thirty-six), "under 37" (she's thirty-eight), and so on. Alternatively, women who choose not to have amniocentesis claim that they are on the good side of the borderline:

> I think I got pregnant when I did [this pregnancy was not consciously planned at that time], because I had this thought that if I waited any longer I would have to deal with the whole

amnio issue—and I did not want to do that —and I think I put
myself into a funny double bind where I had to get pregnant
when I did. I was 35 when she was conceived and 36 when she
was born. I knew every year older, from 36 to 40, I would
have worried more about the possibility of my baby having
Down's syndrome.

Some women felt safe simply because they just *knew* the fetus was okay. Some
women felt they had alternative sources of knowledge. Not all women feel the
need for the scientific verification that amnio provides. One felt that "because I'm
a dancer I feel in touch with my body"; another had an "inner belief in the health
of my fetus"; and still another felt "we were divinely directed not to have it. We
knew that our baby was healthy."

AMNIOCENTESIS AND THE EXPERIENCE
OF MOTHERHOOD

Most women go into pregnancy well aware that lightening does strike even
those who think and feel right. A woman may refuse amniocentesis not because
she thinks it won't happen to her, nor because she rejects abortion as a
possibility, but because she feels confident in her abilities to cope. Just as one
woman felt that a lack of support services in her rural area was a motive for
amniocentesis and selective abortion, other women's experiences of social support may make them feel more ready to deal with what comes:

We felt we could handle a problem if it happened—we have a
close family and good friends for support. Who can expect
perfection? Our two adopted children both ended up needing
extensive orthopedic work after normal adoption physicals.

One would expect that the most significant experience in women's lives that
teaches them whether or not they could cope with the problem of a disabled child
would be motherhood itself. Although some women are having their first
pregnancy after thirty-five, even more women are already mothers by that age.
Does having a child make a woman more or less likely to have amniocentesis
when she has a pregnancy over thirty-five? It seems the whole issue becomes
more complicated when one is already a mother. On the one hand, the experience
of completing a pregnancy changes the meaning of later pregnancies for women.
Many women say that they would have more trouble with an abortion now that
they have experienced a completed pregnancy and birth and know their child, than
they would have had the first time. On the other hand, there is now another child
and another life to consider: the impact of the potential child's disability on the
existing child's needs is a consideration. A decision that is rarely easy is now
that much more complicated.

One woman, who refused amniocentesis with her first pregnancy when she
was thirty-five but had it with her next one a few years later, reported:

> [My] second pregnancy was easier to decide to have amnio—[I] felt the older child, a toddler, would have to give up too much if a younger sibling was retarded.

For many women, however, the experience of motherhood has the opposite effect. Strikingly, a woman who terminated a pregnancy because of Down's syndrome and then went on to have another pregnancy with a healthy child, still struggles with the decision to have amniocentesis with the next child:

> [My husband] and I want to have another baby, and I am having a difficult inner struggle right now. I have to be mentally prepared to have an abortion if the test results are negative, and now that I have had a baby that decision is more difficult for me. I thought it would be easier once I had a baby, but it's just the opposite.

Motherhood changes a lot of things. The woman who would have had an abortion due to fetal defects with a first pregnancy is just not the same woman, not living the same life, once she has had a child. For some women, these changes produce changes in their need or willingness to have amniocentesis.

> If the fetus had been Down's syndrome, I would have aborted for the purely selfish reason of not wanting my possible only child to be less than perfect. At my age, I didn't want my life to be so drastically changed for that. I would have taken the chance of no children. But now that I have a child and a changed life, the decision to abort would be more difficult to make.

Another woman directly addressed the way the experience of parenting can give a woman new confidence in her abilities to cope.

> We had serious concerns about being able to care for a "special child"—physically, emotionally, and economically. As it turned out, the results of the procedure indicated no genetic problems, but she [her child] has had other health problems and we've learned that we can indeed handle these problems and continue to thrive as a "healthy" family.

Thus, some women will abort more readily for fetal defects once they are mothers, and some women will abort less readily.

AMNIOCENTESIS AND THE MEANING OF DOWN'S SYNDROME

What happens to women who have actually faced Down's syndrome? These are the women who are most encouraged of all to have amniocentesis—and many of them do, fully prepared to terminate pregnancies if Down's syndrome is diagnosed. Yet some women choose not to have amniocentesis even with a prior Down's syndrome child:

> I would first say that I never expected to have a child that wasn't perfect and didn't have any fears when pregnant the first time. When I heard my child wasn't normal, I couldn't believe it. I had no experience to compare him so I didn't accept it until 8 or 9 months. I never thought of giving him up. I knew I would love him the same. So when I was pregnant again I knew I could love my next child regardless of how she was born. I also decided, though not a church goer, that I would pray for my unborn child, and I asked others to pray also. The only reason I considered amnio for a little while was because if it came out for the best I wouldn't have to think about it for the rest of the nine months.

Indeed, peace of mind can be the reason that a woman with a prior Down's syndrome child chooses amnio, even if she is not considering abortion.

> Having a Down's syndrome child greatly influenced my decision for an amnio.... If Charles had been a "normal" child, I would never have had amnios performed on my following two pregnancies.... Charles is the love of our lives, a complete joy. I had amnios done so that if I were carrying another DS child I would be warned ahead of time so that the baby's birth could be a happy experience. I could *never* abort a DS child. The amnio does give peace of mind to some extent.

These two women are not dismissing the seriousness of their children's problems—indeed one said that because of her age and of being at risk, she and her husband decided to have no more children, and he had a vasectomy. But neither woman was unwilling to accept a Down's syndrome child with later pregnancies. Differences in available support and, perhaps, the severity of the disability can make a large difference in a woman's feeling about whether she can cope with another Down's syndrome child.

And finally, some women feel that a diagnosis of Down's syndrome is not specific enough to be used for decision making:

> I didn't feel I would have an abortion, give up the baby, even if I knew it was defective, since even the term *Down's syndrome* implies a whole spectrum of possibilities from mildly retarded to severely so, and a similar spectrum of physical ills possible.

THE RISK FACTOR

Running through almost every woman's decision not to choose amniocentesis is a constant refrain—the issue of risk.

> "Risks outweigh the benefits at 35-36."
> "Possibility of injuring, however subtly, the fetus."
> "Why take the risk involved?"
> "I thought amniocentesis might hurt it."
> "Nothing to be gained and possible risk to the fetus."
> "Why take the risk for the baby?"
> "It wouldn't at all be worth the risk."

Over and over, from almost every woman, the same refrain was heard: amniocentesis poses a risk, a risk to the continuation of the pregnancy, a risk to the baby, a risk of hurting the very thing one is trying to achieve—a healthy baby. That risk exists at any age. Risk is almost always cited by women who, for a variety of reasons, do not want to have the test. Their own reasons, their feelings, their intuitions, their sense of discomfort—these are not socially acceptable reasons for rejecting amniocentesis, but risk is.

What would they do, then, if the medical sciences developed an entirely safe, risk-free, early prenatal diagnosis procedure, one that used, for example, a maternal blood sample rather than an amniotic or fetal blood sample? Most women were not altogether sure what they would do if faced with the knowledge that their early pregnancy fetus was damaged, just as most of the women who had amniocentesis were ambivalent about what they would have done if the diagnosis indicated Down's syndrome. "It depends" was the most consistent answer; it depends on the kind of damage, disorder, or disease that is diagnosed; it depends on the life situation of the woman at the time. Risk has provided a convenient rubric for not facing other aspects of the decision to have or not to have amniocentesis.

But if the issue of risk is removed, the value of information, of informed decision making in contemporary American society, comes to the fore:

> If there were a test with no possible risk to the fetus or pregnancy, I would have it and then either relax in the knowledge that my child would not have certain diseases or, if the results showed a problem, wrestle with the moral and emotional question of abortion from an informed position.

That value was put succinctly by one woman: "I believe that the more information I have, the better decision I will make—with less fear and more care." If the technology does develop to the point where risk is removed, the last completely socially acceptable reason for not wanting to know fetal defects will be gone.

THE MORAL QUALITY OF INFORMATION

Once risk is removed as a reason, then the decision to accept or refuse amniocentesis requires phrasing the decision in moral terms, which are far more difficult to explain to others. To reject the test for moral reasons requires what one counselor called "always thinking three steps ahead"—thinking straight to the abortion question. There is not presently even a language of morality that allows us to talk about the moral nature of information itself. Moral questions, as phrased here, come with the problems of what to do with the information. There may be moral (and immoral) decisions to be made, but whether or not to enter into the decision-making process itself is often not recognized as a moral dilemma. This is what enables some counselors to consider themselves *nondirective*: they do not push abortions ("a very personal decision"), though they strongly encourage women to have amniocentesis, get the information, and then decide. Here, information itself has taken on positive social value.

Entry into what has been called the "information era" is reflected in the very way we think. Something beyond knowledge for its own sake is involved: it is the idea that action is based on information and the fullest possible information is needed to responsibly determine action. More than a legal requirement, informed consent is a developing social norm. If information is to be had and decisions made, social value now lies in actively seeking the information and consciously making the decision. To do otherwise is to let things happen to you, to not take control of your life. Such is the contemporary, and particularly the medical definition of mature, responsible behavior. When a wife in a counseling session expressed her discomfort with having to make such momentous decisions, her husband said he'd rather they make the decision themselves "because when we have our baby, having had the amniocentesis or not having had the amniocentesis, we'd have [had] so much more to do with it."

Women who have chosen amniocentesis call upon this same social value to justify their choice. "I feel strongly about the difficult choices amniocentesis presents, but also feel strongly about women having choices and as much knowledge as possible." "Amniocentesis gave control to me—whether I would like the choice or not, I would make the decision." It may not be pleasant, it may not be easy, but individuals are perceived to be better people for making choices: that is the value being put forth. However, those who refuse amniocentesis appear to others as having rejected the socially valued notion of choice, and even more profoundly, appear to have turned away from the use of information in controlling their lives—itself a value in our society.

Certainly within the medical profession's view, and possibly within the culture at large, there is no solid grounding for not wanting to know. According to this value system, if information can be obtained, it should be obtained; if new technologies can make the obtaining of information possible, they should be used. Cultural values stress that one should have all the information, one should be prepared and act rationally, not bury one's head in the sand. The pressure to get information comes from all sides. Even with the problems inherent in amniocentesis—the lateness of the diagnosis, the possibility of miscarrying or damaging a healthy fetus—the pressure was and is there. One woman who refused amniocentesis was made angry by the pressure:

> There's a strong assumption towards it...pressure on the woman to go through with something which would be a horrible experience. People seemed to think it was a normal, okay thing to do. What bothered me was the assumption that it was normal, denying it would be a difficult thing.

When all that a women will need to do to get the information is to have a blood test and "then decide," the pressure to know will be greater. At that point, the underlying belief system will no longer be masked with discussions of risk and risk rates—the moral issues in deciding to obtain information itself will come to the fore. As the technology of prenatal diagnosis continues to advance during the next decade, confrontation with the basic issues raised by prenatal diagnosis—and, indeed, the moral nature of information itself—will enter into the pregnancy experience of the majority of women.

NOTE

This chapter is part of a larger research project on women's experiences with amniocentesis for prenatal diagnosis which has been published as *The Tentative Pregnancy* by Viking/Penguin.

6

THE POWER OF "POSITIVE" DIAGNOSIS: MEDICAL AND MATERNAL DISCOURSES ON AMNIOCENTESIS

Rayna Rapp

> *When we walked into the doctor's office, both my husband and I were crying. He looked up and said, "What's wrong? Why are you both in tears?" "It's our baby, our baby is going to die," I said. "That isn't a baby," he said firmly, "it's a collection of cells that made a mistake."*
> —Leah Rubinstein, age 39

Late twentieth century reproductive medicine offers both benefits and burdens. Its technologies are aimed against maternal and infant mortality and in favor of normal, healthy outcomes. At the same time, however, it controls conditions of pregnancy, birth, and parenting in ways that scientize our most fundamental experiences. Being a woman, becoming a parent, experiencing birth, and sometimes confronting death are processes increasingly organized by reproductive medicine rather than by individuals, families, and communities. Indeed, many of the core experiences of sex, gender, and family formation are now culturally defined by medical science. The access people have to reproductive medicine, as well as its respected or coercive quality, in part defines their experience of pregnancy.

Examining prenatal diagnosis, especially the use of amniocentesis, reveals a great deal about the changing definitions and controls of pregnancy and birth. On this frontier of reproductive technology, medical services are transforming the experience of pregnancy, personhood, and parenthood for the women and their families who use prenatal diagnosis. In offering a test for chromosome anomalies and some other inherited disabilities, amniocentesis holds out the possibility of choosing to carry or not to carry to term a pregnancy in which a fetus will become a child with a genetic disability. That choice is part of the medical definition of what constitutes an acceptable or an unacceptable child in American culture. The choices people make around amniocentesis also reveal the similarities and differences between medical and maternal perceptions of what it means to have a child with a disability.

AMNIOCENTESIS: TECHNOLOGY AND RISKS

The technology of amniocentesis is easily described. Pregnant women who choose the test are screened between the sixteenth and the nineteenth week of their pregnancies. To help prepare parents, genetic counselors provide information about the risks and benefits of the test. A team of doctors and nurses uses ultrasound visualization of the fetus and placenta to guide the insertion of a thin, hollow needle into the amniotic sac, through which about three tablespoons of fluid are extracted. The liquid is cultured in a genetics laboratory, and sufficient fetal cells are usually available in three to four weeks for a diagnosis to be made. At that time, chromosome numbers, shapes, sizes and bands can easily be read. About 98 percent of the women who have amniocentesis will receive the good news that their fetuses are free of the conditions for which they have been tested. The other 2 percent will have to confront the distressing news that their fetus is affected with a disability. These women must weigh the stress and stigma of choosing a late abortion against the choice of having a disabled child.

Three groups of people are usually recommended for amniocentesis. One includes pregnant women and their partners whose families already include someone with an inherited condition for which prenatal screening is now available. The second includes couples from ethnically specific populations in which certain autosomal recessive genetic diseases (for example Tay-Sachs among Ashkenazi Jews; sickle cell anemia among Afro-Americans) are relatively frequent and for which both partners are known carriers. The third is "older" women, who are considered to be at elevated risk for several chromosomal abnormalities, of which Down's syndrome is the best known and most significant one. Older is, however, a social, and not simply a biological construct. While the incidence of Down's syndrome liveborn babies goes steadily up in the 20s, 30s, and 40s, the cutoff age for the test has varied considerably. It was first recommended for women who were 40 years of age or older. Then, the recommendation dropped to 38, and then 35, and it is now moving toward the lower thirties.

The procedures used in amniocentesis are themselves not without risk, and thus the recommended age is identified by the intersection of two epidemiological patterns: one is the safety of the technology itself, the other is the incidence of Down's syndrome in live-born babies of women in different age groups. Amniocentesis adds a small additional risk of miscarriage to the preg-nancies of older women. Three more women per 1000 who have had amnio-centesis will miscarry than will women who have not had the test. The incidence of miscarriage with amniocentesis is thus 1/333. This number approximates the incidence of fetuses with Down's syndrome born to pregnant women who are 35, which is 1/360 (Hook 1981; Hook, Cross, and Schreinemachers 1983; PDL Counseling Protocol n.d.). If the technology improved so that it caused one less miscarriage per 1000, then the recommended age for its use would drop to match the incidence of fetuses with Down's syndrome in that lower age group. We are thus witnessing the intersection of an increasingly routinized technology with the social pattern of delayed pregnancy in some parts of the U.S. population and not any absolute epidemiological threshold of risk.

THE SOCIOLOGY OF AMNIOCENTESIS

The sociology of amniocentesis is more complex to describe. Initially recommended for relatively small numbers of older pregnant women, the test is rapidly becoming a pregnancy ritual for certain sectors of the highly educated, urban middle class. Each year, scores of thousands of women use amniocentesis, but the test is very expensive and unevenly available.[1] Women living in major urban areas, and/or near teaching hospitals, and covered by comprehensive health insurance are most likely to use it. With the exception of a very few states which fund the procedure through Medicaid, amniocentesis remains the prerogative of the well-to-do. Several studies, however, indicate that low income women would use the procedure if it were available to them for a minimal charge. (Marion et al. 1980; Sokal et al. 1980; Joans 1980; Hsu 1982).

The discourse on amniocentesis is filled with the clamor of experts: Health economists tell us that it is cheaper to offer mass screening for Down's syndrome than to support the services disabled children require (Sadovick and Baird 1981; 1982). Geneticists assess the limits and future possibilities of their scientific field, hopeful of screening increased numbers of serious disabilities (Harris 1974; Lipkin and Rowley 1974; Filkins and Russo 1985). Bioethicists comment on the eugenic implications of the technology (Hilton, Callahan, et al. 1973; Powledge and Fletcher 1979). And feminists worry about the effects of sex selection against female fetuses (Hanmer 1981; Corea 1985). But when I entered the discourse as an anthropologist (and in my case, as a pregnant woman), the silence of the women and their families using or refusing the technology was deafening [cf Rothman 1986]. Yet it is precisely those voices which might describe the lived reality of a new reproductive technology that we must make audible if we are to understand its cultural and not simply its medical meaning, probing how the latter may be shaping the former.

A PILOT STUDY

This chapter reports on one aspect of the study of the social impact and cultural meaning of prenatal diagnosis: my initial pilot work with women and their families who received positive diagnoses.[2] In interviews and letters, I asked people to recall the experience of getting a positive diagnosis, making a decision, and coping with its aftermath. My data come from forty women and their families, eleven of whom I interviewed in their homes, five of whom I interviewed by telephone, and twenty-four of whom entered into extensive correspondence with me. All but two ultimately chose to abort affected fetuses. My sample was developed using medical and personal networks and in response to an article I published on amniocentesis in a nationally circulated women's magazine (Rapp 1984). All respondents are self-selected, and the quality of information varies considerably—the telephone interviews yielding the most perfunctory information. Although the letters were written by women from all sections of the United States (in addition to two that came from abroad), recalling experiences with amniocentesis up to a decade ago, the home interviews were all conducted with women who came from the metropolitan New York area and had received a positive diagnosis within the last twelve months. My interview schedule probed for images of fetuses, disabilities, pregnancy, and family life. It asked for information about religious, ethnic, educational, and occupational backgrounds and queried the knowledge people had about the disability diagnosed for their fetus prior to the time that they received their own prenatal diagnosis. It contains questions concerning support and criticism from family and community members, experiences with the medical system, and steps toward resolution and recovery. It is sensitive to the use (or non-use) of medical language in describing this perplexing experience and its aftermath. I have included many quotations from these interviews, changing only the names and ages to protect the women's privacy.

THE PRIVATIZATION OF EXPERIENCE

Although the pilot data are somewhat uneven, three themes appear consistently throughout. The first is the extreme privatization of the experience. Reproductive choices—including abortions—are considered to be personal matters in the contemporary United States, choices conventionally taken by an individual or a couple. Most of the women and their families from whom I gathered information told their immediate families about the positive diagnosis and, usually, about the subsequent abortion. Children of the family received age-appropriate information. Most also told a few close friends. But some told no one, because they lived in communities and in families where strong anti-abortion sentiment was expressed. And virtually all referred to a "miscarriage" or "loss of a baby" in some contexts. The pain of reproductive loss is universal; the boundaries along which people fear they will incur judgment rather than support for a voluntary loss vary considerably. Privatization allows people some control over shaping that boundary between intimate friends who "deserved the truth," and public others who simply "needed some explanation." But privatization also reduces the quantity and quality of social support an individual may receive for her grieving. No one with whom I spoke or corresponded had ever met another woman who had been through the same experience. This new form of intentional pregnancy loss occurs in unknown interpersonal territory. Technology here creates a traumatic experience which is so deeply medicalized and privatized that its social shape has yet to be excavated, and a cultural language to describe it is yet to be found.

The degree of isolation inherent in the experience of receiving a positive diagnosis is in part conditioned by the diagnosis itself. For the more than 80 percent of my respondents whose fetal diagnosis was Down's syndrome, some cultural knowledge was available. Everyone had an image of a child with Down's syndrome. Some had friends, family members, or community members whose children had the condition. While their images of mentally retarded children, especially children with Down's syndrome, were often out of date, they still had a reference point for the diagnosis and felt competent to decide whether or not to end the affected pregnancy. In this pilot study, I had no cases of women continuing a pregnancy after a prenatal diagnosis of Down's syndrome. And medical statistics suggest an abortion rate of about 95 percent after this particular diagnosis (Hook 1981).

Other, more arcane diagnoses were harder to understand, and to judge. Two of my respondents received diagnoses of XYY syndrome, a sex-chromosome anomaly. The diagnosis of XYY includes possible mental retardation, anomalous sexual development, and putative aggressiveness. But the diagnosis is highly controversial and has sparked both technical and popular discussions of whether screening is appropriate or is an artifact of the abuse of minimal scientific information blown out of proportion (see Hook 1973). Both respondents who received this diagnosis spent whole days in a medical library trying to interpret the meaning of XYY syndrome before reaching their decisions. One family's fetus was identified as having a chromosomal tag so rare that a nationally known geneticist could point to only fifteen other reported cases and could only vaguely predict its outcome. Another family received a diagnosis of organ damage and displacement so complex that they consulted with a battery of pediatric surgeons and neonatologists over the course of one month before they reached a decision. Two others didn't understand the language of the diagnosis and had to have it re-explained many times before they could approach their choices. In such cases, unlike Down's syndrome, there is no collective fund of information available, and medical language necessarily dictates the shape of familial understanding.

THE LANGUAGE OF PRENATAL DIAGNOSIS

The use of medical language in itself creates tensions in the discussion of prenatal diagnosis. This is the second theme that runs through all of the interviews and letters. Medical language is not neutral; medical practices are often intentionally distancing, as the quotation that opens this article suggests. Some patients find this distance reassuring in its promise of rationality; others find it cold and denying of their experience. There is a war of words that accompanies virtually all of the stories I have collected. Cells, embryos, and fetuses vie for center stage with babies. "Positive diagnoses" describe the medical discovery procedures, but they painfully reverse and mask the very negative experiences of parents learning that their fetuses have disabilities. In some cases, women literally assume the burden of this impersonal language, speaking in total disconnection from their pregnant bodies:

> So I was in labor for 24 hours and absolutely nothing happened. I mean nothing. A dead fetus, but it wouldn't come out. So I called Dr. X at 8 A.M. and I guess I must have sounded crazy. "Hello," I said, "I'm a demised fetus and a failed

prostaglandin." "Oh no you're not, honey," the nurse said. "You're a lady that's losing a baby, and you'd better stop talking and start crying." (Sandra Larkin, age 36)

Several families mentioned the struggles they had waged to see their dead fetuses or to retrieve them for burial. Usually, fetuses were sent to pathology to confirm a diagnosis. Legal and hospital procedures dictate this practice, which brings the reality of family mourning into conflict with medical protocols. Denied access to dead fetuses, some chose to bury or frame the sonogram visualizations that they had been given during amniocentesis. One family pasted the image into the family bible. They thus created the emotional personification, albeit through technology, that family life required and medical procedures could not grant.[3]

The use of medical language and its accompanying procedures are purposive. As one respondent put it, "This late-abortion business is no picnic for the doctors and nurses." Medical discourse protects medical staff from the sad and disorienting experiences of their patients, allowing the routinization of services. But each woman I interviewed had to perform a complex translation between the medical words she had been given and whatever her own experience of that pregnancy and its ending had been. Often, only medical language seemed legitimate. Many women couldn't use the word abortion, yet hesitated over termination, the term used by medical professionals. Almost all switched from fetus to baby while describing their situations. Yet no one could recall the affected pregnancy without using medical descriptions of its length, dated from last menstrual period rather than by nausea, quickening, or some other intrabody sign. And, of course, the diagnosis itself was always discussed medically. Medical language here reinforces the privatization of the problem, for each woman is seen, and sees herself, as an individual patient rather than as a member of a larger group of women confronting a new technological possibility or coping with grief.

There is an awkward gap between medical and maternal discourses. While some might argue that medical language neutralizes some of the anxiety associated with amniocentesis (Brewster 1984), its function is actually more complex and powerful. Many scholars and activists have noted that medical discourses increasingly define pregnancy itself as a pathological (or potentially pathological) condition, thus justifying professional management and intervention (Shaw 1974; Rothman 1982; Wertz and Wertz 1977). But pregnancy is also an embodied state and a time-framed activity about which a great deal of popular knowledge has been accumulated, often passed down from mothers to daughters, shared among friends, and held by ethnically specific communities (Oakley 1979, 1980, 1981; Snow and Johnson 1978; Thompson 1983). Thus, multiple discourses construct pregnancy as a whole, subdivided among specialists (for example, obstetricians and midwives may think and speak differently about their pregnant patients), and between specialists and pregnant women.

The same cannot be said for prenatal diagnosis, which is constructed as a specifically medical event. The experience itself exists only in relation to the technology, services, and personnel within which it is embedded. Unlike pregnancy, for which a woman has embodied experiences she can and does articulate and share with others (both pregnant and nonpregnant), the event of receiving a positive diagnosis bears no relation to either internal body cues or collective popular knowledge. There is no tradition to call upon in coping with the diagnosis. Acceptance of the test and its results implies a belief in epidemiological statistics, an acknowledgment of risk factors, population parameters, and laboratory procedures all far removed from the individual or the collective sense of pregnancy itself. Those for whom a positive diagnosis is given are thus operating on an unknown terrain, far removed from pregnancy as they have experienced or learned about it. The stumbling words, the gaps of language, the silences surrounding this experience are testimony to its totally medical construction. It is an experience removed from the maternal discourses by which pregnant women gradually become mothers, not simply medical cases.

THE ETHICS OF DECISION MAKING

A third generalization that emerges from these interviews is the ethical complexity and social embeddedness of the decision to abort (or in two cases, not to abort) an affected pregnancy. Five respondents discussed their cases with religious advisors, and six saw psychological counselors in the course of making their decisions. But the majority did not seek nonmedical professional help. They retrospectively identified their decision as having been made in one of two ways: "On the day I decided to go for amniocentesis" (that is, with an almost-conscious knowledge that a diagnosis of any fetal genetic disability would be reason enough to choose abortion); or alternatively, the decision was made "the minute we got the news" (in which case the couple, not the pregnant woman, is recalled as the decision-making unit, and their conversations are recalled ver-batim). In the five cases for which anomalous diagnoses were given, decision making was protracted, involving several rounds of medical consultation and sometimes library research or home visits with families whose living children had the diagnosed condition. Yet even those couples who conducted research before making a decision reported strong leanings toward an abortion as soon as they knew that something was wrong.[4]

Reasons for the abortion decision are often phrased in terms of other family members:

> Some people say that abortion is hate. I say my abortion was an act of love. I've got three kids. I was 43 when we accidentally got pregnant again. We decided there was enough love in our family to handle it, even though finances would be tight. But we also decided to have the test. A kid with a serious problem was more than we could handle. And when we got the bad news, I knew immediately what I had to do. At 43, you think about your own death. It would have been tough now, but think what would have happened to my other kids, especially my daughter. Oh, the boys, Tommy and Alex would have done okay. But Laura would have been the one who got stuck. It's always the girls. It would have been me, and then,

> after I'm gone it would have been the big sister who took care
> of that child. Saving Laura from that burden was an act of
> love. (Mary Fruticci, age 44)

Many families with other children expressed similar concerns, citing the effects
of a disabled sibling on prior children as the reason for choosing abortion. But
over 60 percent of the respondents made an abortion decision during a first
planned pregnancy. They had to take responsibility for the decision on the basis
of their own needs, not an altruistic stance toward dependent children. In these
cases, ambivalence about parenting skills was sometimes expressed:

> So he would have had this sex chromosome thing, he might
> have been slow, and he was going to be aggressive. I didn't
> know how to handle a kid like that. When he got rowdy and
> difficult, could I be a committed parent, or would I have
> thrown up my hands, thinking "It's in his genes"? [Q: What if
> you hadn't known through prenatal diagnosis?] I'm sure if it
> had just happened we would have handled it. But once you
> know, you're forced to make a choice. (David Kass, age 35)

Concern for the marriage, rather than the children, is often identified as a reason
for an abortion decision:

> I talked with this couple who had a kid with Down's, and I
> thought they were terrific. The kid was nice, and they seemed
> like a fine family. But they'd been married almost twenty years
> when it happened, had raised three other kids, and were
> confident of their commitments. Stu and I have only been
> together for two years, and it's our first baby, and what if the
> strain were too great? What if we never got the chance to have
> a normal kid? What if we broke up over it? (Jane Butler,
> age 35)

Altruism toward other household members is central to these descriptions.
Yet two other themes are conspicuous in their absence. One is the fear of
disability, a salient cultural theme for many Americans. The other is the limits
of altruism, the admission that there are specific kinds of children that individual
women would choose not to mother, given a choice. Both absent themes suggest
a wealth of cultural attitudes concerning disability and maternity which
medicalization of the experience masks. Of course, the standards for acceptable
and unacceptable children and the meaning of specific disabilities are always culturally constructed. Some societies prescribe infanticide for those conditions they
label socially inadmissible. In contemporary America, it is a medical procedure
that appears to have become the cutting edge in defining the cultural construction
of disability.[5]

To some degree the decision is diagnosis specific:

> When I heard my obstetrician's voice on the phone, I went
> numb. He told me it was Down's and said "I think we should
> talk about it." "What's there to talk about," I said. "The
> decision comes with the disease." (Leah Rubinstein, age 39)

Others had a harder time, depending on what they knew or could find out about
their fetal diagnosis. Ultimately, however, all had to take responsibility for
ending a pregnancy to which they had already felt a commitment:

> The whole time I was getting ready, the tests, the visits, the
> hospital procedure, I kept thinking, "this is awful, this is the
> most terrible thing." I never, ever wanted to be here. But I *am*
> here, and it's my choice, and I'm the one who's making it. No
> one can explain this to me, not why it happened. No one. I
> have to stop looking for answers out there and trust myself.
> (Michelle Kansky, age 38)

Like David Kass, who doubted his ability to parent a child with a sex chromosome anomaly once he had that information, Michelle Kansky is also expressing
the burdens of individual choice. Informed consent is thought to lead to optimal
individual decision making, which is deemed an absolute good in American legal
and medical culture. Yet this commitment to individual decision making, while
culturally appropriate, increases the burdens of privatization as well. It pushes
people to rely on their own information and feelings, rather than on any larger
social grouping, as they confront the problems and possibilities a new reproductive technology offers.

All respondents described their painful decisions in terms of themselves,
their marriages, their other children—in terms of individuals in nuclear families.
Yet, when we stepped back from these self-descriptions, other sociological facts
weigh heavily in the decision to use amniocentesis and the responses to positive
diagnosis. One is the role of occupation. In a small and totally self-selected
sample, it is striking to find such a large number of helping professionals. Nine
of the forty respondents were teachers, four were social workers, and nine out of
the two groups worked with retarded children, retarded adults, or their families.
How does their commitment to education and to working with disabled people
and families shape their own responses to parenting a potentially disabled child?

Even more striking is the importance of religious background in descriptions of the abortion decision. Nationally, women using abortion services are as
likely to be Catholic as non-Catholic (Petchesky 1984; Henshaw and Martire
1982). But because we do not yet have a general picture of amniocentesis users,
we cannot know if Catholic women and their families are as likely to use these
prenatal services as non-Catholics. Nor do we know if they are as likely to abort
if they receive a positive diagnosis. Yet, six respondents identified themselves as
Roman Catholics, four currently practicing and two raised Catholic. For them,
the choice was very hard and involved a personal exegesis on the meaning of
abortion:

I was raised to take what you get in life, any life you get. If I had stayed at home in Granville, if I hadn't gone to college, if I hadn't married Joe [who is Jewish], I'd still feel that way. I *do* feel that way. But even though I was brought up Catholic to believe abortion is murder, I also believe in a woman's right to choose. In people's right to choose. And that choice is a big part of me now, just as big as my religion. (Terry Hartz, age 34)

I think the hardest problem I faced was confession. I needed to have that abortion, but I also needed to confess, and I couldn't go to our parish priest, even though my mother and my mother-in-law knew, I just couldn't go to him. So I finally went to St. X, across town, where criminals and celebrities go to confess. And that helped a lot. Later, I was talking with the father of an old friend; he's an old man, very conservative, very Catholic. But he was saying how much he admired Geraldine Ferraro for her stand on abortion. "What does the Pope know about these things? Let the women decide on this one, not old men, like me." That helped me, that really helped me, even though he didn't know my situation. Now I say, "Let anyone who'll judge me stand in my shoes first." I'm still a Catholic, but I say Catholics who judge women for having an abortion haven't lived through hard times. Only when you're going to live with the consequences do you get to judge the act. (Marie Mancini, age 38)

For the more than 30 percent of respondents who identified themselves as Jewish, the choice of abortion was philosophically simpler, if still personally painful. Many gave some variant of this account:

You ask why we chose to have amniocentesis and follow through with the abortion. I'll tell you this: If the technology is there, it's better to use it. Better to live with the benefits of modern science, cry over your losses, but use every means science gives you to have a better life. (Michelle Kansky, age 38)

And whatever their religious orientation, almost all felt the need to respond to the abortion controversy which is currently central to United States political and cultural life:

I share a lot of the feelings of the Right-To-Life Movement. I've always been shocked by the number of abortion clinics, the number of abortions in this city. But when it was *my* turn, I was grateful to find the right doctor. I sent him and his staff roses after it was all over. They helped me to protect my own life, and that's a life, too. (Mary Fruticci, age 44)

We baptized our little son [aborted after a diagnosis of trisomy 18], we put the sonogram picture in the family bible. No one can tell us we did the wrong thing, no matter how much they don't believe in abortion. He's gone now. But he *was* real. And abortion is real, and sometimes necessary. (Lena Jarowlski, age 36)

There was no morally correct choice available. Abortion is a terrible choice. But so is the choice to bring a deeply damaged child into this world. People who are anti-abortion can't imagine what this is like. (Carey Morgan, age 36)

AMNIOCENTESIS AND THE PERCEPTION OF DISABILITY

The choice to abort after a positive diagnosis is made, in large part, because of the family's perception of what the child's disability will mean to them. The disability rights movement, however, has made a powerful case for the social, rather than the biological nature of the problems that disabled people face. Whatever their individual medical problems and diagnoses, disabled children and adults—like pregnant women—are more than medical cases. They are people whose access to a high quality of life is limited by the social stigma and institutional barriers they confront. Prenatal diagnosis raises a complex of thorny issues about those prejudices. It is neither appropriate nor realistic to expect individual families to reexamine their attitudes towards disability at the moment that they are being informed that their fetus will have one. But as a society, we need to undertake that reexamination, so that informed consent will include the social realities and not just the medical diagnosis of raising a child with a particular condition.

Many genetic counselors (especially if they work in pediatric, not only prenatal, service units) have information on services and support groups for children with genetic disabilities and their families. This information is rarely requested or volunteered during the crisis and decision making surrounding a positive diagnosis. Only two of the forty families requested visits with families whose live-born children had the conditions that had been diagnosed in their fetuses. In both cases the visit engendered more knowledge about the disability, lessening its mythic terror. Both couples went on to make an abortion decision. In the 80 percent of diagnoses involving Down's syndrome, all respondents could recall seeing children with the condition in their communities, and most had friends, neighbors, or relatives with a child who had Down's syndrome somewhere in their network. Some families were accepting, in principle, of children who were mentally retarded, but grateful to avoid the reality in their own cases. Others expressed more shock, even revulsion, at the idea that their child would be retarded. In almost all cases, their knowledge was outdated and did not usually include information about the accessibility of infant stimulation programs or the high level of function that many children with Down's syndrome now achieve (Garland et al. 1981; Pueschel 1978). Nor did it include a realistic picture of what the emotional or financial costs of raising a child with both physical and mental disabilities were likely to be. This is not to suggest that the decisions were necessarily wrong ones or incorrectly made. I am only suggesting that at the present time, informed consent is a concept which focuses on individual medical knowledge, while social knowledge about the real consequences of disabilities is often underdeveloped.

As long as disabled children (and adults) and their families remain segregated and stigmatized, the knowledge that potential parents might use to decide whether or not to abort a fetus with a diagnosis of disability will also remain unavailable. An individual rights focus is legally and medically appropriate to prenatal diagnosis and is consonant with deeply held American cultural beliefs. But it also masks the larger social attitudes on which knowledge, images, and insufficient services for disabled people are based. To enlarge the scope of informed consent, we must look beyond individual choice toward the sources of com-munity knowledge and prejudice. And here, as with prenatal diagnosis, it is the voices and traditions of the disabled themselves, rather than only the medical and educational professionals, from which we need to learn.

AMNIOCENTESIS AND THE LANGUAGE OF FEMINISM

The language of individualism and pro-choice feminism which is often used in describing the abortion decision after a positive diagnosis grows out of the transformation of work, gender relations, family life, and cultural politics which a generation of women in the United States has recently experienced.

> I've been a woman's-movement activist for a million years; I've counseled abortions; I've helped to set up crisis hot lines for women. And this experience brought me as close to the Right-To-Life Movement as I'll ever come. I'd felt the baby moving; it wasn't a fetus in my mind, it was our baby. Still, I'm grateful to have had the choice. This was devastating, it permanently changed our lives, but then, so would the birth of a kid with Down's. I don't want the Right-To-Life Movement changing my life, I have to do it myself. (Pat Gordon, age 37)

One informant cited Carol Gilligan's work (1982) to me:

> Women are responsible for giving life, not for taking it. Women do have their own morality. Still, I've got to be responsible to myself, Stu, to our future kids, and those responsibilities come first. (Jane Butler, age 35)

These women (and their male partners) are wrapped in the discourses of pro-life/pro-choice politics and mainstream feminism. This language of individual, even feminist, morality seems comfortable to middle-class women, unlike the awkwardness of the medical language, which constructs and constrains their experiences of positive diagnosis. The "second nature" of this discourse is no accident. Mainstream feminism now infuses large sectors of American culture despite its sometimes embattled, oppositional stance. The discourse of maternalism (even medicalized maternalism) *is* becoming more feminist, if by that we mean centered on the expansion of individual women's choices, whether we speak of choices in amniocentesis or styles of birthing babies.

But to examine the cultural imagery surrounding motherhood, it is necessary to shift our focus from the individual woman and her family to the larger community. Because the experience of prenatal diagnosis is so deeply privatized and medicalized, it is easy to miss the gender fault lines on which this new reproductive technology sits. The deeply internalized and socially pervasive imagery of motherhood in American culture is surely shifting. Women who have a choice, including the choice to abort genetically disabled fetuses, are less likely to see themselves, or to be seen by others, as "Madonnas"—long-suffering mothers whose nurturance is unconditional and ever-present. While I would personally argue that freedom from such religiously referential, selfless images of maternity is, on the whole, liberating for women, I would also suggest that we cast a critical eye on the cultural imagery that may replace it—particularly if that imagery is defined in medical terms. For the "new woman" of prenatal diagnosis may feel like an agent of quality control on the reproductive production line:

> I was hoping I'd never have to make this choice, to become responsible for choosing the kind of baby I'd get, the kind of baby we'd accept. But everyone—my doctor, my parents, my friends—everyone urged me to come for genetic counseling and have amniocentesis. Now, I guess I am having a modern baby. And they all told me I'd feel more in control. But in many ways, I feel less in control. It's still my baby, but only if it's good enough to be our baby, if you see what I mean. (Nancy Smithers, age 36)

Neither image—the selfless madonna or the agent of quality control—is constructed by or for women's interests. Both are deeply embedded in patriarchal cultural discourses, the one traditional and religious, the other modern and medically technocratic. The future cultural conceptualization we hold of women as mothers in part depends on turning down the volume of expert voices so that the voices of women themselves may become part of the discourse of prenatal diagnosis.

NOTES

I am deeply grateful to the many women who shared their amniocentesis stories with me. All names and ages have been changed to protect confidentiality. I am also grateful to Dr. William K. Rashbaum, whose concern for his patients led him to recruit women to be interviewed for this study. I hope that he, and they, will find some of this material useful. Carole Browner, Michelle Fine, Susan Harding, Shirley Lindenbaum, and Emily Martin all made suggestions and criticisms on an earlier draft of this article. And Karen Michaelson was a helpful editor. I thank them all and absolve them of any responsibility for the uses I've made of their good ideas.

1. Exact numbers of women using amniocentesis each year are unknown but seem to be growing rapidly. The President's Commission on Bioethics estimated 40,000 tests (1983) at the same time that the Center for Disease Control informally estimated 80,000, and the National Survey on Natality suggested 120,000. The lack of a "ballpark" estimate among government health-policy experts should alert us to the unregulated nature of a service that is available as part of the free-market economy of health care.

2. I am currently doing fieldwork among scientists and support staff of a major genetic laboratory, observing genetic counselors at work with their patients, conducting home interviews with women and their families awaiting the results of amniocentesis, eliciting retrospective interviews with those who received positive diagnoses indicating serious genetic disabilities in their fetuses, participating in support groups for families whose children have the conditions (Down's syndrome, spina bifida) now diagnosable prenatally, and interviewing pregnant women who refused to use the new technology. This research is particularly concerned with differences of class, race, ethnicity, and religion in peoples' cultural construction of pregnancy and childhood disability. I hope it will result in a more complete picture of the social impact of amniocentesis than is given in this brief report of my pilot study.

3. Such technological personifications may be viewed as examples of cyborgs, science fiction chimeras interfacing people and machines, a late twentieth century cultural form insightfully analyzed by Haraway (1985).

4. Anomalous diagnoses are compounded by the newness of the technology and fears—both accurate and exaggerated—of human and technical error in using it. And, as Emily Martin pointed out to me, many more women are told that something *may* be wrong due to technical errors that are later corrected (e.g., maternal/fetal cell confusion in an amniotic sample) than will actually confront a "truly positive" diagnosis.

5. Carole Browner and Shirley Lindenbaum both suggested that the cross-cultural evidence argues for universal constructions of acceptable and unacceptable disabilities. But our current cultural context is one of political struggle over the definitions of disability and social responses.

SECTION II

BIRTH PLACE/BIRTH STYLE

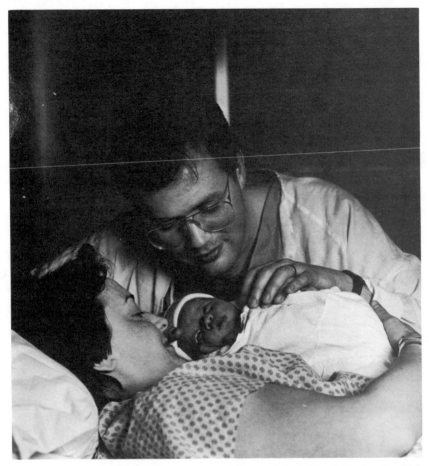

Photograph by LeRoy J. Dierker, Jr., M.D.

BIRTH PLACE/BIRTH STYLE

*Unto the woman He said, I will greatly multiply thy
sorrow and thy conception; in sorrow thou shalt bring
forth children: and thy desire shall be to thy husband,
and he shall rule over thee.*
                                                    —*Genesis 3:16*

*Finally, the unmistakable urge, and Amanda Emily
slowly, beautifully, perfectly entered our world. I lay
weeping with joy, cooing, shaking, blushing at my own
noise, holding her warm wetness to my cheek, feeling
enveloped by deep abiding love*
                        —*Nona McNatt, A Lesson in Empathy*

Although all women come to the birth experience with a similar biological
heritage, they hold, at the time of their infant's birth, different attitudes and
interpretations of that event. Even their experience of pain in labor and delivery
is culturally constructed. Janice Morse and Caroline Park's examination of
cultural differences in the perceived painfulness of birth, in this second section,
indicates the ways that such perceptions can structure the birth experience from
the type of behavior a woman manifests during birth to the selection of those
she wants at her side during labor and delivery. And yet, there are some near
universals in the birth experience. In most cultures women, walk and move
about in early labor, often even in late labor, and they give birth in an upright
position, whether that be kneeling, squatting, standing, or sitting on some culturally acceptable support. Women seek out familiar territory for their births
where they can relax, often returning to their own mother's house to be in the
company of those who love them. The fear or tension of being in a strange place
can slow the course of labor. There is also a preference cross-culturally for
women birth attendants (Jordan 1985).

Robbie Davis-Floyd's chapter in this section gives graphic evidence of how
far American hospital birth diverges from these cross-cultural universals. It is
interesting to compare this description of hospital birth to Trevathan's description (see chapter 14) of birth in a lay-midwife-run clinic, or Lichtman's discussion of medical versus midwifery models of childbirth in chapter 8. Lichtman, a
certified nurse-midwife, continues to work within the framework of the hospital
to humanize the experience of birth, while Trevathan's work describes the
experiences of giving birth with the assistance of lay, or empirical, midwives
working outside of the traditional medical establishment. The differences in these
birth places and birth styles point out the variety of alternatives available to

many American women as they give birth. The authors note that the biomedical model of perinatal care often mandates aggressive intervention into the birth process, and, as Levin points out in Section III, into the postnatal care of critically ill infants. Yet, aggressive medical intervention is differentially valued by women who must try to choose the kind of care that best suits their own physical, cultural, and emotional needs.

Thus, birth alternatives have also been raised as a feminist issue in terms of women's control over their bodies and their reproductive capacity. Lazarus, in the previous section, notes that such concerns have largely been limited to the middle class, where issues such as control by male physicians over women's birth processes have given rise to a gamut of reforms—natural childbirth, alternative birthing centers, and in- and out-of-hospital birthing rooms, beds, and chairs. However, Michaelson and Alvin raise the issue of whether or not such reforms have really given women control over the circumstances in which they give birth. Here, as elsewhere in this book, the critical issue is the appropriate use of technology, played out in the context of the sometimes competing rights of mothers, fathers, physicians, fetuses, and the good of the wider society. Can the court order a cesarean section "for the good of the infant" for a mother who believes she does not require one? Does a woman have the right to satisfy her own needs for a certain type of birth experience, or does society's interest in the infant's safety outweigh her needs? Whose interpretation of relative risk should be used? Just as Rapp and Rothman earlier, and the contributors to the section on neonatal intensive care question whether the very presence of technology must necessarily mandate its use, so do Lichtman, Michaelson and Alvin, and Davis-Floyd in this section question the primacy of technology in controlling birth. The issue is not whether technology is good or bad in and of itself, but under what circumstances should it be used, when does it augment the quality of life of those who use it, when does it detract from that quality, and, perhaps most importantly, who has the power to decide what is appropriate use.

Also raised here is the very real issue of whether such reforms touch more than a handful of women with access to the socioeconomic resources to pay for quality alternative care and the assertiveness to speak out to obtain the care they desire. Poor women, powerless in most contexts, rarely can select alternatives in the care they receive. They may not, indeed, have information that alternatives are available at all.

7

DIFFERENCES IN CULTURAL EXPECTATIONS OF THE PERCEIVED PAINFULNESS OF CHILDBIRTH

Janice M. Morse and Caroline Park

The control and management of childbirth pain has received much attention since the 1950s. In the past three decades, American women have begun to resist using sedatives, anaesthesia, and analgesia to control labor pain and have demanded an increasing role in the control of labor. In spite of the move toward natural childbirth and the self-management of pain, however, in most cases health care professionals still have ultimate responsibility for and control over the mother and infant in the childbirth process.

The assessment of pain in labor and the recognition of patient distress remains one of the most difficult tasks for the labor-room nurse. Although the physiological signs of distress (such as changes in pulse and blood pressure) are well documented, these changes occur slowly, and the primary objective when providing care is to prevent distress before these signs are evident. The task of pain assessment is further confounded by cultural variation in the behavioral expression of pain and by the amount of pain the health professional assumes to be inherent in the process of parturition.

Although some research has examined cultural variation in the behavioral response to pain, less has been conducted on cultural variation in the amount of pain inferred to be experienced by others. Work by Davitz and her colleagues shows discrepancies between the amount of pain experienced by the patient and the amount of suffering attributed to the pain event by the health professional (Davitz, Davitz, and Higuchi 1977a, 1977b; Davitz, Sameshima, and Davitz 1976). As most of the deliveries in North America are conducted in the hospital setting and as the norms in this setting reflect the norms of North American culture, the analysis of the amount of pain attributed to childbirth by different cultural groups will provide important insight into differences in behavioral norms and will identify disparities between client and caregiver during childbirth.

121

CULTURAL VARIATION IN PAIN EXPRESSION

The cultural response to pain and the subjective nature of the pain experience was described by Zborowski (1952, 1969). He suggested that inherent in each culture were patterned attitudes towards pain behavior, such that appropriate and inappropriate expressions of pain are culturally prescribed. By interviewing medical personnel, patients, and their families, he was able to develop cultural descriptions of appropriate pain reactions. When the caregiver came from a cultural background different from the patient in pain, discrepancies in expected behaviors arose, resulting in the rejection of the patient and in value-judgment labels (such as alarmist and nuisances) being given to the patient. Other common labels, such as overexaggerated, overemotional, hysterical, stolid, mature, and masculine, also revealed expected pain behaviors.

Zborowski (1969) also noted that expected pain did not necessarily result in acceptance of that pain. Cultural tradition dictates to the group not only whether or not to expect pain in a certain situation, but also whether the pain is to be tolerated or not and what the expected behavior should be during the painful experience. Culture maintains these norms by using direct and indirect pressure through such means as public opinion, self-control in an effort to conform, and through cultural structures and institutions (such as the health care system). However, the ideal response is rarely attained, and individual differences arise from incomplete compliance and human deviation from the ideal pattern.

By comparing four cultural groups (Italian, Irish, "Old" American, and Jewish), Zborowski was able to demonstrate that similar reactions to pain do not necessarily indicate similar attitudes towards pain, and that a similar pain stimulus may evoke widely disparate reactions in different cultural groups.

Researchers are in agreement with Zborowski (1952, 1969) on the learned nature of pain expression through behavioral and linguistic communication. Behaviorally, Craig's (1978) work on social modeling suggests that pain behaviors are culturally learned and culturally transmitted. Pain behaviors are tolerated or reinforced *if* they are considered culturally appropriate and punished *if* they are inappropriate. Thus, the person in pain may behave expressively or stoically depending on the incentives within the cultural environment. Von Baeyer, Johnson, and McMillan (1984) show that the person in pain communicates nonverbally the amount of distress experienced to the observer, and this in turn affects the observer's concern for the person in pain. Thus, the process of social learning permits individuals to develop evaluations of painful conditions. These evaluations include information on how painful conditions are, even though the painful events have not been personally experienced. Because of this process, males, for example, who will never experience childbirth, may develop some understanding of the nature and intensity of childbirth pain.

Because the expectation and evaluation of pain is culturally specific, Davitz and her colleagues have repeatedly noted that nurses from different cultures attributed different degrees of pain and suffering to the same patients. Conversely, because there are striking differences in the cultural norms surrounding the behavior of laboring women of differing cultural backgrounds, their pain expression may vary from stoical, silent, controlled, and concentrated to restless, vocal, and seemingly uncontrolled behavior. These behavioral differences increase the complexity of the nurses' assessment and recognition of distress in the laboring patient

RACIAL VARIATION IN THE COURSE OF LABOR

Despite differing cultural reactions to and expressions of pain in childbirth, and even though there are significant differences in maternal stature and infant birth weight, investigation into racial variation during the physiological course of labor has revealed no major differences. Duignan, Studd, and Hughes (1975) examined 1,306 parturients from three racial groups: caucasian Americans, Asian immigrants (from India, Pakistan, and Bangladesh), and black African and West Indian immigrants. No significant differences were found in the duration of the first stage of labor, the progress of labor, or the cervical dilation rate. However, slight differences in the duration of the second stage were noted: it was longest in the white group and shortest in the black group. However, these differences were not significant in a second study comparing Malay, Indian, and Chinese women (Lim, Wong, and Sinnathuray 1977); these researchers found only slight differences in the cervical dilation rate, with Indian primiparae experiencing a delay at 5 cm.

In an Israeli study, Melmed and Evans (1976) compared native-born and foreign-born Jews and Arab patients (n=787). They also found no differences in the cervical dilation rate, position of the head at the onset of labor, or in the incidence of the type of delivery (i.e., spontaneous, assisted delivery, or cesarean section). As all of these findings are inconclusive, one can assume that the physiological birth process and the pain stimulus are similar for all groups.

CROSS-CULTURAL STUDIES OF CHILDBIRTH PAIN

Studies examining the cultural perception of childbirth pain are few. In 1978 Jordan reported her observations of birthing in Yucatan, Holland, Sweden, and the United States, emphasizing the different childbirthing "systems" and the justification for each. Inferences about pain perception might be drawn from this data, but they are not specifically addressed. A study by Winsberg and Greenlick (1967) examined the pain response of black and caucasian obstetrical patients using a five-point rating scale to measure the degree of pain, the pain response, and the "cooperativeness" of the patient as rated by the physician, the nurse, and the patient. No differences between the black and caucasian groups were found, but this study used broad levels of measurement, and the distinction between race and culture was not considered.

In 1981 Morse examined the perception of parturition pain in Fijian and Fiji-Indian women. During labor, the Fijian women behaved in a stoic manner and labored silently, while the Fiji-Indians were restless and expressed their pain vocally by calling out. While the Fijian prepared extensively for labor throughout pregnancy and the responsibility for the health of the mother and the infant were considered a community concern, in the Fiji-Indian culture mothers were not prepared for childbirth. There was no dietary supplementation or relief from work, and information was withheld from primiparous women. Measurement of the perceived painfulness of parturition showed that the Fijians rate childbirth highest of all pain events, while Fiji-Indians rate it much lower, second to the pain of a heart attack. In this study, the perceived painfulness was congruent with ethnographic descriptions, so that the Fijians, who had a greater perception of parturition pain, also had the greater number of pain-reducing coping mechanisms, such as belief systems, herbal remedies, support, and comfort measures (Morse, in press).

AMERICAN NORMS OF CHILDBIRTH PAIN

Since the late nineteenth century in America, the pain of childbirth has been increasingly managed medically by removing pain with anesthesia or analgesics. By the early twentieth century, childbirth was considered the purview of medicine and treated as a pathological condition (Hern 1975). More recently, there has been a desire among some groups for the demedicalization of childbirth, for women's increased control over the experience, and for natural childbirth in a homelike setting, such as a birthing room, or even at home. There has been increasing attention to childbirth preparation through classes and a rejection of passive behavioral patterns for a more participatory role in childbirth. These changes include the involvement of the husband and siblings in the birth experience and concern about and provision for support for the woman in labor. Thus, in America, childbirth is in the process of being redefined as a family event, rather than a medical crisis (McClain 1983a).

In the past, the rationale for the medical management of childbirth was the alleviation of pain and the reduction of risk to the mother. However, the pharmacological management of labor pain has some real disadvantages. Because analgesics cross the placental barrier, the infant also becomes sedated and less responsive at birth. The drowsy effect on the mother may dull the emotional experience of birth and interfere with maternal-infant bonding immediately after birth (Affonso 1976). Thus, many contemporary parents choose to use a psychoprophylactic method, such as Lamaze, which focuses on techniques of self-distraction, self-control, relaxation, and the support of a "coach" as a means of alleviating labor pain (Charles et al. 1978; Stevens and Heide 1977).

Within the labor and delivery room in America, there are behavioral norms for the expression of pain that control the introduction of pain-reducing medications. Patients in labor are not to shout or to verbalize their pain constantly. Some soft moaning and muttering is permitted, but this should not disturb others. Patients are expected to obey the instructions of the doctor or nurse and to ring the call bell (not too often) if they suspect that something is wrong. They are expected to be able to relax on command, to push on command, and to pant on command. They must remain supine and are rarely given a choice regarding position for delivery. Usually, one person may stay with the laboring woman to provide comfort.

Behaviors outside this pattern are often met with impatience by the nurse. An overt and emotional expression of pain is considered abnormal, and the patient considered to be inappropriately acting out. Conversely, the patient who behaves in a more stoic fashion and does not display the expected pain cues that are congruent with her progression in labor is perceived to have a precipitous labor and often delivers before the staff are ready. In spite of the difficulty of those who have not experienced childbirth pain (nulliparous women and males) in estimating the amount of pain associated with childbirth, differences between "easy" labors and "hard" labors are noted. Nurses characterize easy labors as those in which the patients are stoical and the labor short or within normative limits. Hard labors are those in which the patient becomes distressed, vocalizes about the amount of pain experienced, and/or has a prolonged labor.

Discrepancies between the patients' rating of the painfulness of childbirth and nurses' and physicians' ratings of the pain have been documented. According to Winsberg and Greenlick (1967), the greatest difference in the amount of pain perceived occurred not between groups, as hypothesized, but between the patients', the nurses', the aides', and the physicians' ratings of the pain, with the health professionals consistently rating the pain lower than the mothers.

When assessing pain, nurses are trained to first evaluate for the physiological indices of pain, such as sweating, flaring of the nostrils, and behavioral signs of distress, such as posturing (Angelini 1978), and then to monitor the patient at regular intervals for physiological indices of distress, such as changes in the blood pressure or pulse (Affonso 1973). The patient's own evaluation of the pain and her verbal behavior may or may not be considered as a valid criterion for pain assessment. That is, the nurse may use the patient's report to confirm her assessment that an analgesic is required, or she may discredit or ignore the patient's pain report if it is in variance with her own assessment. For example, the nurse will state that the pain is "not *that* bad." Thus, it is the nurse, rather than the patient, who determines when an analgesic is administered.

Therefore it is evident that the acceptable behaviors and pain expressions permitted during childbirth are those of the dominant culture, and that the pharmacological management of pain is controlled by these same norms. The inference or the perception of the nurse or physician of the amount of pain that the patient is experiencing determines the control measures instituted, such as the need for medication.

EXAMINING THE PAINFULNESS OF CHILDBIRTH

Many investigators have attempted to quantify the painfulness of parturition by simulating the pain stimulus. Such methods as applying blood pressure cuffs to measure ischemic pain (Mulcahy and Janz 1973; Johnson 1973), putting pressure on the index finger (Manderino and Bzdek 1984), and using cold pressor stimulus (Stone et al. 1977; Worthington et al. 1982) have been used to compare and contrast pain tolerance (timed tolerance), pain threshold (from the time that the subject reported the pain as painful), and self-report of pain intensity. Using such analogues, the investigators have compared the effectiveness of pain-control measures such as various distractions, relaxation, and prepared-breathing techniques used during labor. However, as Beck and Seigel (1980) note, these experiments have several major threats to validity. The context of the childbirth setting and the meaning of the event are removed, and the discomfort from the pain stimulus is not usually timed to resemble the intermittent pain of contractions, nor do they extend over the same time period as labor. Furthermore, as Craig and Best (1977) noted, one of the most distressing components of the pain experience is the feeling of the loss of control and the feeling of being unable to relieve, terminate, or avoid bodily harm, a factor in childbirth that is not present in experimental pain.

The second method of examining pain has been to use psychological rating scales to quantify pain intensity (e.g., the pain thermometer or the McGill Pain Questionnaire) or to elicit qualitative descriptions of different types of pains (e.g., the McGill Pain Questionnaire). Melzack et al. (1981) report that the pain of labor is one of the most intense pains recorded by the McGill Pain Questionnaire. The pain ratings, though widely distributed, were inversely related to the amount of childbirth preparation, to socioeconomic status (Melzack et al. 1981) and to the experience of other painful events (Niven and Gijsbers 1984). They were positively correlated with a history of menstrual difficulties (Melzack et al. 1981) and physiological variables, such as the mother's height-to-weight ratio and the infant's weight (Melzack et al. 1984).

CROSS-CULTURAL PERCEPTION OF CHILDBIRTH PAIN

The study presented here measures the perceptions of the pain of childbirth in four different cultures residing in western Canada: the Canadian-Anglophone the Ukranian, the Hutterite, and the East Indian. For this study, the pain of childbirth was quantified and the differences between groups compared.

Pain was quantified using the technique of paired comparison developed in 1927 by Thurstone (Nunnally 1978). In this technique the pain of childbirth is compared with eight other painful events in all possible combinations to give a total of thirty-six comparisons. The painful events chosen were: heart attack, kidney stone, severe burn, toothache, gallstones, eye injury, broken bone, and migraine. The respondent is asked to choose which is the most painful in each pair of stimuli. For example, the respondent is asked, "Which is more painful, a heart attack or childbirth?" The results are statistically analyzed so that the responses are normally distributed around each stimuli on a continuum and the distributions overlap. This method, however, can only be used when people have difficulty making a choice between the paired items.

RESULTS: CROSS-CULTURAL RATINGS OF CHILDBIRTH PAIN

The Anglophone Canadian sample (N=191) consisted of parents who had elected to have hospital deliveries. They rated the pain of childbirth higher than did members of the other cultural groups (see Figure 1). Childbirth pain scored at 12.9 for the females, 10.55 for the males, and 11.15 for the total group. As previously discussed, the norms surrounding birth for this group are such that they expect childbirth to be painful, and most use a variety of methods to prepare for it (such as childbirth classes). Despite the move towards natural childbirth, this group may be considered to have a relatively passive attitude towards the expected pain. That is, mothers know that if the pain becomes severe and beyond their self-control, they will be offered or given medications to relieve the pain. The lower rating of childbirth pain by males is not surprising, given that fathers' participation in the birth event is a relatively new concept that emerged in the past two decades.

FIGURE 1. Amount of Perceived Pain of Childbirth for Four Cultures: Total Group, Males, and Females

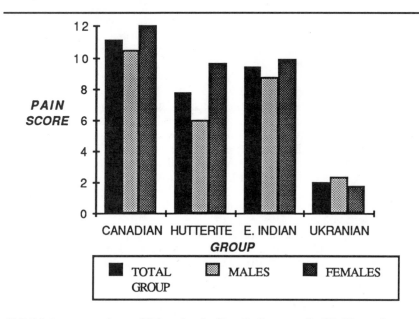

Childbirth was rated next highest by the East Indian sample (N=22; total score 9.52). In this group, males are traditionally excluded from the childbirth setting, and their score was lower (9.16) than the females (10.18). Values of purity and innocence in East Indian culture exclude the overt teaching of females about the process of birth (Morse in press), and during labor these patients express pain by vocalizing continually.

The Hutterite sample (N=41) consisted of all the adults in one colony, a farming community of about 100 members. The Hutterites maintain a patriarchal society that rigidly restricts a woman to the maternal role. Once married, a woman is expected to bear children throughout her childbearing period (Schludermann and Schludermann 1971). Contraception is considered to violate divine will unless maternal health is threatened (Converse, Buker, and Lee 1973), and therefore family size averages 10.4 children (Hostetler 1974). During pregnancy, there is no change in the woman's work role or diet. Women are accepting of their pregnancy, and perceive the pain of childbirth as coming from God. There is, however, some ambivalence towards the pain of childbirth, for the women reported that "if one worked hard, the pain was less." In traditional Hutterite settings, the husband is excluded from the delivery. The males rated the pain of childbirth much lower than did the women (5.88 and 9.93 respectively, with a total group score of 7.92).

The last group, the Ukranians, immigrated from Europe during the Ukraine famine of the 1930s. They settled on the Canadian prairies, forming strong ethnic communities. Though the Russian Orthodox Church permits the use of contraceptives, children are highly valued. Large families were considered essential and were required to assist on the farm. In this sample (N=48), childbirth pain was rated lowest (total score 2.14). The males rated childbirth pain higher than the females (2.4 and 2.11 respectively), and this low score is consistent with female reports that "the pain [of childbirth] isn't that bad." Nevertheless, it is im-portant to note that, though childbirth pain has been rated low, it is not con-sidered pain free. Males are not encouraged to remain with their wives during labor, as this is considered to cause unnecessary stress. One Ukranian woman who shared her birth experience with her husband was asked, "Why did you put him [the husband] through all that?"

A comparison of the cultures that rated childbirth pain highest (the Anglo-Canadians and the East Indians) and lowest (the Ukranians and the Hutterites) shows important differences in the attitudes toward childbirth. The two groups that rated childbirth pain highest do not consider childbirth to be a natural event. The medicalization of childbirth in Anglo-Canadian culture and the withholding of information about birth in East Indian culture are reflective of this attitude. On the other hand, the Hutterite and the Ukranian cultures consider childbirth more of a natural event which does not have to be extensively managed or purposefully ignored.

However, the relationship between the evaluation of painfulness of childbirth and ethnographic analysis of childbirth attitudes and practices must be explored further. The most important point made here is that the norm for the amount of pain attributed to childbirth varies markedly between cultures and can be quantified.

CONCLUSION

In this study, the amount of pain attributed to childbirth was distinctly different in four cultural groups. It is important to recall that this study did not measure how painful childbirth *actually* is, but rather how painful it is *thought to be*. As previously discussed, this has important implications for the pain expectations of the mother as she approaches delivery and it may affect the amount of anxiety experienced during labor and delivery. These perceptions also have important implications for the management of childbirth and the care of the pregnant woman within the culture.

An important area to consider is the cultural differences in pain inference, particularly when a nurse or physician is from a cultural background different from that of the patient. Although thus far, studies have not measured the relationship between the pain inferred and the behavior of the laboring patient, or the relationship between pain inference and empathy, these are questions that must be addressed in future research.

This chapter has argued that not only are culturally appropriate pain behaviors communicated, but also the perceived intensity of the pain is taught. The expectations of the painfulness of childbirth are culturally determined. Because this information is learned by others, including males, others are able to form a support system and provide empathy for the person in pain. However, if the mother's behavior is not within cultural norms, the undesirable behavior is censored. Problems occur in the health-care setting when the nurse and/or physician are from different cultural backgrounds than the patient and the patient's behaviors are thus contrary to the health professionals' expectations. In these cases, patient distress and the need for analgesic may be hard to assess. Understanding the amount of pain attributed to childbirth by various groups will assist with pain assessment.

NOTE

The authors wish to acknowledge the assistance of Jane Buchan, R.N., M.N., Pat Chern, R.N., B. Sc.N., Taynez Kanji, R.N., and Olga Chittack, R.N., B.Sc.N. for their assistance with the collection of data, and Robert Morse, M.Sc., M.Ph. for his statistical advice and expertise. This article was prepared with the assistance of a National Health and Research Scholar Award to Dr. Morse.

8

MEDICAL MODELS AND MIDWIFERY: THE CULTURAL EXPERIENCE OF BIRTH

Ronnie Lichtman

All participant observation is colored by the researcher's prior experiences and by her or his attitudes and beliefs. In this case, the observer's bias is clear. I am a certified nurse-midwife and as such have a deep commitment to practicing according to what I will call the "midwifery model" of obstetric care rather than what is usually termed the "medical model." Although there is no universally accepted theory of midwifery, most practitioners would agree that there are several differences between midwifery and the medical model of birth as practiced by most physicians. The most widely accepted distinction is that midwives see pregnancy and birth as normal processes, as part of the life cycle, not as illnesses or disease states. In practice, midwives allow nature to run its course unless intervention becomes a necessity. Most midwives consider psychological, emotional, interpersonal, family, and spiritual needs as essential parts of health care. Finally, most believe in each woman's right to maintain control of her body and of her care. This is accomplished through informed decision making, which mandates a great deal of teaching and information giving by midwives.

The data for this article were gathered by participant observation (as care provider, birth attendant, and instructor of midwifery) in two distinct hospital settings. Despite a consistent belief in these principles, in the two settings in which I have been a birth attendant I have had profoundly different relationships to my work and to childbirth. The structure, policies, and power relationships within these two settings have affected and, in fact, determined, the way I have been able to practice and my perception of myself as a practitioner, as well as the way that the women and families in my care have experienced their births.

TERMINOLOGY

Before describing the two hospitals in which I worked, it is important to discuss terminology. Vocabulary choice can reflect attitudes toward pregnancy or toward women. I have heard the words "patient," "client," "consumer," "woman," "lady," "girl," and "mother" used to refer to pregnant persons. The word patient usually refers to someone who is sick. In the American medical system, this often implies dependency. Client is usually associated with a more equal relationship between a professional (e.g., a lawyer) and a recipient of her or his services. The professional is, in a sense, the employee of the client; a contractual relationship exists between them. This latter term has come into use by nurse-midwives (and some physicians) to express their belief that pregnant women are not ill and not dependent or powerless. It rings, however, of a somewhat impersonal relationship and overlooks the difference in the quality of emotional content of health care as compared to other services. The word consumer implies a buying and selling relationship—which only represents a part of what is involved in health care interactions. Moreover, in municipal hospitals women (and men) do not really have consumer power, and contracts with providers are at best verbal, more often unspoken or nonexistent. None of these terms is really adequate. I will, however, use the word patient rather than client or consumer, despite its unpopularity in progressive childbirth movements. I will use the term woman rather than lady or girl.

Language also becomes a major concern when referring to hospital policies. Descriptions of policy often use the terms "permitted" or "allowed" as in: "Fathers are permitted to attend labor and normal vaginal deliveries." This language depicts the hospital as a beneficent parent rather than an institution in the employ of its users. This terminology has therefore been avoided, although this avoidance somewhat distorts the reality that hospital policy is very often patronizing and, especially in the municipal system, beyond the control of patients.

INSTITUTIONAL DIFFERENCES

Institutional characteristics affect the experience of birthing women in a number of ways. They affect the subjective perception of pregnancy and birth and, in a more total sense, of self, of control over one's body. The two institutions are both municipal hospitals. The women presenting themselves for care at both North and South Hospitals accept the need for medical supervision during pregnancy. Therefore, to a large extent the association of pregnancy with illness is unavoidable, despite most midwives' firm conviction that pregnancy is a normal event, an event whose deep personal connotations far exceed its medical impact. Yet the vast majority of patients at North Hospital never see a physician during their pregnancy, while physician care is the norm at South Hospital.[1]

Most women who come for care at these institutions are poor, from an ethnic minority, and likely to have no more than a high-school education—frequently they have less. Many speak little or no English. Although in modern-day obstetrical thinking there is an assumption that all women of such "low" socioeconomic status have greater risk in childbirth, in North Hospital the implementation of high-risk procedures must be based on an individualized assessment of such risk; in South Hospital high-risk procedures are routine. These procedures include uncomfortable but rarely dangerous interventions, such as enemas, pubic shaves, and intravenous feedings, as well as those that are more invasive, such as the insertion of electronic monitors directly onto the fetal scalp, artificial rupture of membranes, and lithotomy position for birth using high, widely spaced stirrups—any of which can potentially lead to complications.

The major difference between the two hospitals is that North Hospital's labor and delivery units are staffed primarily by certified nurse-midwives, while South Hospital's are staffed by obstetrical resident physicians. Both services have attending obstetricians as back up. Although South Hospital does have a small staff of midwives, they see a relatively small number of pregnant women and do not provide 24-hour, seven-day-a-week coverage in labor and delivery as do the midwives at North Hospital. The midwives at North Hospital have some responsibility for all women in the obstetrical service, functioning with physicians as co-managers of care when a medical problem arises or is anticipated. Thus, midwifery philosophy permeates the care of every pregnant woman—healthy or ill, with or without problems—at North Hospital. At South Hospital, the midwives' presence has not significantly influenced the overall experience of childbirth except perhaps for the few women they attend.

Management choices and treatment of women at the two institutions reflect the different training, philosophies, and personal characteristics of care providers and the power relationships among them, as well as institutional goals secondary to health care. Although the main purpose of both hospitals is to provide direct patient care, South Hospital is also a training center for medical-school graduates who wish to specialize in obstetrics, while North Hospital is a demonstration project utilizing nurse-midwives as primary care providers.

Differences in Patient Care

Prenatal Care. Pregnant women at North Hospital see the same midwife in clinic throughout their pregnancy, generally establishing relationships with their midwives on a first name basis. The midwives value the personal components of interaction with patients and emphasize health maintenance. Nevertheless, many women view hospital-based midwives as very much a part of the medical system. When I was a staff midwife at North Hospital, I had several patients who consistently called me "Dr. Ronnie" regardless of my careful and repeated explanation that I was not a doctor and my assurrance that they could see a doctor if they preferred (an option rarely exercised at North Hospital). Still, any cursory review of prenatal charts at the two hospitals attests to differences that begin in the prenatal period—despite the system recently established at South Hospital in which a consistent caregiver is provided for all prenatal visits. Most physician notes are short and refer only to the woman's physical condition: "24 weeks by size and dates, no problems" is a typical sort of entry. Midwifery notes tend to be more detailed and include references not only to physical but also to psychological and personal concerns, such as family relationships, childbirth class registration, and preparation for labor and delivery. Even notes about the physical aspects of pregnancy refer to topics such as nutritional intake and common discomforts of pregnancy often ignored or devalued by physicians. From such notes one can infer a very different focus at prenatal visits. Although two conference nurses are on staff at South Hospital, and a nurse-practitioner works as patient-care coordinator and counselor in the high-risk clinic, their care is not always ongoing, and since their responsibility is for all clinic patients, counseling is necessarily brief.

Such differences in prenatal care can certainly affect the cultural patterning of pregnancy. What happens at prenatal visits can determine how much attention is paid to diet, how involved other family members become with the actual processes of pregnancy and birth and with health maintenance in this period, how much time is devoted to preparation for the event of labor, and who participates directly in that event. This may be especially true for women such as those at North and South Hospital who do not, as a group, read extensively about pregnancy and birth and who do not come prepared to present caregivers with their own requirements.

Labor. In labor and delivery, differences are even more apparent. It is quite rare to see a woman laboring at North Hospital without the presence of a support person of her choice. It is a given policy, established by the director of midwifery when the service was opened several years ago, that every woman has the right to labor accompanied by a person of her own choosing—not necessarily her husband. Most North Hospital midwives believe that it is a woman's right to choose to have more than one person with her, including appropriately supervised siblings. Although opposition to that policy has come largely from nursing, individual nurses often support this more permissive approach. Two or three support persons are not uncommon at North Hospital, and occasionally, a child participates in labor and birth.

Conversely, until two years ago it was rare to see a woman at South Hospital who was not alone. The policy there required that in order to attend labor and delivery, a person had to have completed a series of childbirth-education classes and be able to produce a certificate as evidence of such completion. Many midwives (myself included) resorted to dishonesty in the face of powerlessness to change this policy by falsifying certificates for women who came into the labor unit with partners whom they wanted to remain with them. The rule was finally revoked at the insistence of a new director of midwifery, who has since left the service. Despite the policy change, however, more pregnant women are alone in labor at South Hospital than at North Hospital; perhaps this is due to differences in prenatal teaching and preparation. Midwifery students are taught to discuss childbirth education classes with all women during prenatal visits and to encourage their attendance at such classes. Indeed, many midwives teach childbirth classes, and most midwifery schools offer teacher-training courses. This is not a part of medical education and is not stressed in obstetrical residency training programs.

An observant guest wandering through the labor units at these two hospitals would be struck by the contrast. At South Hospital, all laboring women are in bed with intravenous tubing and attached to fetal monitoring machines either externally via abdominal belts or internally via fetal scalp electrodes. I have witnessed scenes that, except for the human pain involved, would be comic: a woman comes to the labor floor fully dilated, almost ready to deliver, yet the intravenous is started before she is instructed to push. She may be told to stop her pushing efforts, which is not an easy task. This is all done without assessing the risk factors that might necessitate an intravenous, though most of these can be automatically ruled out just by the fact that the woman had gotten to this point in labor. Many women at South Hospital are medicated, though this in no way makes for painless childbirth; sounds of pain, varying in type and degree, often permeate the labor area.

At North Hospital there is greater diversity in the patterns of labor. Laboring women who have no complications often choose to walk around. Couples—composed of a pregnant woman and either her male partner or another, often older, woman—can be seen wandering about. Occasionally a group of three or more are encountered. Contractions are dealt with in a variety of ways. A woman may lean up against a wall, against her support person, or continue moving. Rocking back and forth is not uncommon. Some women spend part of their labors sitting in chairs. Others remain in bed, in semi-sitting positions, lying on their sides, or assuming a hands-and-knees position to relieve back pressure. Of those women in bed, some are connected to fetal monitors, others are not. Most commonly, the machine is used intermittently.

Another noticeable difference between North and South Hospitals is the amount of privacy afforded patients. In neither institution is privacy considered a priority. Staff members value their right to freely enter any room at any time. At North Hospital, however, there are attempts made to safeguard privacy. As a practitioner at North Hospital, I felt comfortable closing doors; at South Hospital I knew that sooner or later someone—a nurse or a resident —would come in, not necessarily to provide patient care but to check on what was going on "behind closed doors." I remember one day working in the admitting room at North Hospital when an older, well-dressed gentleman approached the door. I was with a woman whose legs were in stirrups on the exam table. The man started to enter, announcing, "It's all right; I'm a doctor." "I'm sorry," I told him, "there's a woman being examined in here. I'd like you to wait please." He did. I later found out that he was the service's newly appointed director of obstetrics. I was quite pleased with myself and never heard any more about the incident. I must admit that at South Hospital I would have been much more hesitant in the same situation, and I don't know what the reaction or repercussions would have been.

Seasoned practitioners, myself included, can easily lose sensitivity to the need for privacy. To understand how important it might be to a woman, I have to remember my own shock and outrage in my first obstetrical-nursing job at another city hospital—quite similar, in many aspects of its functioning, to South Hospital—at the complete inattention paid to the rights and needs of women for privacy. Over the years, my horror has diminished, much to my own chagrin. For each woman, the feeling of intrusion must be like my own initial reaction except that, in a very real sense, it is her body that is being assaulted.

Birth. Deliveries provide another area of contrast. With a few exceptions, births at South Hospital take place in the delivery room, which looks like a standard operating room with its steel tables and imposing lights. Women are moved from their beds to a narrow, flat table. Their legs are generally placed in stirrups and covered, along with their abdomens, with sterile towels. The women are told not to touch the towels. The baby is born into the hands of the obstetrician, held aloft so that the mother can identify its sex, and quickly placed in a warmer, which the mother, lying on her back, cannot see. Eventually, after the baby is footprinted, identified with wristbands, and has had medication placed in its eyes, she or he is given to the mother for a brief period. The newborn is soon transported to the nursery. It is several hours before the mother will see her child again.

This scenario is sometimes played out at North Hospital—in the event of a baby with a problem—although even then the delivery table is only used in the rare event that forceps are anticipated. Instead, most North Hospital births are done in the labor room, in the labor bed. Even when there is a problem that may require infant-resuscitation equipment, available only in the delivery room, the laboring woman usually remains in her bed, which is wheeled to the delivery room. This has several advantages: she need not move at a time when moving is awkward and uncomfortable; she need not have her legs in stirrups which puts undue pressure on the perineum (and may cause trauma to the legs, especially in heavy women); she can sit up or lie on her side. Both these positions facilitate pushing efforts far better than lying flat. In the sitting position, the woman can sometimes see her baby emerge or touch its head as it is crowning. Although some hospital delivery tables have elevated backrests and mirror arrangements to enable women to watch their babies emerging, South Hospital uses neither of these.

Many midwives place the baby on the mother's abdomen once it is born, if she wants this immediate contact. Although the North Hospital nurses will take the baby away for a while for identification and medications, the period of initial contact is much longer than at South Hospital. The mother is in a more comfortable position to hold, cuddle, and often breastfeed her newborn.

Patients and Staff

Another difference, perhaps not perceptible from casual observation, is the relation between staff and patients—the extent to which patient needs and desires are solicited and incorporated into the management plans for each individual labor. Management is a broad term which relates to the treatment of labor and birth: what is done for the woman and her baby. In midwifery practice, the management of labor involves several aspects: the physical care of the laboring and birthing woman and her newborn, her emotional care, and the involvement of her family and/or friends. In each of these areas, the input of the woman is implicit. Ideally, this input begins with pregnancy and continues during labor and through the actual birth. In North Hospital, this is modified by the constraints of a busy service and by the fact that the birth attendant usually meets the woman and her support persons for the first time when they arrive in labor since the midwives work in scheduled shifts rather than on-call. In South Hospital, midwifery management is modified by rigid hospital protocols and hierarchical relationships among staff members that place the patient—along with the midwife—at the bottom of a long chain of command.

An anecdote involving my interaction with a resident at South Hospital well illustrates this relationship to patients. A midwifery student and I were caring for a woman who was quite uncomfortable and was having a long and difficult labor. During contractions she was loudly making her discomfort known, but between contractions she was alert and lucid. We discussed the possibility of medication with her, outlining its pros and cons. We explained that it might relax her and relieve some, but not all, of her pain and it would make her feel more distant from the pain. We told her that we would give her a dose that would not harm the fetus or, since it was early enough in her labor, produce a sleepy baby, though subtle effects on the newborn were possible. Although her labor was sufficiently established so that it would not be stopped entirely with medication, we presented the possibility that it might slow down. The woman asked a few questions and decided against the medication. She did not want to risk prolonging her labor at all. Shortly afterward, a senior resident entered the room. He checked the woman's monitor print-out and suggested that we consider medication. I told him that we had just discussed it with her and she had decided against it. "You discussed it with her?" he asked in a puzzled voice. "With whom? With Dr. M? She didn't want to prescribe medication?" (Dr. M. was the junior resident who happened to be female.) "No," I replied, "with the patient. The patient doesn't want medication." His face showed his clear surprise. It obviously had not occurred to him that we had negotiated our care with its recipient. I was not sure if he would order the medication anyway, but he did not.

I had a similar experience with a physician at North Hospital; the difference was not in the doctor's attitude, but in my own attitude and behavior. I was with another young woman, also vocal in her contractions, but relaxed, comfortable, and aware between them. We had a similar discussion about medication and she made the same choice—to get through labor without it. A few moments later, I overheard the attending physician ordering 50 milligrams of a narcotic commonly used in labor. I had a hunch it was intended for that patient. I knew she was the noisiest woman on the floor, and doctors (and midwives) are troubled by noisy patients. It makes us feel that we have somehow failed in making their labor comfortable. Anyway, I confronted the attending physician. I told him about my conversation with the woman and asked if he had discussed the order with her. He had not. I informed him that the patient was not to have medication at that time. He admitted that the need was more his own than hers. The crucial difference was that I knew that my decision to accept the patient's wishes would not be superceded at North Hospital and that I could tell the physician my plan without being put in the position of needing his approval.

Professional Identity

For me, working at these two institutions has been like having two professional identities—and at times, two selves. What I could offer to women in terms of their childbirth experience, how much decision-making power I had, how confident I was in my own abilities to make judgments and carry them out, how competent I felt as a teacher, and even how secure I felt in my hand skills have all been determined by the institutional settings in which I have had to function. At North Hospital I could work with women and with families to make childbirth humane and satisfying, even in the face of complications. There was the possibility of preserving dignity for birthing women and for myself as a birth attendant with knowledge and skills. I felt I could pass this sense on to students and teach them how to make safe judgments and to individualize labor and birth management in ways that they could carry with them wherever they worked.

At South Hospital I saw my role as an attempt to make the experience of childbirth as humane as possible given the circumstances and to teach as well as possible, helping students to see beyond the situation at hand. In my teaching I used the technique of creating fantasy situations. "Pretend you were free to use midwifery management for this woman," instructors might say to a student; "what would you do?" This is a poor substitute for reality since belief and philosophy in health care must be based on what is actually experienced, but it was the only way to educate students at South Hospital to be creative and flexible practitioners whose care would be based on the safest management for each woman, rather than on routines learned by rote.

Although the basis for routine care, especially in busy institutions, is to avoid danger through omission, the implementation of particular routines in certain situations can itself create problems. Whenever a student and I cared for a woman at South Hospital, I would make certain that one of us was in the room at all times so that the residents would not come in and change our management. We would devise strategies to avoid their intervention. For example, even in situations where frequent vaginal exams are contraindicated, as in ruptured membranes, the routine at South Hospital is to examine everybody every two hours. The residents would insist on knowing how our patient was "progressing." They would not accept indicators other than pelvic findings, such as changes in contraction pattern or behavioral clues. We would thus anticipate their queries and come up with reasons to prolong the time between exams. "We were just about to examine her, but she needed to use the bedpan. We'll be examining her as soon as she's finished," would be a typical excuse. Such conniving was not needed at North Hospital, where midwife management and judgment were accepted.

Cesarean Rates

The actual physical event of childbirth differs between these two institutions. At South Hospital, birth is far more likely to become an operative procedure with its attendant risks. The published cesarean rate for North Hospital is below the national average (NICHD 1980:5), while staff report of South Hospital's cesarean rate indicates that it is generally above the national average. According to the *Draft Report on Cesarean Childbirth* (NICHD 1980) maternal mortality and morbidity rates are significantly higher following cesarean birth than after vaginal deliveries. Although there is no single reason for the difference in cesarean rates at the two hospitals, there are several possible explanations. Some involve factors that are institutionally determined, other explanations have to do with population variables independent of hospital control. All are speculative and until research demonstrates their relative worth, individuals will base their acceptance or rejection of each on personal values and beliefs.

One possibility is that because midwives do not perform cesareans, they have a vested interest in helping achieve vaginal birth. This attitude may lead to greater willingness to extend the time limits of what is medically considered normal in labor. At South Hospital, the residents need to learn to do cesareans. Although I have never seen a cesarean performed merely for a resident's education, there can be an unconscious desire for such experience that may subtly affect management. For example, the recommendation to perform a cesarean if the labor is longer than "normal," even if there are no other problems, often feeds this need. Furthermore, high risk procedures applied to low risk women have the potential to create risks. One example of this is the artificial rupture of membranes relatively early in labor to apply a monitor to the fetal scalp. Since such internal monitoring is the policy at South Hospital, membranes are generally ruptured by at least 4–5 centimeters or shortly after admission if a woman comes into the labor unit at a more advanced dilation. Such treatment forces women to stay in bed. This can slow labor and increase the likelihood that exogenous hormones will be needed to stimulate contractions. The result can be a labor so powerful that it leads to fetal distress. Another example is the more routine use of medication which may slow labor.

Looking at the situation from a different perspective, it can be claimed that South Hospital is located in a neighborhood whose population is less healthy than that of the community surrounding North Hospital and that this explains some of the disparity between cesarean rates in the two institutions. Another explanation is that a lack of prenatal care leads to increased risk, necessitating operative deliveries. According to figures compiled by the state department of health, the proportion of women receiving late or no prenatal care in the area served by South Hospital is higher than that in the area served by North Hospital. Interestingly, it is not known how much of this difference in prenatal care is due to population characteristics and how much is due to institutional factors, such as the amount of time spent in and the quality of interaction during prenatal visits.

The differential education of practitioners may also play a role in accounting for cesarean rates. Medical education, and hence practice, differs greatly from midwifery education. There is often a value placed on aggressive action in modern medicine. This is particularly evident in surgical specialties, of which obstetrics is one. I have heard physicians at continuing education conferences declare that there is absolutely no reason to avoid gathering as much information as possible about labor if the technology is available. This translates into the use of electronic fetal monitors throughout labor for everybody. Such an attitude ignores the possible dangers of continuous monitoring for women who have no medical indication for the procedure. Midwives, however, are taught to watch nature work, to use non-invasive measures to observe progress in labor. Many midwives refer to themselves as guardians of nature's processes.

DISCUSSION

Education, and its attendant socialization, can only be a partial explanation of the many institutional differences described here. After all, there are physicians at North Hospital. Indeed, without medical support, the midwifery service could never have been established. Ultimately, the doctors control obstetric policy. Furthermore, some of the physicians at South Hospital are willing to step back so that the midwives can care for patients with little interference. Various human factors also have an impact on differences in care. Personal characteristics obviously play a role. Flexibility, security, ego strength, and a willingness to relinquish power are rarely found in new medical-school graduates. Attitudes toward women are also significant. Surprisingly, perhaps, this is not necessarily determined by sex. Women in obstetrics are, as a group, more in philosophic agreement with their male medical colleagues than with female midwives. They are not even necessarily more polite to patients or more willing to accept the patient's having an active role in her own care. This may be due to a number of factors: the selection process of medical schools; the socialization process during medical education; psychological factors related to the choice of obstetrics as a specialization; the stress inherent in obstetric residency programs; and the fact that women in medicine comprise a small minority. Like other minorities, they may feel that in all aspects of achievement they have to outdo the dominant group—males—on male terms. It remains to be seen if obstetrics will change significantly if women become the majority of its practitioners.

The most compelling and pervasive explanation for the differences seems to be a structural one. The organization of South Hospital to achieve its secondary goal—physician training—is most responsible for the role delegated to its midwives. The organizational chart of that hospital's obstetric service presents a clear hierarchy. At the top are attending physicians—those who have already progressed through the various steps and are certified as obstetrical specialists. Beneath them are senior residents, those in their last year of post-medical-school training. Obstetrics is a four-year program so that the residents' hierarchy has four distinct categories. Each year is directly responsible to the ones above it, with the chief resident (chosen from among the seniors) directly responsible to the attending physicians on staff. Junior (first- and second-year) residents are subject to continual surveillance, though senior residents are not above supervision either. Yet, because this supervision is not always available on a one-to-one basis, even junior residents are often in a position to make important decisions. Such a system makes independence, flexibility, and creativity in management virtually impossible. Rules must be rigidly adhered to.

Theoretically, the midwives, who, unlike the residents, have completed their training, are not a part of this hierarchy; they are perceived as being on a level with the senior residents. And in theory, only the senior residents and attending physicians are consultants to the midwives. In fact, this does not always represent reality. The junior residents often regard the midwives as being on the bottom of the hierarchy and may take control of the supposed midwifery patients, especially if there is relatively little else for them to do at any particular time. Furthermore, the midwives must negotiate with the resident in charge for the right to take care of a given patient. In contrast, because the secondary function at North Hospital is to provide a model for midwife-based care, the personnel structure at that hospital is, in fact, quite different from that at South Hospital. In North Hospital the midwives assign patients to themselves or to co-management, if a problem arises or is anticipated. It is a rare doctor at North Hospital who does not accept the midwives' word "She's normal" and refrain from actively involving himself or herself in that patient's direct care.

There are similarities, of course, between North and South hospitals. Both are busy municipal hospitals and share many of the same problems: there is a lack of calm and peace; practitioners are often harried; tempers can be short; women are frequently left too long without professional attention; and laboratory reports are often missing. In addition, South Hospital has made some changes in the seven years since I first worked there as a midwifery student. Support persons are no longer required to take educational classes to be with a woman in labor. Some midwives do bed deliveries, and some protocols—such as a two-hour limit on the pushing (or second) stage of labor—have been relaxed. Perinatologists have joined the staff, and the quality of medical care, as reflected in better statistics in important obstetrical indicators such as perinatal mortality, have improved.

CONCLUSIONS

For women who can afford private care, the childbirth of their choice can sometimes be purchased. Midwives need not be a part of this package; an increasing number of physicians in private practice are attempting to meet consumer demand by changing the patterns of childbirth to provide what has become known as "family-centered care.[2] But the care seen at North Hospital is rare in municipal hospitals where most poorer women must go. The quality of that care is directly related to the fact that midwives are responsible for the day-to-day running of the service.

There is a contradiction inherent in this model, however. Nurse-midwifery as it exists today is dependent on medicine—its beneficence in "allowing" midwives to practice or its acquiescence to consumer demand by including midwives for birth care. Rothman (1982) calls midwifery "almost a profession," because it does not adhere to the sociological definition of a profession as "an occupation that has social power and thereby social control." The midwifery model as practiced at North Hospital will thus not be widely accepted as the standard for municipal hospital obstetric services as long as those who espouse the medical model remain in power.

REMAINING QUESTIONS

This chapter raises many issues that warrant further research. The impact of an alternative model for the delivery of maternity care in the public sector needs to be examined from the medical perspective in terms of maternal and newborn outcomes. But just as important, it must be examined from the perspective of social science. How, for example, do perceptions of the experience of childbirth differ between women delivering at a midwifery-model hospital and a medical-model hospital? How do these hypothetically different perceptions affect other attitudes? How do they influence a woman's sense of control over her own body, her sense of self-respect? Do differing family roles in childbirth affect family roles in childrearing? How does the experience of childbirth relate to future health-related behaviors and interactions with the health care delivery system for the indigent? These questions have significant policy implications.

On a macro level, there are economic and political questions to be explored. What is the economic impact of midwifery-run services? Are they cost effective? If so, at what other cost is this economic benefit maintained? Why, for example, is one of North Hospital's perpetual problems a high turnover rate among midwives? Do midwives work too hard for too little money? In this era which espouses equal pay for equal or equivalent work, how can midwives, who are predominantly women, continue to accept salaries far lower than those paid to physicians,who are predominantly men? Could midwifery survive if midwife salary scales become equivalent to those of physicians? Would that be equitable? What political strategies can women and midwives use to change the power relationships in the health services? How can those women who are without economic purchasing power effect change in the health care systems that serve them? Can midwifery ever become a true profession? What can be done to make that happen, and what would be its effect on the overall structure of health care delivery? These compelling questions, which have potentially far reaching implications, must be explored by future investigators.

NOTES

1. North Hospital and South Hospital are ficticious names that indicate only a geographic relationship between the two hospitals.

2. I would prefer woman-centered care with the family included to the extent that the woman chooses, but this is not what childbirth activists have been promoting.

9

TECHNOLOGY AND THE CONTEXT OF CHILDBIRTH: A COMPARISION OF TWO HOSPITAL SETTINGS

Karen L. Michaelson and Barbara Alvin

A mother-to-be selects the place she will give birth for a variety of reasons. Chief among these is her perception that the location will be safe and that it will be a place where she can have the birth experience she desires. For women who choose an in-hospital birth, the choice of hospital includes such factors as convenience, cost, whether her caregiver practices at that location, and the types of birth alternatives available.

In most parts of the United States, both large tertiary-care hospitals with their high-technology profiles and smaller community hospitals have begun to offer alternative birthstyles in response to increased competition in the "obstetric market place" (Dobbs and Shy 1981). These efforts to attract new patients are largely aimed at women who are at low risk of complications of labor and delivery. In areas where several hospitals offer obstetric services, options may range from labor in the labor room and delivery in the delivery room birth to home-like birthing rooms or single-unit delivery systems (where women remain in the same room from labor through their postpartum hospital stay). Some hospitals offer champagne dinners for the new parents or birth-day parties during which the whole family can get to know their new member.

Yet, a woman's choice of birth options and, indeed, her entire experience of her infant's birth is structured by the hospital she chooses. That choice, at times, may mean that she does not have the birth experience she expects. There is increasing evidence that despite the availability of family-centered birthing alternatives for low-risk mothers, in hospitals where the latest high technology obstetric procedures are available, they are used. "With increased specialization and the availability of obstetrical resources, there is a pattern of increased obstetrical intervention.... The availability of technology for high-risk patients may lead to its utilization on low risk patients" (Adams 1983:31). This is true even though there is no evidence of better neonatal outcomes for low-risk births with the application of more technology (Adams 1983). In fact, studies comparing births in alternative birthing units with traditional medical methods of delivery indicate that the alternative units have as good or better results for mother and baby (Goodlin 1980). Although the use of sophisticated technology may be appropriate for some high-risk births, few interventions have been proven effective in routine use (Brody and Thompson 1981). Moreover, the use of such sophisticated technology in cases where it may not be necessary is costly, not only in terms of sheer economics but in terms of the physiological and psychological effects on the parturient woman. For, though there appears to be no difference in neonatal outcome in such births, there is certainly an increase in maternal morbidity for women who have been subjected to anesthesia, cesarean section, or other aggressive obstetrical interventions.

The primary reason for this tendency to use the most advanced technology available in the management of birth is what has been called the "maximin strategy" in obstetrics (Brody and Thompson 1981). This approach to childbirth dictates that the physician expect and prepare for the worst possible outcome with every birth. The fear of a malpractice suit, pressure from other physicians, and, for some, the sincere belief that treating all pregnancies as high risk is good obstetric practice, supports this worst-case approach. Although alternative-birth options are intended to "increase the individual's participation in medical care and recognize the importance of social and psychological support in medical treatment" (DeVries 1983), the maximin strategy gives precedence to physiological over psychological variables in weighing risks and benefits. Thus, even when a woman has selected an alternative birth style, the physician's interpretation of the progress of labor and delivery determines whether or not she will have the birth experience she desires.

THE PRESENT STUDY

The research described here is part of a study that compared the birth experiences of rural and urban women in northeastern Washington. Twenty women from a rural county north of Spokane and twenty urban Spokane women were interviewed within the first six weeks postpartum. The urban women were selected by a random sample of births announced in local newspapers; the rural population was drawn from the total number of births to women in Stevens County during a six-week period in May-June 1983, and included both registered births and those not-yet-registered births that were identified by word of mouth.

The women were asked questions from an open-ended questionnaire which was designed to gather data on their overall experience of pregnancy, childbirth, and early postpartum adjustment. They were asked about their social world, about their health before, during, and after pregnancy, about their preparation for childbirth, their concerns during pregnancy, and the changes that took place in their lives once the baby was born. Each woman described her labor and delivery and discussed her feelings about the experience and her expectations. The data were coded for computer entry and analyzed using SPSS-X (a commonly used statistical package for social scientists), thus providing both a quantitative and a qualitative perspective on the birth experiences.

Characteristics of the Women

The women were all married, had from a high school to a postgraduate education, and were between twenty years old and their mid-thirties. Twenty-one of the women were giving birth to their first child; nineteen had prior children, ranging from one to seven previous live births. All but one of the women had taken a childbirth-education class for this or a prior birth; most took what they described as Lamaze classes, which consisted largely of descriptions of the physiological aspects of pregnancy and birth and breathing exercises based on the Lamaze method. Several women also took other classes, such as exercise classes. Almost all of the women read books on childbirth; those who expressed a desire to control their birth experience reported reading extensively about birth alternatives.

In each population, there were two home births and one birth in a free-standing birthing center located in Spokane. The remaining urban women and two of the rural women (totaling nineteen) gave birth in one of Spokane's two large tertiary-care hospitals. The remaining rural women (totaling fifteen) gave birth in a community hospital located in Colville, the largest town in the rural county. Of the two rural women who chose the Spokane hospitals, one was a repeat cesar-ean and both made disparaging comments about the quality of care at the com-munity hospital.

For purposes of this analysis, the women were divided into two groups, dependent upon whether they had given birth in the community hospital or either of the Spokane hospitals. The out-of-hospital births were excluded. Because the tertiary-care hospitals care for many birthing women whose infants may be at real risk of damage or death and thus may require aggressive intervention into the birth process, it was necessary to determine whether the two groups of women were, in fact, similar in terms of risk and thus might be expected to be similar in terms of expected interventions. Chi-square tests were used to test for association between type of hospital and the women's report of the presence of several common primary risk factors: problems with a previous delivery, diabetes, high blood pressure, spotting during pregnancy, toxemia during pregnancy, and premature delivery. There were no significant differences between the two groups, and they appeared to be in good health and relatively low risk. Chi-square tests were also performed to test for association between hospital type and a series of other factors that might possibly have an effect on obstetric risk. These included smoking during pregnancy, use of alcohol, whether or not a patient was overweight or underweight, presence of anemia during pregnancy, excessive weight gain in pregnancy, swelling of the upper or lower limbs in pregnancy, mother's age, and length of labor. There was only one factor for which there was a significant difference: the women at the larger hospitals appeared to be slightly younger then the community-hospital group. However, they fell within an age range (20–35) that is not usually considered a risk factor in obstetric management. Overall, the women appeared to be at low risk for complications of labor and delivery and had prepared for their births.

Characteristics of the Hospitals

The city of Spokane has a large medical complex which serves the needs of a huge, predominantly rural area covering several western states. There are approximately 6,000 births per year in Spokane county, most of which take place in one of the two large hospitals represented in this study. These two hospitals have taken part in nationwide efforts to regionalize and stratify obstetric care. They both provide extensive high-risk maternal and infant care, have neonatal intensive care units, and participate in a maternal and infant transport program (by helicopter, if necessary) for at-risk mothers and babies from an area that extends from the rural regions of eastern Washington east of the Cascade mountains, through eastern Oregon and northern Idaho, to remote areas of Montana and Wyoming. At present, twelve out of every 1,000 births in Spokane are classed as high risk, higher than the state average of 7.1 births per 1,000. This, no doubt, reflects the influx of high-risk women from outside the county who come to Spokane for specialized care.

Both of these hospitals are equipped with the latest in obstetric technology, from ultrasound imaging to sophisticated monitoring equipment. Both obstetricians and family practice physicians deliver infants at the hospitals. The majority of doctors are committed at a minimum to the routine use of a fetal heart monitor during labor and delivery (some do not even consider this to be an intervention), and many routinely perform other interventions, such as episiotomy. In order to attract urban low-risk patients as well as the high-risk patients who need specialized care, both hospitals have installed birthing rooms, which have a slightly more homey atmosphere, and both permit delivery in the labor room if the mother's condition permits. Both allow fathers to be present at normal labors and deliveries and, if requested, allow babies to room-in with their mothers.

The hospitals are also somewhat different from one another in their practices. One is somewhat more restrictive about allowing different birth options, and, in the public image, its nurses are deemed both friendlier and more prone to administer analgesia or request anesthesia for the laboring mother. The other hospital is thought to be more liberal in allowing alternative birthstyles, and discussions with a number of women of childbearing age and with area childbirth educators indicates that they believe that if the parents argue their case well at this hospital, they can get many options as long as their caregiver agrees to them.

The rural hospital in this study is similar to many that serve small, somewhat isolated regions. It has an obstetric unit, and cesarean sections can be performed in the surgical unit if necessary. The hospital has a birthing room. High-risk cases needing highly specialized care are referred to the Level III hospitals in Spokane. Births at the community hospital are usually attended by family practitioners. Women who choose to give birth in the hospital come from the surrounding rural area, which is sparsely populated, often isolated by geography and weather, and economically distressed. The hospital has the reputation of being a convenient place to go for care rather than going all the way to

Spokane (a one-to-two hour drive in good weather) to give birth, although there are some residents who put greater trust in the urban hospitals.

RESULTS

The initial conceptualization that informed the collection of data on birth interventions was that women giving birth in large urban hospitals would be offered more options in birthstyle, in keeping with the hospitals' desire to attract new patients, while women giving birth in smaller community hospitals would have few options, and the small hospitals would opt to use whatever technology they had on hand to counter the impression that they were not as up-to-date as Spokane hospitals. The results were diametrically opposed to this conceptualization. Chi-square tests were performed to test for differences in the frequency of various interventions in labor and delivery by hospital type. These included cesar-ean section, the use of forceps, electronic monitoring (internal and external), the use of anesthesia, induction of labor, and episiotomy. There was a significantly higher level of use of anesthesia (p<.01) at the Level III hospitals than at the community hospital. All but one woman giving birth at the urban hospitals had some form of anesthesia; only six out of fifteen women (including three cesarean sections) giving birth at the community hospital used anesthesia. Most women reported the use of epidural anesthesia, though paracervical blocks and local anesthesia (for episiotomy) were also mentioned by a few. In addition, while only six out of fifteen women at the community hospital used an electronic monitor during labor and delivery, sixteen out of nineteen at the Spokane hospitals did (p<.05). There was, however, only a slightly higher percentage of cesarean births at the Spokane hospitals (31.6 percent) than at the community hospitals (20 percent), a nonsignificant difference. The length of hospital stay was also longer at the Spokane hospitals.

It is also interesting to examine the place of birth within each type of hospital, as both the larger hospitals and the community hospital have alternative birthing rooms designed to provide low-risk women with a more personalized family-centered birth. Of the nineteen women who gave birth at the Level III hospitals, six delivered in what they referred to as the "C-section room," thirteen delivered in the regular delivery room, and one delivered in the labor room. *Not one* delivered in the birthing room, though most would have been eligible to do so, and some had expressed a desire or planned to deliver there. Of the fifteen women giving birth at the community hospital, eight delivered in the birthing room. Four delivered in the regular delivery room including two grand multiparas (having their fifth and eighth child respectively), who wanted to use the delivery room because it was familiar, and two women who were transferred out of the birthing room because of complications. The three cesearean sections (including two repeat cesareans) delivered in the hospital's surgical unit.

DISCUSSION: THE EXPLANATION OF DIFFERENCE

Explanations can be given at a number of levels for the difference in rate of intervention and use of alternative birthing facilities at the two types of hospital.

Caregiver Factors

Women in this study giving birth at the Level III hospitals were cared for by private physicians who worked in groups and/or had other physicians covering for them when they were not on call. Many women reported that the doctor who delivered their baby was not the same one they saw throughout their pregnancy, because their own doctor was not available at the time they went into labor. Some of the women had met the covering physician prior to the birth, but many had not. Thus, desires for an alternative birthstyle worked out with their own physician may not have been honored as often by the new physician. Moreover, a physician covering for another, not knowing all of the details of the mother's physiological and psychological experience of pregnancy and birth, might choose to intervene more quickly in the birth process, to err, as it were, on the side of caution when dealing with an unfamiliar patient. The presence of an unfamiliar doctor may also have made the parturient women somewhat more tense, possibly slowing their labor. Certainly, even for those whose own physicians attended their births, entering the hospital meant having no caregiver at their side throughout the labor and delivery who had been familiar with them during pregnancy, for doctors primarily attend the laboring woman only for an occasional progress check and the delivery itself.

At the community hospital, however, a different pattern of physician care existed. All of the physicians who delivered babies at that hospital had joined in a single cooperative practice. During pregnancy, a woman was followed by a single physician but usually had occasion to meet the other doctor partners. More importantly, most of these women reported seeing the same nurse practitioner for the majority of the prenatal visits. When a woman came to the hospital in labor, the nurse practitioner, a person familiar with the woman's physiological and psychological needs, came to the hospital and stayed with the laboring woman throughout labor, providing guidance and comfort. The doctor came to attend the delivery or, in the case of complicated labors, might come earlier to manage the labor and delivery to a successful outcome. Because the presence of a supportive person at birth often contributes to a more positive experience, this pattern of care may have contributed to the women's sense of well-being during their labor and delivery, and thus encouraged low-intervention births. In fact, many of the women in this study mentioned the presence of the nurse practitioner, the supportiveness of the medical staff, and the continuity of care as important factors in their satisfaction with their birth experience.

Cultural Factors

It is useful also to consider cultural differences between the two areas, for health care is an arena that is mediated by the individual's network of family and friends. "Women do not make birth decisions based upon medical risk and benefit perceptions alone; rather the decisions are made in concert with other considerations, including perceptions of social risks and benefits connected with place of birth" (McClain 1981a:1034). Choices in health care are structured by the opinions of family and friends, community values, and prior experience as well as the actual facilities and options available.

Spokane is a fairly stable urban community. While it is growing slowly, most of the Spokane women in this study were long-time city residents whose families lived in the area. A few had spouses from outside of the area, but many had their in-laws nearby. Social interaction in Spokane takes place very much along family lines. Casual observation as well as the reports of the women surveyed indicates that interaction with family is frequent. Respondents reported visiting with their families several times a week or even daily. They shared meals, television watching, and card playing, and, in summer, they often retreated in larger family groups to one of the many lake resorts or cabins in the area. Often, families lived in the same neighborhood, and in at least one case they lived just across the street. Thus, family opinion and tradition had a great deal to do with the choice of birthplace and birthstyle. One woman reported that both she and her husband had been born at one of the Level III hospitals, and they had no doubt that it was the place they wanted to deliver their child. Another had been delivered by the same doctor that she chose to deliver her baby. For most, any birth but an in-hospital birth was almost unthinkable. Women reported that their families supported their choice of a hospital birth and that they would have faced opposition if they had tried any other alternatives. In fact, one woman, who began her labor at a free-standing birthing center but had to be transferred to a Level III hospital because of complications, said that she met with great opposition and lack of understanding for her original choice and heard many "I told you so's" over her unexpected hospital delivery.

The opinion of family and friends is also important in selecting in-hospital alternative birth procedures. Several women reported family opposition to natural childbirth; one woman said her mother-in-law thought Lamaze classes were "nonsense." Others said their friends told them to be "knocked out" for the birth. These opinions have an effect on the woman's expectations of her birth experience. Despite the fact that all of the women took Lamaze or "natural" childbirth classes, they expected to have conservatively managed births, expected to have some anesthesia, and were by and large not disappointed when it was given. At least one woman wanted a cesarean birth because she felt she could not bear the pain of labor. This attitude toward childbirth reinforced the tendency of many physicians to admit technological interventions into the birth process. In addition, the high rate of intervention, particularly electronic fetal monitoring and anesthesia, reinforced most women's view that this was the "right way to have a baby."

Even those women who stated that they expected to have some control over birth and selected the birthing room and other birth-style alternatives (often over family opposition) felt the pressure of community standards on obstetric care. Many women said that childbirth classes did not prepare them adequately for interventions or give them the knowledge they needed to make choices about which interventions were appropriate when complications arose. One said that she was not prepared enough "for when things went wrong." Thus, they were not prepared to defend their choices of childbirth options when faced with hospital staff who implied that a given intervention was best for the baby. They found, as well, little support for their opinions within the broader set of community values that informed the management of birth at the Level III hospitals.

The rural county in this study also has a large, stable population of long-time residents with nearby kin. But there was also a substantial influx of outsiders to the area in the late 1960s and early 1970s when the panhandle of Idaho and the remote and rugged countryside of northeastern Washington became a haven for those seeking alternative life-styles. Young people came to the region from various parts of the United States seeking cheap land and the isolation that would permit them to live their lives in the way they saw fit. Even some of the offspring of the region's existing population joined the movement toward alternative life-styles. The life-style that the newcomers desired emphasized self-sufficiency and living off the land. Things natural were to be valued, things technological to be eschewed. The values of naturalness and simplicity espoused by these new residents were not, in reality, far from the values held by long-time residents, who took pride in their rural life-style and independence. Over time, as the newcomers became more integrated into the region's social and economic life, many of these values were shared.

As the newcomers began to have families of their own, they chose a natural course, and a tradition of lay midwifery arose in the area. But for those who wanted a physician-attended birth, many of the same desires for a natural birth were part of their decision making. Most of the rural women in this study reported that they expected to have a natural birth with little or no intervention. There was a premium put on a drug-free birth which was expressed as "a natural drug-free birth produced a bright, alert, happy baby," or "if a mother takes care of herself and eats the right foods, she shouldn't need anything at birth." These expectations for childbirth were supported by family and friends. Indeed, one woman said she was criticized by her friends for not trying home birth, as it was "even more natural." These community values have also influenced the pattern of care provided by medical personnel, who themselves emphasize a relatively intervention-free birth and provide childbirth education and a birth-support system that encourages natural birth. Indeed, the physicians have, since the time of this study, added a certified nurse midwife to their practice to meet community desires and needs.

Hospital Factors

Patterns of physician care and cultural values provide a reasonably satisfactory explanation of why there was less use of anesthesia and fetal monitoring and more use of the birthing room at the community hospital. But they do not adequately account for the higher rate of intervention at the Level III hospitals or the lack of use of the birthing room by these seemingly low-risk women. After all, there are at least some women in Spokane who espouse a natural life-style and advocate an intervention-free birth. And, there are some physicians who are liberal in their practice and claim to use few interventions in low-risk births. In addition, the hospitals themselves have set up birthing rooms to attract just such women.

Because Level III hospitals are set up to assist in high-risk births, they are equipped with sophisticated technology. Such technological innovations as electronic fetal monitoring are valuable in high-risk births, where the infants well-being may be compromised in labor and delivery. They are of far less value in low- or moderate-risk births. "Fetal monitoring has met with an acceptance out of proportion to its documented or expected benefits" (Brody and Thmpson 1981:982). But hospital staff, trained to use fetal monitors in high-risk births and enculturated to a birth-management strategy that treats every case as if the worst possible outcome might happen, tend to use them for all births "just in case." The problem is that obstetrical interventions form an interconnected system, so that a particular intervention brings in new risk factors which in turn require new interventions (Brody and Thompson 1981). For example, monitoring, which requires the mother to remain relatively still in bed, may slow her contractions. This, in turn, may encourage the use of pitocin to speed the contractions and then anesthesia to reduce the pain brought on by the induced, rapid contractions. Sometimes, this may lead to a reading of apparent fetal distress and finally to a cesarean section, thus fitting the hospital model that the worst can indeed happen.

In Level III hospitals with their commitment to high-risk care, it is difficult for physicians and staff to make a commitment to alternative birth styles. There is an ambivalence to patients controlling their own normal labor and deliveries. Patients are rarely presented with treatment choices as their labor progresses but are given generalized reassurances that their labor is going as it should (Danziger 1979). Requests for alternative birth styles are often disregarded because they may interfere with established hospital routines or because it is assumed that parents do not know what is best for themselves and their infant. If a parent is assertive and questions an intervention, physicians refer to their years of experience in managing births (Danziger 1979) and question the parent's responsibility toward his or her infant. Thus, even well-informed women who have made a choice as to the type of birth experience they want, may yield to hospital staff because they are anxious about their infant's well-being.

The pattern of low usage of alternative birthing rooms and high transfer rates out of those facilities is common (DeVries 1983), especially in Level III hospitals. Despite their provision of such family-centered facilities for low-risk mothers, they remain committed to a physician-managed birth policy which derives from their acute-care orientation.

IMPLICATIONS

One characteristic of this acute care, or maximin, orientation to the management of childbirth is that it focuses primarily on perceived physiological needs and not on the social or psychological needs of mothers. Attending physicians and hospital staff are fearful of sacrificing safety for "mere emotional satisfaction" (Brody and Thompson 1981:985). Yet, emotional satisfaction with childbirth can have important consequences for the mother's own feelings of self-worth, and the record of most alternative birth options indicates that they do not compromise safety. There are a number of important emotional components in childbirth, including the woman's feeling of joy in her accomplishment of mastering pain and fear ("getting through it"), and her joy after the birth in her relationship with her newborn baby (Cox and Smith 1982). "If a woman feels she does not perform well at birth, [her] perceptions of her capabilities in other mothering behaviors may be doubtful" (Mercer, Hackley, and Bostrom 1983:207). Women who have had an unexpected cesarean section, for example, experience a loss of control over their birth situation. Some feel guilty because they are dissatisfied with their birth experience even though they have a healthy baby, or they may feel frustrated because they are unable to mother their infants as they would like to do because of the need for healing (Erb, Hill, and Houston 1983). Similar feelings were expressed by women in this study who had unexpected cesareans and even by those whose births had more interventions of other kinds than they expected. Several women were angry with themselves because they had failed at "natural birth," and even those who expected some intervention were at times disappointed at the high level of intervention that took place.

One must take care to not overdraw the relationship between medical intervention in the birth process and the subsequent maternal/infant relationship. Reports of increased child abuse of infants born of a cesarean section may not be measuring the impact of that intervention but rather the factors that may have led to the cesarean section, such as poverty and subsequent premature birth, substance abuse, or other factors in the parents' lives. Moreover, studies have indicated that the mother's negative feelings about her birth experience are not often reflected in her feelings toward the child (Bradley 1983) unless other factors intervene. Still, medical intervention into the birth process can have an impact on a woman's sense of self-worth. It is difficult for a woman to maintain a sense of mastery over the birth experience when she is treated as if she were not competent to decide what that experience should be.

In addition to the emotional implications of intervening in low-risk women's birth processes, there is also the issue of the possibility of iatrogenic effects to mother and infant. Infection from incision, the depression of infant functioning as a result of anesthesia, and other negative effects can result from routine use of technology. Indeed, the use of technology in routine obstetric cases may not necessarily be quality care but poor clinical judgment (Brody and Thompson 1981). Added to these effects are the increased costs such interventions incur. High-technology births are expensive and often require longer hospitalization for the mother and/or infant.

It is, in fact, possible to identify low-risk pregnant women and provide them with a birth experience that is safe, reduces apprehension, and provides a positive beginning for both mother and baby. The presence of sophisticated technology need not dictate its routine use. The community hospital in this study, after all, was able to use anesthesia and electronic fetal monitoring in some cases without their routine use for all low-risk patients.

A POSTSCRIPT

Hospitals change in the light of consumer demand and the need to compete for patients in the obstetric marketplace. Dobbs and Shy (1981) note that with increased competition from alternative birth settings, such as the home, hospitals increase their availability of options such as birthing rooms. This is especially true of large urban hospitals that may have to compete with a number of other institutions that care for pregnant women. Since this study, the obstetric marketplace in Spokane has witnessed increased competition, particularly for low-risk women. The free-standing birthing center has closed in the face of increased insurance costs, but some smaller hospitals in Spokane have opened the doors to family-centered in-hospital birthing units which feature homelike rooms where the mother can stay all through labor, delivery, and recovery, have implemented liberal policies as to who can be at the birth, and have added other amenities such as champagne dinners for the new parents. One of these small hospitals has an aggressive advertising campaign which encourages pregnant women to join their mother-to-be club and receive newsletters, merchant discounts, and the like.

In response to this competition, at least one of the Level III hospitals has with great fanfare converted the majority of its labor rooms into an in-hospital birthing center and modified its obstetric policies to allow more flexibility in who may stay with the woman in labor and delivery. The hospital has altered its nurse staffing so that a single nurse stays with a laboring woman through labor, delivery, and recovery, and has added other niceties, accompanied by an extensive advertising campaign, to enhance the image of its obstetric service. It would be interesting to see if along with stated changes in policy, the reality of a lower level of intervention for low-risk women has also occurred in the face of competition, or if the combination of physician preference, cultural factors, and the hospital's acute-care philosophy still dictates a high level of intervention at birth.

NOTE

This research was supported by a grant from the Northwest Institute for Advanced Study.

10

BIRTH AS AN AMERICAN RITE OF PASSAGE

Robbie E. Davis-Floyd

In any society, "the way a woman gives birth and the kind of care given to her point as sharply as an arrowhead to the key values in the culture" (Kitzinger 1980:115). By making the naturally transformative process of birth into a cultural rite of passage, a society can ensure that its basic values will be transmitted to the three new members born out of the birth process: the new baby, the woman reborn into the new social role of mother, and the man reborn as father. Most especially, society must make sure that the new mother is very clear about these values and the belief system that underlies them, as she is generally the one most responsible for instilling this belief system in the minds of her children—society's new members and the guarantors of its future. This goal is accomplished through the ritualizing of the birth process.

It is commonly held that the transfer of the birthplace from home to hospital which has taken place in American society has resulted in the de-ritualization of what in other, more "primitive" societies has traditionally been a process laden with superstition and taboo. On the contrary, the placement of birth in the hospital has resulted in a proliferation of rituals surrounding this natural physiological event more elaborate than any heretofore known in the "primitive" world. In the United States, childbirth has been transformed into a rite of passage designed to initiate the birthing woman into the dominant core value and belief system of American society.

BIRTH AS A RITE OF PASSAGE

I didn't know I was an adult until I had a child. (Linda)

Some of the pride I had was having felt that I'd crossed a barrier, that I had joined the rest of the mothers in the world, and that I had joined my mother, in a sense. And that was an

153

experience that nobody could ever take away from me. (Constance)

A rite of passage is a series of rituals designed to conduct an individual (or group) from one social state or status to another, thereby transforming both society's perception of the individual and the individual's own perception of her- or himself. Rites of passage generally consist of three stages, as outlined by van Gennep (1966): (1) separation of the individuals from their preceding social state or status; (2) a period of transition in which they are neither one thing nor the other; and (3) an integration phase, in which through various rites of incorporation they are absorbed into their new social state. In the year-long pregnancy/childbirth rite of passage in American society, the separation phase begins with the woman's first awareness of pregnancy; the transitional phase lasts until several days after the birth; and the integration phase ends gradually during the newborn's first few months of life, when the new mother begins to feel that she is "mainstreaming it again" (Davis-Floyd 1986b).

The most salient feature of all rites of passage is their transitional nature, the fact that they always involve *liminality* (from the Latin *limens*, or threshold), the stage of being betwixt and between, neither here nor there (Turner 1979). In the liminal phase of initiatory rites of passage, "the ritual subject passes through a realm that has few or none of the attributes of the past or coming state" (Turner 1979:237). One of the primary characteristics of this liminal period is the gradual psychological opening of the initiates to profound interior change. In many initiation rites involving major transitions into new social roles (such as Marine basic training), this openness is achieved through a ritualized combination of physical and mental hardships that serve to break down the initiate's belief system—the internal mental structure of concepts and categories though which she/he perceives and interprets the world and his/her relationship to it. The breakdown of her belief system leaves the initiate profoundly open to new learning and to the construction of new categories.

Ritual serves a number of purposes in effecting the transition intended by rites of passage:

> (1) It provides its participants with a sense of control over natural processes that may be beyond their control, by making it appear that these natural transformations (e.g., birth, puberty, death) are actually effected by society and serve society's ends (Malinowski 1954).
> (2) It conveys, through the emotions and the body, a series of repeti-tious and unforgettable messages to the initiate concerning the core values of the society into which she/he is being initiated, through the carefully structured manipulation of symbols (Turner 1979).
> (3) It promotes ideal conditions in its participants for the full reception and incorporation of these messages by (a) breaking down the category systems of the initiates through "hazing" and "strange-making" (Abrahams 1973); and (b) "tuning" in

the initiates to the new messages through the use of specific techniques such as rhythmic repetition and intensification.

(4) It protects the group's belief system by fencing in or out the dangers perceived to be present in transitional periods (when individuals are in-between social categories and thus call the reality of those categories into question), while at the same time allowing those conducting the ritual to gain access to the revitalizing power of these transformative events (Douglas

(5) It renews and revitalizes these values for those conducting as well as those participating in or observing the rituals, so that both the perpet-uation and the vitality of the belief and value system of the society in question can be assured (Turner

THE CHARACTERISTICS OF RITUAL

A ritual may be defined as a patterned, repetitive, symbolic enactment of a cultural belief or value; its purpose is to effect some type of transformation. Such enactments may be both ritual and instrumental or rational-technical (Leach 1979 [1966]); Moore and Meyerhoff 1977:15). In my analysis of hospital birth as a rite of passage, I shall show that the obstetrical routines applied to the management of normal birth are also transformative rituals that carry and communicate meaning above and beyond their ostensibly purely instrumental ends. Certain of ritual's primary characteristics play critical roles in this transformational process. These include redundancy and intensification, symbolism, order and formality, a cognitive matrix, the production of an affective state, transformation, and preservation of the status quo.[1]

Redundancy and Intensification. For maximum effectiveness, a ritual concentrates on sending one basic set of messages which it will repeat over and over again in different forms and in a gradually building crescendo.

Symbolism. Ritual works by sending messages, in the form of symbols, to those who perform and to those who receive or observe it. A symbol, most simply, is an object, idea, or action that communicates multiple cultural meanings (Turner 1967). Symbols are effective vehicles for ritual's messages because they are received by the right hemisphere of the brain, where they are interpreted as a *gestalt* (Luria 1966:90; Ornstein 1972; Lex 1979: 124–30; d'Aquili and Laughlin 1979:173–77). In other words, instead of being intellectually analyzed, a symbol's message will be *felt* in its totality through the body and the emotions. Although the individual may be only dimly aware of his/her incorporation of the symbol's message, its ultimate effect on the recipient may be extremely powerful, acting to "map changed or adjusted perceptions of the possibilities inherent in a situation onto the actor's orientation to it" (Munn 1973:593), thereby gradually drawing individual belief and value systems into alignment with that of the larger society.

Order and Formality. Its exaggeratedly precise order and formality set ritual apart from other modes of social interaction, enabling ritual to establish an atmosphere that feels both inevitable and inviolate. According to Moore and Meyerhoff, "in its repetition and order, ritual imitates the rhythmic imperatives of the biological and physical universe, thus suggesting a link with the perpetual processes of the cosmos. It thereby implies the permanence and legitimacy of what are actually evanescent cultural constructs" (1977:8).

A Cognitive Matrix. Through ritual, the belief system of a culture is enacted (Wallace 1966; McManus 1979b); thus, an analysis of ritual can lead directly to a profound understanding of that belief system. For example, analysis of the rituals of hospital birth reveals their cognitive matrix to be the technological model of reality which forms the philosophical basis of both Western biomedicine and American society.

Production of an Affective State. Behavioral psychologists have long understood that learning is far more likely to be imprinted on the human mind if it is accomplished in an emotional context. Recent research in the health sciences has succeeded in defining the physiological chain of events through which emotional learning takes place:

> Highly charged emotional experiences...are transferred electro-chemically (acetycholine is the neuro-transmitter) through the hippocampus which acts as a bridge between the limbic system and long-term memory storage. If events are not perceived as carrying value or significance to the individual the data are kept approximately seven hours, never to be encoded in long-term memory storage (Peterson and Mehl 1984:194).

Collective rituals, including those of hospital birth, create the kind of "highly charged emotional experience" which can lead to long-term memory storage through careful staging, "evocative presentational style," and "careful and precise manipulation of symbols and sensory stimuli" (Moore and Meyerhoff 1977:7).

Transformation. According to Moore and Meyerhoff, "a transformation occurs when symbol and object seem to fuse and are experienced as a perfectly undifferentiated whole...and insight, belief and emotion are called into play, altering our conceptions at a stroke" (1977:11). In hospital birth, this fusion occurs when reality as presented by obstetrical procedures and reality as perceived by the birthing woman become one and the same, thereby making her birthing process one of cognitive, as well as physiological, transformation.

Preservation of the Status Quo. Through explicit enactment of a culture's belief system, ritual works both to preserve and to transmit that belief system and so becomes an important force in the preservation of the status quo in any society. However, ritual must also continually work to renew and revitalize the belief system that underlies it.

One technique available for such revitalization is *symbolic inversion* (Babcock 1978). The natural process of birth stands our everyday category system on its head: one becomes two, females produce males, cultural beings emerge from the natural realm. When everyday norms are turned upside down through such symbolic inversion, the energies released through the "power attendant upon confusion" (Abrahams 1973) become available to help cultures combat the constant erosion of entropy. Hospital birth rituals work to channel this energy to the hospital personnel who "deliver" the baby, so that birth's transformative power serves as a constant source of revitalization to the medical subculture surrounding birth.

THE TECHNOLOGICAL MODEL AND THE RITUAL ENCAPSULATION OF BIRTH

The effectiveness of ritual as a didactic tool is extremely important to its cultural use in birth, for the technologically based belief and value system which birth rituals are designed to transmit runs contrary to the conscious set of beliefs in individualism, democracy, and the right to self-responsibility which many U.S. citizens hold. In the United States today, our core values constitute an oppositional paradigm—a model of reality based on an inherent tension between two sets of categories. In this paradigm, the interests of science, technology, patriarchy, and institutions are held above, and are often imposed on, those of nature, individuals, families, and women. The belief system underlying this set of oppositions is based on what Carolyn Merchant (1983) terms the "mechanical model" of reality inherited from the Scientific Revolution in Europe. This model assumes that the universe is mechanistic, following predictable laws that can be discovered through science and manipulated through technology in order to decrease human dependence on nature. In the twentieth century, this model has been transformed into what I label the "technological model of reality" (Davis-Floyd 1986b), a paradigm that surpasses the promised increased independence from nature with the promise of ultimate transcendence over nature.

Yet childbirth constitutes a visible and constant reminder that our survival as a species still depends on the natural world. As such, birth presents an especially serious conceptual challenge to our culture, for it threatens to undermine this technological model. A common cultural response to this type of conceptual challenge is to wall it off from the mainstream of social life by creating special categories of "taboo" that are often reflected in actual social spaces designed to contain the conceptual danger (Douglas 1966). The conceptual bomb can then be defused through the careful and consistent performance of rituals designed to mold the inconsistent phenomenon into apparent compliance with society's official belief system, a technique that Evon Vogt (1976) labels "encapsulation."

American culture uses ritual encapsulation to cope with the conceptual threat presented by natural birth. We have surrounded the birth process with "taboo" and have removed it from the mainstream of social life by walling it off in hospitals. The first step in this process of the ritual encapsulation of birth under the technological model was the metaphorization of the human body as a machine.

THE TECHNOLOGICAL MODEL OF BIRTH

The interpretation of society and the universe as purely mechanistic necessitates the perception that the human bodies which comprise society are also mechanistic—a problematic conceptual task, since in reality bodies are not machines. It is up to Western medicine, as the branch of society officially in charge of the body, to accomplish this by treating the body as if it *were* a machine. Because the technological model had its beginnings at a time in history when the prevailing world view held that women were inferior to men, closer to nature, with less developed minds, and with little or no spirituality (Merchant 1983; Ehrenreich and English 1973), it was the *male* body which set the standard for the proper form and functioning of this body-machine (Rothman 1982:37). The female body, insofar as it deviated from this standard, was considered an inherent-ly defective machine, a concept which formed the philosophical foundation of modern obstetrics (Rothman 1982:39). The rising science of obstetrics was thus enjoined from its beginnings to develop tools and technologies for the manipulation and improvement of the inherently defective and therefore dangerous process of birth. To obstetrics, society also assigned the formidable task of making childbirth—heretofore the primary symbol of culture's dependence on nature for its perpetuation—support rather than threaten the emerging promise of the technological model to master the forces of nature. Obstetrics ultimately accomplished this goal by adopting the model of the assembly-line production of goods as its base metaphor for hospital birth.[2]

In accordance with this metaphor, in the hospital a woman's lower half is treated like a birthing machine by skilled technicians working under semiflexible timetables to meet production and quality-control demands. The most desirable product is the new social member: the baby; the new mother is a secondary by-product of this process. Birth is a technological service that obstetrics supplies to society—the doctor delivers the baby to society. (Traditionally he hands the baby to the nurse, not the mother.) If the product is perfect, the responsibility and the credit are his; if flawed, the responsibility will transfer to another technical specialist up or down the line. Any blame will be categorically assigned to the inherent defectiveness of the mother's birthing machine. With this metaphor as their conceptual guideline, obstetricians were able to develop ritual procedures to transform the natural process of birth into proof of the accuracy and superiority of the technological model and of the values and behaviors it justifies.

STANDARD PROCEDURES FOR NORMAL BIRTH: A SYMBOLIC ANALYSIS

In most hospitals in the United States, "standard procedures for normal birth" include placing the laboring woman in a wheelchair and transporting her to labor and delivery where she is "prepped"—a multi-step procedure in which she is separated from her husband; her clothes are replaced by a hospital gown; her pubic hair is shaved (or clipped); and she is given an enema. She is then reunited with her husband, if he chooses to be present, and put to bed. Her access to food is limited or prohibited, and an intravenous needle is inserted in her hand or arm. She is administered some type of analgesia, and often pitocin, a synthetic hormone used to speed labor, as well. An external fetal monitor, which records the strength of her contractions and the baby's heartbeat, is attached to the woman by means of a large belt strapped around her waist. If there is a reason to suspect fetal distress, the amniotic sac is ruptured and an internal monitor is attached through electrodes inserted into the baby's scalp. And usually at least once every two hours the laboring woman's cervix is checked for degree of dilation. These procedures may be performed at varying intervals over a variable time period, depending on the length of the woman's labor and the degree to which it conforms to hospital standards. The less conformity the labor exhibits, the greater the number of procedures that will be applied to bring it into conformity.

As the moment of birth approaches, there is an intensification of actions performed on the woman. She is transferred to a delivery room, sometimes given some type of anesthesia, often an epidural or spinal block, placed in the lithotomy position, covered with sterile sheets, doused with antiseptic, and given an episiotomy. After the birth, she will be handed the baby for a specified amount of time, her placenta will be extracted if it does not come out quickly on its own, her episiotomy will be sewn up, her uterus will be palpated, more pitocin will be administered to assist her uterus in contracting, and finally she will be cleaned up and transferred to a hospital bed.

The baby, too, receives a good deal of procedural attention during a hospital birth. While still in the womb, she may be viewed with ultrasound; her heart tones will be monitored; sometimes an electrode will be stuck on or into her head. As the baby emerges from the birth canal, her head will be supported and turned, her shoulders may be twisted slightly, and the mucus will be suctioned from her mouth and nostrils. Immediately after her birth, the newborn's umbilical cord will be cut. She will be rated with an Apgar chart at two different times, washed, weighed, diapered, and wrapped; silver nitrate or an antibiotic substitute will be put into her eyes, and she will be given a Vitamin K injection. She may then be handed to her mother for a brief period of time, after which she will be transferred to the nursery and placed in a plastic bassinet for about four hours. When it is "time" to go home, a wheelchair will carry the newborn and her mother to the hospital door.

These interventions are not only instrumental acts but also serve ritual purposes: to mold the natural processes of birth into conceptual compliance with the technological model and to inculcate birthing women (and their attendants) with the core values of American society as encoded in this model. In doing so, these rituals fulfill the ever-present need of the wider culture to ensure the effective socialization of its citizens and thus its own perpetuation. Individual analysis of these birth rituals will demonstrate precisely how this socialization is accomplished.[3]

Wheelchair. Under the technological model, labor is viewed as a mechanical process that takes place inside a machine inherently predisposed to malfunction. It is thus incumbent upon the hospital to assume that malfunction may occur at any time and to be constantly prepared for its occurrence—an assumption which has led to what Suzanne Arms has called "just-in-case obstetrics" (Ettner 1976: 38). It is also incumbent upon the hospital, as we have seen, to make the premises of the technological model appear to be true and to map the reality contained within this model onto the birthing woman's perceptions of her situation so skillfully that she will be able to perceive her experience in these terms *only*.

The wheelchair is an effective first step in this process. To place a healthy woman in a wheelchair, rather than allowing her to walk on her own, is to tell her that at the very least the hospital thinks of her as disabled and weak. Although she may reject this message on a conscious intellectual level, its passage through her body and into the right hemisphere of her brain will guarantee that, on an unconscious level, she will receive the message, "you are disabled"; in other words, she will receive what one psychologist has called a "felt sense" (Gendlin 1980) of her body as suddenly weak and unable to walk. Thus, from the moment of her entry into the labor and delivery unit, the laboring woman is marked as someone who cannot or should not walk. As in any initiatory rite of passage, this estranging, or "strange-making" device is employed at the very beginning to start the breakdown of the initiate's category system which is necessary to ensure her openness to new learning:

> I can remember just almost being in tears by the way they would wheel you in. I would come to the delivery or into the hospital on top of this, breathing, you know, all in control. And they slap you in this wheelchair! It made me suddenly feel like maybe I wasn't in control any more. (Suzanne)

Some women accept the message sent to them by the wheelchair, as did Suzanne, while others invert its symbolism and so avoid internalizing its message:

> The maternity room sent somebody down with a wheelchair. I didn't have any need for a wheelchair so we piled all of the luggage up in it and wheeled it up to the floor. (Pat)

The "Prep." In the separation of husband and wife during the multi-step procedure called the "prep," we see the continuance of the conceptual demarcation of boundaries begun with the wheelchair, as the woman's body is claimed for the institution by its representative, the nurse. This "standard hospital policy" sends two powerful messages: (1) the hospital has the right to separate husband and wife and thus holds an authority higher and greater than the family; and (2) the laboring woman now conceptually belongs to the institution and must be marked as such.

This marking is accomplished by the prep itself. A woman's clothes are her markers of individual identity; removing them is an effective way of communicating the message that she is no longer autonomous, but dependent on the institution. Like the identical uniforms of Marine basic trainees, the hospital gown indicates the woman's liminal status:

> Liminal entities, such as neophytes in initiation or puberty
> rites, may be represented as possessing nothing. They
> may...wear only a strip of clothing, or even go naked, to
> demonstrate that as liminal beings they have no status,
> property, insignia, secular clothing indicating rank or role....
> Their behavior is normally passive or humble; they must obey
> their instructors implicitly, and accept arbitrary punishment
> without complaint. It is as though they are being reduced or
> ground down to a uniform condition to be fashioned anew
> (Turner 1969:95)....

The gown's openness intensifies the message of the woman's loss of autonomy:
not only does it expose her most private parts to institutional handling and
control, it also prevents her from simply walking out the door anytime she
chooses. Like a prison inmate, she is now marked in society's eyes as belonging
to a total institution—the hospital.

Further intensification of this ritual marking of the woman as hospital
property is accomplished by the shaving of the pubic hair and the administration
of an enema. The shaving of a laboring woman's pubic hair separates her from
her former conceptions of her body and, like the gown, further marks her as
being in a liminal state. But the hospital gown, the shave, and the enema do
more than that. They also (1) ritually establish a boundary separation between
the upper and lower portions of a woman's body; (2) strip the lower portion of
her body of its sexuality, thus returning the woman to a conceptual state of
childishness with its accompanying characteristics of dependency and lack of
personal responsibility; and (3) begin a powerful process of the symbolic inversion of the most private region of the woman's body to the most public.
Moreover, the enema, readily recognizable as the obligatory ritual cleansing of
the initiate traditional in many rites of passage, sends the clear message that the
woman's most private parts were internally dirty while they were private and that
it is the institution which made them clean. Underlying this message is the
deeper message that individuals are impure, while society is pure.

Confinement to Bed. Many a laboring woman wearing a hospital gown at
this moment would perhaps tell us that she believes herself to be healthy and
strong. But this conviction, which the hospital staff may verbally reinforce, is
steadily undermined by the messages with which the woman's environment
bombards her. Being put to bed intensifies messages already communicated by
the wheelchair and the gown: that she is a patient, that she is sick. Or more
precisely, it tells her that the hospital conceptualizes her as sick—a message
which, as time passes and labor becomes more intense, becomes more and more
likely to be internalized as "I am sick." As Elizabeth perceived it:

> It's funny—it seems so normal to lie down in labor—just to
> be in the hospital seems to mean "to lie down." But as soon as
> I did, I felt that I had lost something. I felt defeated. And it
> seems to me now that my lying down tacitly permitted the

> Demerol, or maybe entailed it. And the Demerol entailed the pitocin, and the pitocin entailed the cesarean. It was as if, in laying down my body as I was told to, I also laid down my autonomy and my right to self-direction.

In contrast, Paula said:

> I walked the halls for most of my labor. It just hurt more when I laid down. And I felt strong and in control when I walked, even though it still hurt, so I kept on walking, because that was a lot better than being in bed and feeling like a little sick kid.

Although today in many hospitals women may choose to walk around during labor, still the bed and its messages remain their locus, the point to which sooner or later they must return.

In the responses of individual women to the procedures thus far analyzed, we can begin to detect a process at work that I have called "conceptual fusion of the laboring woman's beliefs with the technological model" (Davis-Floyd 1986b). For example, Suzanne's response to the wheelchair was that she suddenly began to feel that maybe she was not "in control any more"; Susan's response to being separated from her husband during the prep was similar: "By the time my husband was allowed in the labor room, so many things had happened and so many people had tried to help as his substitute that I was confused and losing control." In the responses of these individual women we can detect the beginnings of the cognitive disorientation that is a prerequisite for the reconstruction of their individual belief systems in conformity with the technological model.

A further example of this process is Charlene's response to the enforced fast that generally accompanies hospital birth:

> I went into labor just after dawn. I called my OB, and he said not to eat, so I skipped breakfast and went on in to the hospital. By that evening, when things were getting really intense, I was so weak from hunger I thought I would die.... It wasn't till I had the epidural that I started to feel like I could make it.

Birth rituals thus often function like "cranking gears": as they work to map the technological model onto the laboring woman's perceptions of her birth experience, they also set in motion a physiological chain of events that will make this model *appear* to be true and their intensified performance to be both appropriate and necessary. When I interviewed Elizabeth and Charlene some months after their births, they had become consciously aware of this cranking gear process and pointed out how one procedure had inevitably led to another in their labor and birth experiences.

Fasting and the IV. According to Feeley-Harnik, "Persons undergoing rites of passage are usually prohibited from eating those highly valued foods that would identify them as full members of society" (1981:4). In rites of pregnancy and birth in all cultures, food taboos serve the purpose of marking and intensifying the liminal status of the pregnant woman. To deny a laboring woman access to her own choice of food and drink in the hospital is to confirm her initiatory status and consequent loss of autonomy and to tell her that only the institution can provide the nourishment she needs—a message that is most forcefully conveyed by the IV.

The intravenous drips so commonly attached to the hands and arms of birthing women make a very powerful symbolic statement: they are umbilical cords to the hospital. The long cord connecting her body to the fluid-filled bottle places the woman in the same relation to the hospital as the baby in her womb is to her. She is now dependent upon the institution for her life and is receiving one of the most profound messages of her initiation experience: we are all dependent on institutions for our lives. But this message is all the more compelling in her case, for she is the real giver of life. Society and its institutions cannot exist unless women give birth; yet the birthing woman in the hospital is shown not that *she* gives life, but rather that the *institution* does.

The "Pit Drip." Under the technological model of reality, time—mechanical and linear—is viewed as being measurable in discrete, almost weighable units, so we say that something should take place within a specific "amount" of time. As the process that re-produces society, birth must set the standard for the general cultural handling of time: birth must be culturally shaped to occur within specific amounts of time, just like the production of any factory good. When a woman's labor fails to conform to production timetables (labor time charts), it will be speeded up with the drug pitocin, a synthetic form of the hormone oxytocin.

> The quality and quantity of uterine contractions are greatly affected when oxytocin is infused. The contractions tend to be longer, stronger, and with shorter relaxation periods between. As a result, the fetus is compromised—stressed, before its first breath. With each uterine contraction, blood supply to the uterus is temporarily shut off. If deprived of blood supply, a fetal bradycardia (decreased fetal heart rate deceleration) follows with oxygen deprivation and cerebral ischemia causing the grave possibility of neurological sequellae. Truly the fetus has been challenged, and the EFM dutifully records the stressed fetal heart rate. With suspicions confirmed, a diagnosis of fetal distress is noted and an elective cesarean section is the treatment of choice (Ettner 1977:153).

The tendency of pitocin to set in motion the above chain of events is entirely in keeping with the structuring and ordering characteristics of ritual and with the sense of inevitability—the conceptual cranking gears—that ritual's consistent performance can invoke. The administration of pitocin through the umbilical IV sends several messages to the laboring woman: (1) that our cultural concept of time as linear, measurable, and a valuable commodity is right and true; (2) that her body is a machine; (3) that her machine is defective because it is not producing on schedule; and (4) that the institution's schedule is much more important than her body's internal rhythms and her individual experience of labor. Moreover, the increased pain during contractions that results from the administration of pitocin serves the ritual purpose of hazing—that is, of speeding up the breakdown of the initiate's category system through the intensification of physical stress.

External Electronic Fetal Monitor. A common feature of all rites of passage is the ritual adornment of the initiates with the visible physical trappings of their transformation. In primitive (i.e., low technology) societies, these adornments usually consist of objects representing the most deeply held values and beliefs of the society, such as "relics of deities, heroes or ancestors...sacred drums or other musical instruments" (Turner 1979:239). This perspective provides a fascinating insight into the symbolic significance of the electronic fetal monitor (*EFM*)—a machine which utilizes ultrasound to measure the rate of the baby's heartbeat through electrodes belted onto the laboring woman's abdomen. The EFM has itself become *the* symbol of high-technology hospital birth. Observers and participants alike report that the monitor, once attached, becomes the focal point of the labor, as nurses, physicians, husbands, and even laboring women themselves become visually and conceptually glued to the machine, which then shapes their perceptions and interpretations of the birth process:

> As soon as I got hooked up to the monitor, all everyone did was stare at it. The nurses didn't even look at me anymore when they came into the room—they went straight to the monitor. I got the weirdest feeling that *it* was having the baby, not me. (Diana)

In Diana's response to the electronic fetal monitor, we can observe the successful outcome of the conceptual fusion between her perceptions of her birth experience and the technological model. So thoroughly has this model been mapped onto Diana's birth that she, reduced to a mere onlooker, has begun to *feel* that the machine itself is having the baby. In contrast is Pat's response:

> [They put me in bed] and put on the fetal monitor..."just to check"...that was kind of fun. I could watch and my husband could tell when a contraction was starting sooner than I could, so he could help me get ready.... Then around seven, I got real uncomfortable. I said "Get this thing off me," because I needed to rub—you know, do that Lamaze rub on my stomach. Well, if the fetal monitor is on, you can't rub. That's where I wanted to rub, so I said, "Get it off me." They said, "Fine, we'll get it off."

In Pat's response to the fetal monitor, as well as her earlier conversion of the wheelchair into a luggage cart, we can observe that by maintaining conceptual distance from the technological model, she is able to avoid the conceptual fusion which obstetrical procedures seek to achieve. Conceptual distance can be maintained when the woman places technology and the institution at *her* service instead of the other way around.

If we stop a moment now to consider the visual and kinesthetic images that a laboring woman will be experiencing—herself in bed, in a hospital gown, staring up at an IV pole, bag, and cord on one side and a big whirring machine on the other and down at a steel bed and at a huge belt encircling her waist—we can see that her entire visual field conveys one overwhelming perceptual message about our culture's deepest values and beliefs: Technology is supreme; you are utterly dependent upon it.

Internal Electronic Fetal Monitor. To this profound message, the internal fetal monitor adds a further note: your baby is a technological artifact, too. And as such, it is the institution's product, not yours (the woman's). In fact, *your* machine is so defective that society's product may be in danger from its potential malfunction, so it is necessary to apply a special machine to monitor the product's progress in order to protect it from potential harm caused by *you*. Here we can see clearly how conceptually essential is this metaphorizing of the baby as a mechanical product—to screw an electrode into an infant's scalp must be an easier task if one holds the belief that, being an object, the not-yet-born does not feel any pain:

> At Doctor's Hospital I learned to screw a monitor lead into the scalp of a baby not yet born.... Was the baby frightened? Does this baby still want to be with us? What have we taught this new person about what life is like? At Doctor's Hospital I attached the woman to the monitor and no one looked at her anymore. Held in place by the leads around her abdomen and coming out of her vagina, the woman looked over at the TV-like screen displaying the heartbeat tracings. No one held the woman's hand. Childbirth had become a science (Harrison 1982:91).

Cervical Checks. Frequent cervical checks drive home to the laboring woman the physical significance of the messages about time, about the suspected defectiveness of her own body, and about her lack of status and lack of power relative to the hospital staff (the institution's representatives) and the institution (society's representative). When they are painful, cervical checks also function as part of the impersonal hazing of the initiate. They intensify the process of symbolic inversion begun with the prep—to have a series of strangers sticking their hands through a woman's vagina and deep into her cervix approaches the extreme of opposition to a woman's usual conceptions of appropriate relations between herself and society, an extreme that will ultimately be reached on the delivery table with the lithotomy position.

Analgesia/Epidural Anesthesia. The many and varied forms of analgesia and anesthesia received by most laboring women intensify the message that their bodies are machines by adding to it the message that their machines can function without *them*. In particular, epidural (or caudal) anesthesia, which completely numbs a woman from the chest down, puts the final seal on this message, dramatically illustrating to the woman the "truth" of one of Western society's fundamental principles—the Cartesian maxim that mind and body are separate.

Yet to fully understand the symbolic significance of the epidural in hospital birth, we need to consider the meaning of its replacement of scopolamine and general anesthesia as routine procedures in most hospitals. Although "scope" did serve to reinforce the technological model of birth, in that it told women that their machines did not need them to produce a baby, it did not make women act like machines but like wild animals—an uncomfortable metaphor that undermined society's attempts to make birth appear to be mechanical enough to conform to the reality created by the technological model. Furthermore, any type of general anesthesia meant that the woman would miss many of the important messages she could be receiving. The "awake-and-aware" Lamaze patient with the epidural fits the picture of birthing reality painted by the technological model much better than the "scoped out" or "gassed out" mother, for the epidural makes a physical reality out of the conceptual separation of mind and body, a reality that the woman will grasp precisely because of her awareness.

"Now Push!/Don't Push!" If the birthing woman's body is a machine producing a product, then it makes perfect sense that once the opening is sufficiently large for that product to pass through, it should immediately be produced, given that time is of the essence if production schedules are to be maintained. And, given the constant danger of damage to the product from maternal mechanical malfunction, it seems in the product's best interest as well to get it out as soon as possible.

Thus, in most United States hospitals, once full cervical dilation is reached, the nursing staff immediately begins to exhort the laboring woman to push with each contraction, whether or not she actually feels the urge to push. But when the baby is near to being born, the woman must be transported to the delivery room. So that the baby will not be born en route, the laboring woman in transit will be exhorted *not* to push with as much vigor as she was previously commanded *to* push.

To have a number of people commanding her either to push or not to push constitutes a complete denial of the validity of the natural rhythmic imperatives of the laboring woman's body and intensifies the messages of the mechanicity of her labor and of her subordination to the institution's expectations and schedule:

> The obstetrician reported that the cervix was fully dilated and I should begin voluntary pushing with subsequent contractions. Shortly thereafter, though, I didn't perceive the contractions to be as intense as before, nor at the same rate, all of which was confirmed on the monitor. Having finally arrived at the second stage, it seemed as though my uterus had suddenly tired! When the nurses in attendance noted a contraction building on the recorder, they instructed me to begin pushing, not waiting for the urge to push, so that by the time the urge pervaded, I invariably had no strength remaining, but was left gasping,

dizzy, and diaphoretic. The vertigo so alarmed me that I became reluctant to push firmly for any length of time, for fear that I would pass out. I felt suddenly depressed by the fact that labor, which had progressed so uneventfully up to this point, had now become unproductive. (Merry)

In Merry's response, we can observe her internalization of the message that her machine was defective. She does not say "The nurses had me pushing too soon," but "My uterus has suddenly tired," and labor "had now become unproductive." These responses reflect a basic tenet of the technological model of birth—when something goes wrong it is the woman's fault:

Yesterday on my rounds I saw a baby with a cut on its face and the mother said, "My uterus was so thinned that when they cut into it for the section, the baby's face got cut." The patient is always blamed in medicine. The doctors don't make mistakes. "Your uterus is too thin," not, "We cut too deeply." "We had to take the baby" (meaning forceps or cesarean), instead of, "The medicine we gave you interfered with your ability to give birth" (Harrison 1982:174).

Lithotomy Position. The vast majority of hospitals and obstetricians in the United States insist on a birthing position that quite literally makes the baby, who follows the curve of the birth canal, be born heading upwards. According to one obstetrical text:

The lithotomy position is best. Here the patient lies with her legs in stirrups and her buttocks close to the lower edge of the table. The patient is in the ideal position for the attendant to deal with any complications which arise (Oxorn and Foote 1975:110).

This lithotomy position completes the process of symbolic inversion that has been in motion since the woman was put into that "upside-down" hospital gown. Now we have the woman's normal bodily patterns of relating to her world quite literally turned upside down: her legs in the air, her buttocks at the table's edge, her vagina totally exposed. As the ultimate symbolic inversion, it is ritually appropriate that this position be reserved for the peak transformational moments of the initiation experience: the birth itself. The official representative of society, its institutions, and its core values of science, technology, and patriarchy, now stands not at the mother's head nor at her side, but at her bottom, where the baby's head is beginning to emerge. Structurally speaking, this puts the woman's vagina where her head should be, a total inversion which is perfectly appropriate from a social perspective, as the technological model promises us that we can have babies with our cultural heads instead of our natural bottoms.

The overthrow of the initiate's category system is now complete: this position marks and reinforces her total openness to the new messages she is about to receive and itself constitutes one of those messages, as it speaks so eloquently to her of her powerlessness and of the power of society at the supreme moment of her own individual transformation.

Sterile Sheets and Antiseptic. The sterile sheets with which the birthing woman is draped neck to foot reinforce this inversion, as the one part that is always covered in public is now the one part left uncovered. The sterility itself carries a profound series of messages. Besides intensifying both society's purification of the initiate begun during the prep and the message of her fundamental irrelevance to the birth, the emphasis on sterilizing the area around the vagina graphically illustrates to the woman that she and her sexuality are fundamentally and conceptually dirty, while her baby—society's product—is pure and clean.

Episiotomy. Besides episiotomy's obvious function of hazing and ritual mutilation of the initiate (episiotomy is a surgical incision of the perineum to make more room at the vaginal opening), this procedure, which is used on over 90 percent of first-time mothers delivering in major United States hospitals (Thacker and Banta 1983), conveys to the birthing woman the value and importance of one of the most fundamental markers of our separation from nature: the straight line. The vagina constitutes the cross-cultural symbol par excellence of the natural, creative, powerfully sexual, and male-threatening aspects of women (long honored in myth as the *vagina dentata*, the vagina with teeth which threatens to consume or castrate the impotent male). Through episiotomy, physicians, as society's representatives, can deconstruct the vagina (and by extension, its representations), then reconstruct it in accord with our cultural belief system. Episiotomies are performed in part because doctors are taught that the straight cut heals faster than jagged tears—a teaching that is in accord with our Western belief in the superiority of culture over nature.

The episiotomy is also conceptually useful to obstetrics. From its inception, the obstetrical profession was constrained to justify itself as being of equal value to the other branches of medicine in which the inherent pathology of the disease or accident being treated was perhaps clearer than is the inherent "pathology" of natural birth (Wertz and Wertz 1977). Since surgery constitutes *the* central core of Western medicine, the ultimate form of manipulation of the human body-machine, the legitimization of obstetrics necessitated the transformation of childbirth into a surgical procedure. Routinizing the episiotomy has proven to be an effective means of accomplishing this transformation.

On top of that, the episiotomy reinforces and intensifies the messages of the other procedures about the importance of on-time production, the inherent defectiveness of the female birth machine, and the supremacy of the male over the female in our society and in society's production of the baby.

All of these messages are, of course, reinforced if the baby is pulled out with forceps. The application of forceps shows the mother that her machine is indeed defective and brings home the message that the lives of the mother and her baby are truly dependent on the institution and its technology. However, the use of forceps is no longer routine in many hospitals, as this procedure is rapidly being replaced by the cesarean section, the operation that is increasingly moving childbirth into the real sanctum sanctorum of modern medicine: the operating room. A recent editorial in the prestigious *New England Journal of Medicine* considers the potential advantages of universal prophylactic cesarean section (Feldman and Freiman 1985). The possibility of the routinization of delivery "from above" is the most extreme manifestation of the cultural attempt to use birth to manifest the superiority and control of Male over Female, Technology over Nature.

Washing the Baby. Blood and vernix are natural substances which must immediately be removed from society's product because their presence threatens the fragile conceptual framework, so painstakingly established and guarded through hospital birth rituals, within which birth takes place: the framework which claims that the institution produces the baby. To wash the baby before giving it to the mother is in part to remove it conceptually from its natural origins and to begin immediately the process of enculturation.

Prophylactic Eye Treatment and Vitamin K Injection. The placing of silver nitrate drops or an antibiotic substitute in the baby's eyes once again tells the mother that she—and the father—are impure in society's eyes and that they have potentially polluted society's product, which science and technology must now restore to purity: a purity that *only* society can bestow. The vitamin K injection—indeed, all the routine procedures performed on the newborn baby— reinforce the message to both baby and mother that nature does not work right, that they are dependent on science and technology for their lives and health. These procedures form the modern structural equivalent of the medieval Catholic rite of baptism: they symbolically enculturate the newborn, removing her step- by-step from the natural realm through restructuring her very physiology in accordance with the dictates of the technological model.

Bonding. The fact that the baby is handed by a hospital staff member to the mother for a time-limited "bonding period" conveys the message that society gives her baby to her. At the same time, it constitutes a powerful ritual ac- knowledgment on the part of society that she is now a mother, that her trans- formation is complete. Holding and touching the baby shortly after birth—while the new mother is still physically and psychologically at her most open—enable the mother to incorporate her new baby physically and emotionally into the transformed identity with which she will emerge from her initiation experience. To the woman, the baby constitutes a powerful symbol of her motherhood, her individuality, her new family, the beauty and wonder of nature, and the perfection of her own body and her procreative powers. To hold it unhindered against her body is to internalize its messages; often these are powerful and positive enough to entirely override, in the mother's conscious perception of her birth experience, any negative feelings of powerlessness, humiliation, and pain she may have experienced before her baby's birth. The presence of the father at these very special moments of highest affectivity ensures that he, too, will be incorporated into the mother's new sense of her identity, and she and the baby into his.

Four-to-Twelve-Hour Separation. What society gives, society can take away. The four-to-twelve hour ritual separation of mother and child after birth and bonding that is common in many hospitals powerfully reminds the mother that her baby belongs to society first. By sending the mother this message now, separation interrupts the powerful natural feelings generated in her by holding the newborn baby, working to ensure that she will be willing to give her baby over to society's institutions (hospitals for its medical care, schools for its socialization) for the rest of its life.

Bassinet/Incubator. The hospital bassinet with its clean straight lines, its see-through plastic walls, and its soft blankets gives a special message directly to the newborn baby. A symbol of society itself, the bassinet tells the baby that it belongs to society more than to its mother and that the only sure comfort, peace, and warmth in life will come ultimately not from people but from society and its products. The incubator, when used, intensifies this message by adding to it the additional message that machines are more reliable than mothers. The mother's womb is replaced by the womb of culture which, comfortably or uncomfortably, cradles us all.

Wheelchair. Just as the woman in labor, in transition from one social identity to another, undergoing one of the most profound transformations she may ever experience in her cultural life, enters her place of initiation, so she will leave it—in a wheelchair:

> It's almost like programming you. You get to the hospital. They put you in this wheelchair. They whisk you off from your husband. And I mean just start in on you. Then they put you in another wheelchair and send you home. And then they say, well, we need to give her something for depression. [Laughs] Get away from me! That will help my depression! (July)

The message going out of the hospital was the message coming in: a final reminder of exactly where she stands in society's eyes and of what her role is to be.

SUMMARY: BIRTH RITUALS AND SOCIETY

These obstetrical procedures fully satisfy the criteria for ritual as described above. They are patterned and repetitive; they are profoundly symbolic, communicating through the body and emotions messages concerning our culture's deepest beliefs about the necessity for cultural control of natural processes.These procedures provide an ordered structure to the chaotic flow of the natural birth process; in doing so they both enhance the natural affectivity of that process and create a sense of inevitability about their performance. Obstetrical interventions are also transformative in intent; they attempt to contain and control the inherently transformative processes of birth, and to transform the birthing woman into a mother in the full social sense of the word—that is, into a woman who has internalized the core values of American society: one who believes in science, relies on technology, recognizes her inferiority (either consciously or unconsciously), and so at some level accepts the principles of patriarchy. Such a woman will tend to conform to society's dictates and meet the demands of its institutions.

These birth rituals also transform the obstetrical resident, who is taught to do birth in no other way, into the unwitting ritual elder who performs them as a matter of course (Davis-Floyd 1987a):

> No, they were never questioned. Preps, enemas, shaves, episiotomies—we just did all that; no one ever questioned it....And I'd say that about 80 percent of the doctors in this town still do all that, all the time. That's just the way it's done. (male obstetrician, age 42)

Of course, there are many variations on this theme. Many younger doctors are dropping preps and enemas from their standard orders (although several complained to me that the nurses, themselves strongly socialized into the technological model, frequently administer them anyway). Increasing numbers of women opt for delivery in the birthing suite or LDR (labor-delivery-recovery room), where they can wear their own clothes, do without the IV, walk around during labor, and where the options of side-lying, squatting, or even standing for birth are increasingly available. The fact that many of the procedures analyzed above can be instrumentally omitted, however, underscores my point that they are rituals.[4]

Yet in spite of these concessions to consumer demand for more "natural" birth, a basic pattern of consistent high technological intervention remains: most hospitals now *require* at least periodic electronic monitoring of all laboring women; analgesics, pitocin, and epidurals are widely administered; and one in five will be delivered "from above"—by cesarean section. Thus, while some of the medicalization of birth drops away, the use of the most powerful signifiers of the woman's dependence on science and technology intensifies.

The transformative process at work in hospital birth is neither inherently negative nor inherently positive; every society in the world has the need to thoroughly socialize its citizens into conformity with its norms and has developed rituals to do just that. Yet human beings are not automatons, and the extent to which this type of ritual succeeds in such thorough socialization depends a great deal on the individual involved, as is evident in the women's responses that do not conform to desired societal goals. Pat, for example, turned the wheelchair with its message of infirmity into a luggage cart and maintained her autonomy by demanding the removal of the fetal monitor when that technology no longer suited her needs. In doing so, she demonstrates some elements of the process by which women can, should they so choose, rewrite the messages of hospital birth (Davis-Floyd 1986b:256–347).

Through hospital ritual procedures, obstetrics deconstructs birth, then reverses, inverts, and reconstructs it as a technological process. But unlike most transformations effected by ritual, birth does *not* depend upon the performance of ritual to make it happen. The physiological process of labor itself transports the birthing woman into a naturally liminal situation that carries its own affectivity. Hospital procedures take advantage of that affectivity to transmit the core values of American society to birthing women. From society's perspective, the birth process will not be successful unless the woman and child are properly socialized during the experience, transformed as much by the rituals as by the physiology of birth.

NOTES

1. The characteristics of ritual described here are adapted from the following sources: Moore and Meyerhoff 1977:7–8; d'Aquili, Laughlin, and McManus 1979; Geertz 1973; Munn 1973; Redfield 1960:358; Malinowski 1954; Turner 1967, 1968, 1969, 1974; Rappaport 1971; Burns and Laughlin 1979; Douglas 1973; Vogt 1976; Abrahams 1973.

2. More explicit and detailed versions of what I label the "technological model of birth" can be found in my Afterword to Rima Beth Star's *The Healing Power of Birth* and in Davis-Floyd (1986b:87–93; 1987b).

3. An abbreviated version of this analysis also appears in "Routines and Rituals: A New View" (Davis-Floyd 1986c).

4. A growing body of medical research now provides scientific and statistical substantiation of what midwives have been saying all along: hospital procedures cause far more physical and psychological harm than good, and hospital birth, instead of being safer than planned home birth, is more dangerous and more likely to result in injury or illness of mother and child (Burnett et al. 1980; Hinds, Bergeisen, and Allen 1985; Tew 1985; Mehl et al. 1977). Not only is this research reported in medical and scientific journals, but a number of excellent summaries have also provided the lay public with this evidence (Brackbill, Rice, and Young 1984; Inch 1984; Parfitt 1977; Stewart and Stewart 1977).

SECTION III

BABIES IN CRISIS

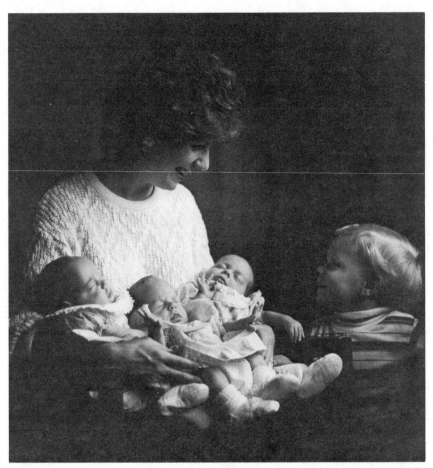

Photograph by LeRoy J. Dierker, Jr., M.D.

BABIES IN CRISIS

States...must...have programs or procedures in place...for the purpose of responding to reports of medical neglect, including instances of the withholding of medically indicated treatment (including appropriate nutrition, hydration and medication) from disabled infants with life-threatening conditions.
—Federal Register 50(72): 14878

But I must say it was a very small child; for, though it ought to have been born in the eighth month, it was born indeed in the sixth.... As we had been told that he must be kept very warm, because he was only a seven months' child, it was decided that he should be kept in the bosom by day as well as by night. Next day...at half-past six o'clock in the afternoon he suddenly died.... Only for one day to be called a mother! To have a child born only to see it die!... Surely, I thought, if a child must die within two days after birth, it were better that it should never be born....
  Now while the husband and wife,
  each clasping the hands of the other,
  make lament together,
  if anyone pausing at the entrance
  should listen to their sorrow,
  surely the paper window
  would be moistened by tears from without.
—A Woman's Diary 1866-1900, (Japan)

Many of the critical decisions that must be made in the prenatal period occur again postpartum, particularly in those cases where the infant is in a crisis state. The same radical advances in technology which make early prenatal diagnosis of fetal problems possible also now make it possible for younger, smaller, and more critically ill infants to survive outside of the womb. Through aggressive intervention, the number of premature and low birthweight infants who remain alive has increased dramatically. Yet many of the same questions about quality of life and quality of care which arose in pregnancy arise here again. Both Guillemin and Levin talk about the rights of the parents, of society, of the infant, and

175

of the medical practitioner in treating the critically ill newborn. Like Rothman in chapter 5, the authors in this section question whether the simple existence of technology, which makes certain acts possible, requires that such technology be put to use. Here, too, information itself takes on a moral quality—once a parent or physician knows a treatment is possible, must it be applied? At what point will the fetus's pain and suffering as well as the quality of its later life be considered? Levin, like Rapp who examined prenatal diagnosis and Davis-Floyd who described the ritualization of hospital birth, shows how the language of physicians describing both the condition and the treatment of the critically ill newborn defines the context for decision making about the infant's care. Thus the discourse on the appropriate use of technology is largely shaped by those who control the technology.

It is useful to look at the aggressive intervention of technology to insure infant survival in a cross-cultural context, for the very definition of when an infant (or a fetus) becomes part of a society, with rights therein, is culturally defined. In some parts of India, for example, a child is not considered a full part of society until its naming ceremony at about two weeks after birth. If the child is frail and thought unlikely to survive, the naming ceremony is put off, ostensibly to avoid the attention of evil spirits who would be attracted by the celebration, but also so that the greater mourning required for a named member of society can be avoided. If the infant dies, certainly the parents' sorrow is great, yet the infant is not cremated like a full member of society, but buried instead. In Brazil, impoverished mothers may not fight against the deaths of children who may be weak but, perhaps sadly yet with necessary resolve, withdraw care from that infant, focusing their limited resources on their other children who have a better chance of survival. Mothers feel that it is best that such weak infants die without a prolonged and wasted struggle for life and fear those conditions that would leave the mother with a permanently disabled, frail, or dependent child (Scheper-Hughes 1984). Western agents who work in these societies and introduce programs for child survival no matter what the long-term prospects for the child, are introducing their own values into a cultural context that has allowed the poor to use their limited resources on the children they feel will be productive members of society. What does this "non-altruistic" model of child survival (Cassidy in press) say about the ethical issues raised in neonatal intensive care? Both Rapp and Guillemin make a plea for consideration of the long-term consequences of intervention or non-intervention strategies. How can one resolve the conflict between a family looking at a lifetime of life support for a severely handicapped infant and a medical team whose reputation rests on the infant's survival (Newman 1984)? Parents have different definitions of what is actually a handicap, and these are dependent upon their own life experiences and their economic resources and social support. As in each of the preceding sections of this book, in this section the authors consider the issue of whose rights predominate in mandating the level of care.

The view that society has the right to mandate treatment for its members was put into law as the *Baby Jane Doe* rules: public policy demanding that catastrophically ill infants be treated. Although these regulations were denied by the United States Supreme Court in the middle of 1986, many state laws and hospital policies continue to mandate aggressive care. These same policies may deny support to the pregnant woman at a point where intervention in her pregnancy might have avoided the premature birth or low birthweight infant. Here, again, the issue of access arises. Critically ill, low birthweight infants are often the infants of those who received the poorest prenatal care. Do such infants have the same access to aggressive immediate postnatal interventions as do middle-class newborns? What of followup care for the frail infant returned to an impoverished or otherwise stressful home environment? Newborn intensive care is costly. The sicker the infant, the more expensive the days, weeks, and months of care become. Where in society does the responsibility fall for bearing the cost of such care? Some critics have said that public monies should be spent in the prenatal period to avoid the circumstances described by Boone, Poland, and Lazarus in the first part of this book which result in poor reproductive outcome

For the infant itself, the meanings of this period of crisis for long-term development must be raised. Newman describes the environment of low birthweight infants being treated in newborn intensive care. That environment, and its implications for sensory and affective development, must be compared to the immediate postnatal environment of infants; this is done in the chapters by Trevathan and Breisemeister and Haines in the final section of this book. For the latter infants, integration into the social world of parents, friends, and kin occurs soon after birth. The kind of social learning the critically ill newborn begins and when such learning occurs may be issues in the postpartum adjustment of parent to child.

11

THE CULTURAL CONTEXT OF DECISION MAKING FOR CATASTROPHICALLY ILL NEWBORNS: THE CASE OF BABY JANE DOE

Betty Wolder Levin

On October 11, 1983 a baby was born who came to be known as Baby Jane Doe. She had a number of major birth defects including spina bifida, and her parents and physicians decided against neurosurgery. Someone informed a "right-to-life" lawyer, who went to court and involved the federal government in an effort to make surgery mandatory. Her case became part of the growing national debate about decision making for catastrophically ill newborns.[1]

Decision making for catastrophically ill newborns has recently emerged as a public issue. Few people in the United States had heard of neonatal intensive care as recently as five years ago, and few were aware that decisions were sometimes made to withhold treatment from seriously ill newborns. Today, most people are aware of neonatal decision making because of publicity surrounding the cases of a number of infants such as Jane Doe. Individuals from the right-to-life movement, and the disability rights movement, civil rights advocates, health professionals, religious leaders, bioethicists, and policy makers have been debating the questions "Who should be treated?" and "Who should decide?"

The issue is sometimes presented either as a direct result of technological advances or as a result of a change in traditional values. Both of these views, however, oversimplify a complex issue, which can only be understood by looking at the cultural context in which it takes place. The interaction of technological, social, and ideological factors has affected the provision of care on a number of levels.

Since 1977 I have been doing research on decision making in neonatology including participant observation in the neonatal intensive care unit (NICU) at Columbia-Presbyterian Medical Center, a large teaching hospital in New York City. I also visited and conducted interviews with staff from over a dozen other NICUs and conducted a survey on neonatal decision making (Levin 1985). This research has primarily focused on how treatment decisions for catastrophically ill infants have been conceptualized.

THE RISE OF NEONATAL INTENSIVE CARE

The outstanding improvements in the ability to treat catastrophically ill newborns reflect the systematic direction of modern Western medicine. Since the late nineteenth century, the dominant paradigm has been the biomedical model, which focuses both the etiology and treatment of health problems on the individual, biophysical level. It has been primarily oriented towards cure rather than prevention. The pattern of resource allocation, the growth of medical specialization, the status system, and the compatibility with other aspects of contemporary ideology encouraged the trend towards emphasis on acute, technology-oriented care, especially sophisticated "rescue medicine" for critically ill patients (Brown 1979; Fabrega 1972; Sidel 1981; Hahn and Kleiman 1983). The phenomenal development in the ability to care for catastrophically ill newborns in many ways epitomizes the trend.

Efforts to Reduce Infant Mortality 1945–1965

Following World War II, concern with the nation's health was seen as an important component of the Cold War strategy because it would build up America's strength and demonstrate humanitarian concern. The "war against disease" used the same means that had brought the U.S. victory in war, the "massive mobilization of enormous material assets and a rapid increase in technological development" (Silverman 1980). Science was "the new frontier."

Previously, the federal government had spent little on health; after World War II, however, the government began to invest millions and then billions of dollars in the health field. The 1946 Hill-Burton Act provided money for hospital capital expenses and encouraged investment in expensive hospital equipment (Richmond 1969; Starr 1982). Federal expenditures increased from $3 million for medical research in 1941, to over $75 million by 1951, and to well over $1.5 billion by 1965. Some of the federal money went to preventive health programs and the delivery of primary health services, but the major thrust of the funding was directed to acute care. It primarily stimulated research on hospitalized, critically ill patients. (Starr 1982; Richmond 1969)

Before World War II, much of the concern in maternal and child health focused on the safety of the mother. In 1935 maternal mortality was almost 6 per 1,000. With the wartime development of antibiotics and blood banking, maternal mortality fell sharply to less than 1 per 1,000 by 1949 (Devitt 1977). A study at the time, however, noted that for every two soldiers killed overseas during World War II, three babies under one year had died at home (Corwin 1952). Newborn mortality had become a major area of concern.

From the beginning of the twentieth century, largely because of improvements in living conditions and public health measures which resulted in the reduction of deaths from contagious diseases, infant mortality fell dramatically. In New York City, for example, deaths of infants under one year fell from 136.7

per 1,000 births in 1898–1900 to 26 per 1,000 in 1946-50 (Department of Health, New York City 1982). After the war a new system of record keeping was initiated in which both length of gestation and birthweight were recorded. This led to the realization that, though deaths of children above one month had sharply decreased, deaths of newborns under one month had hardly changed at all (Corwin 1952); most of the deaths occurred in premature, low birthweight babies (under 5 1/2 pounds). The development of glass-walled incubators, which allowed clinicians to observe the troubled respiratory efforts of unswaddled premature infants, combined with the new statistical awareness led to both a literal and a statistical visibility of the problem of prematurity (Silverman 1980:70–71). The high death rate of premature babies was addressed by efforts to centralize their care. Special premature centers were built, some with the help of Hill-Burton funding. Some cities, such as New York, organized infant transport systems and subsidized care.

Some pediatricians started to specialize in the care of critically ill infants. They conducted research on newborn physiology, about which little was previously known, and applied developments from other fields, such as antibiotics and plastics. This improved the care of most babies. Many survivors, however, were left with impairments, such as blindness or cerebral palsy (Lubchenco et al. 1963; Silverman 1980; Budetti et al. 1981). In the early 1960s, adaptations of technological and organizational developments characteristic of intensive care for adults (Russell 1975) transformed premature centers into NICUs (Hilberman 1975). Changes included the use of respirators and electronic monitors, analysis of small blood samples, and a specialized staff of highly trained nurses.

While the quality of care delivered to infants in the NICUs improved, there was still little decline in overall rates of infant mortality. Premature babies continued to be born at a high rate, and most did not receive intensive care. In 1960, for example, the infant-mortality rate of New York City was still 26.0 per 1,000. The infant mortality rate fell to sixteenth among industrialized nations in 1965, an embarrassment to the United States as infant mortality rates had become an accepted indicator of the quality of a nation's medical care and the health of a society (Richmond 1969; Miller 1985; Newland 1981).

Efforts to Reduce Infant Mortality: 1965 to the Present

Since the mid-1960s, there has been a dramatic decrease in the overall infant-mortality rate and improvements in the care of critically ill infants. This is due to a number of factors, including biomedical advances, changes in the organization of services, such as "regionalization," and an increase in third-party coverage. Third-party payments from Medicaid, Blue Cross, and other private companies provided the funds that allowed for the development of expensive, sophisticated equipment and of methods to treat catastrophically ill infants. The costs of care were not limited to what families could afford to pay. From 1940 to 1980, medical expenses paid by third-party plans increased from under 20 percent to over 70 percent, of which more than half came from government sources (National Center for Health Statistics, 1984a). In some states, Medicaid subsidizes neonatal care for others beside the poor, because infants can become

Medicaid eligible without their families having to deplete their resources to poverty level in order to qualify. The structure of third-party payments has provided relatively little for preventive services and moderate amounts for ambulatory care, but it has been most comprehensive for acute hospitalized care, such as intensive care. One study found that third-party payers covered 85 percent of the costs for neonatal care, hospitals absorbed an additional 11 percent, and individual families paid only 4 percent of the costs (Budetti et al. 1981).

Regional networks were organized to coordinate services for obstetrical and newborn care. Regional centers developed services specializing in high-risk births and the care of sick infants. Mothers and infants were transferred to these centers for tertiary care. These centers were also responsible for training clinicians from community hospitals and specialists in neonatology (Committee on Perinatal Health 1976). Neonatology became a Board Certified Subspecialty in 1975. Neonatologists developed and used even more sophisticated technology, and private companies selling specialized equipment and supplies began to aggressively market products for use in the NICUs. Because people in the United States have traditionally looked towards technological solutions to problems, hospitals that had the latest equipment were able to attract staff and patients who wanted the "best" facilities. NICUs, with their sophisticated biomedical equipment, became showcases for the capacity of modern medicine.

Survival rates for premature infants rose dramatically as infant care was revolutionized due to further development of respirators and other respiratory support devices, new methods of feeding, and other techniques. The change was most striking for the treatment of *very* premature infants. Infants born after less than twenty-eight weeks gestation used to be considered "non-viable fetuses" and were usually classified as miscarriages; now they are considered "live births," and many premies born between twenty-four and twenty-eight weeks have been treated successfully (Budetti et al. 1981; Driscoll et al. 1982; Stahlman 1984).

In 1985, at Columbia-Presbyterian Medical Center, over 60 percent of all infants 500–750 grams (1-1 1/3 lbs) survived, as did over 90 percent in the 750–1000 gram range (Driscoll et al. n.d.).

TABLE 1. Infant Survival (%) by Birthweight Group: New York City, 1950–80

Weight		Year			
Grams	Approx. lb.	1950	1960	1970	1980
<1000	<2 1/4	3.2	6.8	18.9	39.0
1001–1500	2 1/4–3 1/3	53.7	52.4	64.6	83.6
1501–2000	3 1/3–4 1/2	82.3	82.5	88.1	94.4
2001–2500	4 1/2–5 1/2	95.1	95.6	96.7	97.9
>2500	>5 1/2	98.9	98.9	99.2	99.4
	TOTALS	97.5	97.4	97.8	98.4

Data Source: Department of Health, New York City, n.d.

The overall United States infant-mortality rates have been sharply reduced from 24.7 per 1,000 in 1965 to 10.9 per 1,000 in 1983 (Miller 1985). Part of the reduction is due to greater availability of family planning and abortion services which have lowered the rate of birth to high-risk mothers (Lee et al.

1976), but most of the reduction results from better treatment of premature and other acutely ill infants (Budetti et al. 1981).

Surgical techniques were developed to treat babies born with many congenital anomalies. Open-heart surgery and new drugs enabled treatment for infants with many cardiac defects. For babies such as Baby Jane Doe who were born with severe spina bifida (a defect in the formation of the spinal column which causes damage to the spinal cord and other anomalies), new neurosurgical techniques could be used to close the spinal lesion and shunt excess fluid from the brain. Over two-billion dollars are spent on the provision of care for the 6–7 percent of all babies born in the United States who are admitted to over 600 NICUs each year (Budetti et al. 1981; Institute of Medicine 1985). In addition to saving the lives of many critically ill infants, NICU care has prevented impairments for many others who would have survived even without intensive care, but who would have had disabilities. Although infants who were in an NICU have a higher incidence of impairments than other children, the vast majority of NICU survivors have no lasting impairments (Shapiro et al. 1983; McCormick 1985).

Some people have suggested that medicine is approaching a theoretical limit, beyond which developments in acute care may be unable to lower infant mortality, but such a limit has not yet been demonstrated. During the last twenty years the ability to save infants formerly thought to be untreatable has continued to increase.

PREVENTION VERSUS ACUTE CARE

One factor not adequately addressed in the struggle to reduce infant-mortality rates has been the continued birth of many premature and low birthweight infants— the group of infants most likely to die. Of all babies born in the United States in 1981, 6.8 percent were low birthweight. Therefore, despite advances in technology which greatly increased the rate of survival for low birthweight babies, the United States infant mortality rate still ranks seventeenth among industrialized nations (Miller 1985).

The association of socioeconomic factors, including race and social class, with the rate of birth of preterm and low birthweight infants has been well documented (Antonovsky and Bernstein 1977; Miller et al. 1985; Institute of Medicine 1985). Infant-mortality rates among blacks, at 19.6 per 1,000 are nearly twice as high as among whites. In 1982, 124 out of 1,000 black babies were low birthweight while the rate for whites was 56 per 1,000 (Miller 1985). In some areas, the sociodemographic difference is even more striking. For the primarily poor residents of Central Harlem, the 1983 infant mortality rate was 21.2 per 1,000, while for the primarily prosperous residents of Manhattan's Upper East Side the rate was only 7.2 per 1,000 (Department of Health, New York City 1984).

Because the primary thrust of expenditures for health care has been to cure rather than to prevent, less has been done to prevent the births of infants at risk than to cure them once they are born. Research has shown that increased use of prenatal care would be cost effective by reducing the number of low birthweight infants born and thus reducing the very high health-care expenditures for such infants (Institute of Medicine 1985). Improvements in the standard of living and the provision of better primary health-care services would also decrease the infant-mortality rate. In fact, recent increases in infant mortality rates in some areas have been shown to be associated with cutbacks in programs for mothers and children and increased economic stress (Newland 1981; Miller 1985; Miller et al. 1985). While social and health services have not been adequate to significantly affect the risk of low birthweight associated with sociodemographic characteristics (Institute of Medicine 1985), high quality neonatal intensive care has been made available to infants of all social classes. A recent study showed that in New York City, the chance of babies in a given weight category surviving the neonatal period did not vary significantly with socioeconomic factors (Paneth et al. 1982). However, sociodemographic characteristics are strongly associated with postneonatal infant mortality rates. For example, the 1983 death rate of infants one month to one year was only 1 per 1,000 on the Upper East Side of Manhattan, but 11.7 per 1,000 in Central Harlem (Department of Health, New York City 1984).

THE RISING CONCERN WITH BIOETHICS

For most babies, neonatal intensive care is clearly beneficial. For some, however, new treatments lead to survival with brain damage and other severe impairments or the prolongation of the dying process. In the late 1960s and early 1970s, at some regional centers where treatment for such babies was concentrated, clinicians came to see severely impaired and dying babies not as isolated cases, but as part of a group of cases for which newly developed treatments might be doing more harm than good. Whereas previously an isolated practitioner and/or family might have privately decided to withhold treatment to allow an individual baby to die, practitioners at some regional centers now began to discuss such treatment decisions. Some felt that policies should be devised to identify and withhold treatments that would do more harm than good.

In the late 1960s and early 1970s, articles about such practices began to appear in the clinical literature. From the beginning, much of the debate focused on decision making about infants with spina bifida (see Zachary 1968 and letters in response to his article in *The Lancet*). Selective non-treatment was also discussed for babies with other anomalies and very low birthweight premature infants. Some clinicians saw such decisions as based on scientific criteria and argued that only physicians should make them (Lorber 1971). Others, recognizing the social and ethical components of such decisions, argued that parents should make the decisions (Duff and Campbell 1973).

In the past decade, philosophers, clinicians and others have joined the debate over neonatal decision making. (For more information see: Bell 1975; Colon 1981; Fox, et al. 1986; Gustaitis and Young 1986; Infants 1978; Jonsen 1976; Kuhse and Singer 1985; Lyons 1985; Magnet and Kluge 1985; Murray and Caplan 1985; President's Commission...1983a; Shelp 1986; Stinson and Stinson 1983; Swinyard 1978; Weil and Benjamin 1987; and Weir 1984). Social scientists have also examined the bioethical issues, including the decision to withhold treatment (c.f. Anspach forthcoming; Barber 1978; Clausen 1985; Fox 1976; Frohock 1986; Guillemin and Holmstrom 1983, 1986; Mumma and Benoliel 1984; Parsons, Fox, and Lidz 1972; Weiner et al. 1979). The most comprehensive examination of the treatment of the critically ill, which included information on the treatment of newborns, was based primarily on a survey of physicians' attitudes. It indicated that physicians are moving from a physiological toward a social definition of life; they feel they should not treat all patients, but only those who will have the potential to interact meaningfully with others—"those who have the capacity to fulfill social roles" (Crane 1975).

The public is itself split in attitudes towards neonatal decision making. A Gallup poll found that when asked what they would do as parents of a "badly deformed baby who would only live a few years," 40 percent said they would ask doctors to keep the baby alive, 43 percent took the opposite view, and 17 percent reported no opinion (*New York Times* 1983).

CLINICIANS' CONCEPTUALIZATION OF TREATMENT CHOICE FOR CATASTROPHICALLY ILL NEWBORNS

In order to understand the decisions that are made concerning the treatment of catastrophically ill infants, it is necessary to understand how clinicians conceptualize the issue. It is important both in those situations in which clinicians alone make decisions and also in those in which parents, judges, or others are involved in decision making. Many clinicans believe that patients or family members should make the important decisions about treatment for family members, including newborns. Even in such cases, clinicians define the areas that are considered legitimate domains for family decision making, outline the treatment options, and provide most of the information to the family on characteristics of patients and treatments. Clinicians have also played an important role by defining the issues in cases brought to the courts.

Although clinicians may talk about a decision concerning a catastrophically ill newborn as if the decision being made is to treat or not to treat, my research indicates that in today's modern hospital, a patient is virtually never not treated, if this means that absolutely no treatments are given. Rather, decisions about withholding treatment involve decisions about giving some treatments and withholding others out of the range of possible treatments. Therefore, in these cases it is not only a question of who should be treated and who should decide, but which treatments should be given and which should be withheld.

Since clinicians give some treatments to patients from whom they withhold other treatments, they make distinctions based on characteristics of treatments as well as characteristics of patient condition (Levin 1982; President's Commission 1983a). Clinicians categorize patients and treatment options along a number of dimensions that may be labeled by a number of different terms, but may be understood by using the analytic model of the clinicians' conceptual system in Figure 1.

Although each of the dimensions is sometimes used as if it involved a dichotomous distinction (eg. good/poor quality of life; ordinary/extraordinary treatment), each may be seen to form a continuum. And though there is agreement among most clinicans that all of the dimensions outlined in Figure 1 are to be addressed in decision making, there is variation in how particular patients and treatments are evaluated and in the relative importance of various dimensions in particular cases.

These categorizations reflect, in part, objective technical criteria, such as those based on the results of diagnostic tests. However, categorizations involve evaluation using subjective, culturally defined criteria as well. This may be most obvious for categorizations about quality of life, but even the distinction between withholding and withdrawing has culturally defined dimensions. Each of these categories will be explained in more detail below as part of the discussion of the case of Baby Jane Doe.

FIGURE 1. Conceptual Categories for Clinical Decision Making about Withholding Treatment

Patient-Condition Characteristics	
Quality of life	Physical impairment
	Mental impairment
Uncertainty	about being "normal"
	about severity
Nature of the critical condition	Salvageable/unsalvageable
	Acute/chronic
Social value/costs	To family
	To clinicians
	To "society"
Treatment Characteristics	
Aggressiveness	
Ordinary/Extraordinary	
Withholding/Withdrawing	
Active/Passive Euthanasia	

The goals of treatment also affect decision making. The classical goals of clinicians are (1) To preserve life; (2) To provide care; and (3) To do no harm. In cases where these goals are felt to be in conflict, clinicians may choose to maximize one of them or may seek to find means to balance two or three. One way in which this is accomplished is to choose treatments that are seen as commensurate with the patient's condition. The categorizations of patient condition and treatments discussed above are considered and an appropriate level of "aggressiveness" of treatment is chosen (Levin 1985). In most cases, even when the patient is probably dying, everything possible is done to preserve life (Mumma and Benoliel 1984). If the patient is felt to be suffering, however, the goals of "doing no harm" and of "providing care" are sometimes considered primary. A level of treatment may be chosen that will soon lead to death.

A very small, premature baby with respiratory problems who has suffered severe brain damage may be taken off the respirator. But if there is more uncertainty regarding outcome and/or there is more emphasis placed on the sanctity of life, a level of care may be chosen for which the outcome is uncertain. In such a case, the baby may be left on a respirator, but a decision may be made not to increase respirator settings if the baby needs more oxygen and not to resuscitate the baby if his or her heart stops. In these cases, though "treatment is withheld," the patient may live. In such a situation, clinicians may feel that their choice allows "a baby to declare herself," "nature to take her course," or "God to decide." As with characteristics of patients and treatments, the categorizations of a treatment choice intended for comfort or cure, evaluated as doing good or harm, may vary.

THE CASE OF BABY JANE DOE

It is possible to illustrate some of the ways that social and ideological, as well as technical factors, influence decision making by examining available information about Baby Jane Doe (*New York Times* 1983, 1984; Lyons 1985) and data from my own case observations and interviews. Baby Jane Doe was the first child born to a young Catholic couple who lived on Long Island, New York. She was born with spina bifida (a L-3 to L-4 myelomeningocele) resulting in substantial paralysis of her legs and incontinence of bowel and bladder. In addition, she had hydrocephalus and microcephaly, indicating a high probability of severe mental retardation, a condition which prevented her from completely closing her eyes or from using her tongue properly to suck, spasticity of the upper extremities, and a thumb abnormality indicating that she would not have full use of her hand. Shortly after birth, she developed meningitis, a critical infection of the central nervous system which sometimes leads to lasting brain damage (Lyons 1985:45–46). The decision-making process in her case can be elucidated by consideration of the characteristics of patient condition and treatments outlined in the above model.

Patient Condition Characteristics. When Baby Jane Doe was born, her parents, in consultation with her doctors, decided against neurosurgery to close her spinal lesion or shunt the excess fluid from her brain. They believed that because of the multiple anomalies, she could only have a poor quality of life. Because of the level of the spinal lesion, they knew that she would definitely have paralysis and incontinence. In addition, the brain malformations almost certainly meant that there would be some developmental delays, with a high probability of severe retardation. Although the defects were not themselves critical, their presence was likely to lead to complications, such as meningitis, urinary-tract infections, and uncontrolled hydrocephalus, that would lead to critical conditions. The press reported that without surgery she would probably die within two years; with treatment she could live for twenty. (Knowledgeable clinicians felt that without treatment she could die sooner and with treatment she could live longer).

During the weeks following her birth, neither her parents nor the clinicians apparently felt that surgery to close her back would have social value. I find it useful to distinguish here between *quality of life* and *social value*, for the terms are used a number of ways and the concepts are often confused. Quality of life refers to the benefits versus the burdens of life *to the baby*, while social value is used here to refer to the benefits versus the burdens *to others*. The implications of these terms will be further discussed below.

Other people might have made a different evaluation concerning her condition. Some feel that any sort of noncomatose existence is a life with sufficient quality to justify treatment, while others believe that even minor impairments can lead to a poor quality of life. The stigma against those with disabilities in United States society is strong; many new parents and clinicians know little about the lives of people with disabilities. Judgments about quality of life are sometimes made based on little information on the actual quality-of-life implications of particular impairments. The degree of impairment is a technical fact, but the degree of handicap depends on social conditions, including the resources available for treatment and education and the barriers presented by both attitudes and the physical environment (Goffman 1963; Gliedman and Roth 1980; Asch and Fine 1984). There is debate concerning the appropriate role of quality-of-life considerations in life and death decision making (Arras 1985; Rhoden and Arras 1985).

Some people, including Surgeon General Koop, suggested that there was more uncertainty about Baby Jane Doe's condition than her physicians presented. These critics posited that she might indeed enjoy an acceptable quality of life. Some felt that her back lesion presented a critical condition which needed immediate surgery. Additionally, opinions of physicians and bioethicists varied about the social value of surgery. Some believed that, though the continuation of life may not be of benefit for the patient, the social costs of tolerating nontreatment would be too high for society. They believed that not treating would show a lack of respect for the value of human life or would undermine the traditional ethics of clinical care. The financial cost of immediate or life-time care for a patient may be mentioned, but it is rarely an important factor in the clinical-decision making process about an individual newborn.

Treatment Characteristics. In addition to considerations about patient-condition characteristics, her parents and clinicians considered treatment characteristics. While Baby Jane Doe's caretakers withheld the neurosurgical procedures to close her back lesion and shunt fluid from her hydrocephalic brain, they gave antibiotics to treat her meningitis. They also presumably provided such "treatments" as a sterile environment by putting her in an isolette and covering her lesion with sterile dressings and gave regularly scheduled feedings.

The same treatment decisions would not have been made by all decision makers. Some would have recommended neurosurgery, others would have withheld antibiotics, and, at least in other countries, some might have placed such a patient in an open bed, given her sedatives, and fed her only on demand

(Lorber 1971). It is important to note that the decision to withhold neurosurgery but not other treatments could not have depended on differences in patient condition characteristics alone. The severe impairments, which led the decision makers to feel that it would be in her best interest if she died, would not have been alleviated by any of the treatments.

One way that clinicians differentiate between treatments is in terms of their *aggressiveness*. Treatments, such as those which produce large physiological effects, involve the use of high technology, and are experimental, invasive, and/or costly in terms of staff time or monetary costs, are considered more aggressive than treatments that do not have such attributes. For example, neurosurgey constitutes a very aggressive treatment, though the administration of antibiotics is seen as not very aggressive. And, such practices as keeping a baby in a sterile environment may not be conceptualized as a treatment at all. Some people feel that very aggressive treatments may be optional, but that non-aggressive treatments *must* be given. In Baby Jane Doe's case, even when the decision was made to withhold aggressive treatments, other, less aggressive treatments were given

Many people writing about bioethical decision making have made a distinction between *ordinary* and *extraordinary* care. The concept was first developed in Catholic moral theology. A distinction was made between ordinary (obligatory) and extraordinary (optional) treatments based on the value of the treatments for patients. Ordinary treatments were defined as those that would "offer a reasonable hope of benefit to a patient" and "could be obtained and used without excessive expense, pain, or other inconvenience" (Kelly, quoted in Beauchamp and Childress 1979). Extraordinary treatments were those that did not have these characteristics. The terms are now used in a number of different ways (President's Commission 1983a:82–89). Ordinary is used to refer to treatments that are (1) used frequently; (2) not very aggressive; (3) of benefit to the patient; or (4) a combination of these criteria.

It is possible that Baby Jane Doe's caretakers believed that though neuro-surgery constituted extraordinary treatment and could therefore be withheld, anti-biotics constituted ordinary treatment which had to be given. Others would have categorized the treatments differently. Some would consider antibiotics to be extraordinary and would have withheld them, feeling they would be of no benefit. Nevertheless, even clinicians who considered such treatments as antibiotics to be extraordinary generally consider such routine procedures as maintaining a sterile environment to be ordinary—such practices are almost never withheld. Others, who saw benefit to neurosurgery, may have categorized even neurosurgery as ordinary treatment and recommended surgery. Clinicians vary markedly in how they categorize specific treatments in specific cases and in how they believe such categorizations should relate to treatment recommendations (Levin 1985).

When making treatment decisions, clinicians often distinguish between *withholding* treatment (not starting a new treatment) and *withdrawing* treatment (stopping an ongoing treatment). Some clinicians and bioethicists feel that withholding a treatment is more acceptable than withdrawing one because it does not involve active intervention. Although I do not know why Baby Jane Doe received antibiotics for meningitis, the following example from my case material illustrates the way that the distinction between withholding and withdrawing influenced clinical decision making for another child born with spina bifida.

Antibiotics were started soon after birth for a child who had a high-level spinal lesion. The clinicians discussed the case with the baby's parents, who at first were unsure if they wanted the baby to be treated. After meeting with physicians, nurses, social workers, and other people familiar with the outcome for babies with such problems, they decided that treatment should be withheld. The following morning, the social worker was suprised to find that the baby was still being given antibiotics. When she questioned the resident, he said that treatment would be withheld but not withdrawn. He would continue the antibiotics for a seven-day course, for he felt that not to do so would constitute withdrawing treatment. Although the social worker would not have removed the current I.V. bottle containing medication, she would not have added more antibiotics to the next I.V. She conceptualized that as withholding, not withdrawing treatment.

The final distinction, and perhaps the most important factor governing treatment choice, is a distinction between *active* and *passive euthanasia*. While there has been a growing acceptance of the practice of passive euthanasia, there is still a strong sanction against active euthanasia. Passive euthanasia is often defined as "allowing a natural death to occur" or "not prolonging the dying process." Active euthanasia is seen as "causing death." Most clinicians conceptualize active euthanasia as an immoral means even if it would serve a "good" end, ending a life characterized only by pain and suffering (President's Commission 1983a; "In the Matter of Claire C. Conroy" 1985).

While there is growing consensus surrounding the norms allowing passive euthanasia, there is little consensus about the categorization of some treatment practices. Some clinicians and bioethicists, for example, feel that withholding an extraordinary treatment constitutes passive euthanasia and is therefore acceptable, while withdrawing an ordinary treatment constitutes active euthanasia and is therefore unacceptable. (For a discussion of this position and critique, see "In the Matter of Claire C. Conroy" 1985). There is, however, no consensus about what constitutes ordinary or extraordinary treatment in some cases nor about the distinction between withholding and withdrawing. Therefore, there is controversy about whether some treatment choices entail active or passive euthanasia. Although many feel that withholding neurosurgery in the case of Baby Jane Doe was passive euthanasia, many would feel that withdrawing antibiotics, a less aggressive treatment, would have been active euthanasia. Others, however, would consider withholding any treatment, including antibiotics, as passive euthanasia.

Such distinctions have real life-and-death consequences. For example, in one case I observed a baby who had a problem soon after birth that led to the loss of almost all of his small intestine. A decision was made not to give hyperalimentation (intravenous feeding of fats, proteins, and other nutrients). His physicians knew of no infant who had survived for a long time on such feedings alone. Although I.V. feedings were withheld, I.V. fluids were given. When I asked a nurse why he was not getting the hyperalimentation, she said it would be extraordinary treatment and would only prolong his suffering. She was emotionally attached to the baby but felt that the decision was in his best interest; she said she hoped he would not suffer for long. When I asked why they did not also withhold I.V. fluids, she said, "We couldn't do that, that would be murder." A day or two later, one of his physicians found a report on another baby, with even less intestine, who had eventually been able to digest some food. After reading the report and consulting with the parents, hyperalimentation was started. If the baby had not been getting I.V. fluids, he might have already died. He did well for a long time, but could never successfully be weaned from the hyperalimentation. Despite aggressive efforts to treat all complications, he died when he was about two and a half.

In Baby Jane Doe's case, also, the outcome might have been different if other treatment choices had been made. Without antibiotics, she probably would have died quickly from meningitis. She recovered from the meningitis and remained in the hospital for about six months. Her back lesion closed, reducing the chance of a subsequent infection. When her hydrocephalus progessed and caused discomfort, her parents agreed to neurosurgery to shunt excess fluid from her brain. After the surgery her parents brought her home. Her neurologist says that he sees no reason to revise his original prognosis; he thinks she will be severely retarded and will remain bedridden for her whole life (Lyons 1985).

DECISION MAKING FOR CATASTROPHICALLY ILL NEWBORNS AS A POLITICAL ISSUE

Decision making for catastrophically ill newborns has recently gained prominence as a public issue. Beyond its importance for the babies, their families, and their caretakers, decision making for newborns is important because it involves a number of issues which are of critical concern for society. These include the proper use of technology—especially high-cost technology; the conception of humans' relationship to God or nature; moral obligations and human rights, particularly the rights of the handicapped and those of children and parents; and the authority of the state and federal government. These issues all have political as well as philosophical significance. Decision making for catastrophically ill infants receives much public attention, not only because it is the focal point where a number of these issues come together, but also because it is used as a metaphor for debating these other issues (Fox 1980).

The many-faceted nature of this issue leads to political alliances that cut across traditional liberal and conservative boundaries. This can be illustrated by the debate surrounding the "Baby Doe Directives" (Department of Health and Human Services 1982–1984b; Rhoden and Arras 1985). Right-to-life advocates have long seen the issue of withholding treatment from newborns as part of a continuing assault on the sanctity of life. Speaking against abortion before he became surgeon general, Everett Koop said:

> The first domino to fall was abortion on demand, and it has
> split this country as no other social issue since the practice of
> slavery. The second domino to fall was infanticide. It fell
> silently because unlike abortion, which is a public issue,
> infanticide is practiced behind the shielding facade of the

hospital. The third domino is euthanasia: it has been struck and is falling (Brozan 1979).

After publicity about a child with Down's syndrome who died in 1982 because relatively routine surgery had been withheld, the Reagan administration issued a directive stating that "discriminatory failure to feed and care for handicapped infants..." is prohibited by federal law "in institutions receiving federal financial assistance" (DHHS 1982). The regulation was based on Section 504 of the Rehabilitation Act of 1973, civil rights legislation designed to protect the right of the handicapped to education and employment. For this regulation, the administration took a broad view of federal law in order to deal with an issue usually considered to be either under the jurisdiction of state governments or not subject to government interference by defining Medicaid and Medicare funds to hospitals as federal financial assistance and withholding treatment as discrimination.

The "Baby Doe Directives" were applauded by "right-to-life" advocates as well as by some liberals—members of civil rights organizations and others active in the disability rights movement. They felt that this interpretation of the law would obligate hospitals to abide by all other civil rights statutes as well. Most health-care professionals, bioethicists, and civil rights advocates, as well as people active in the women's health movement, however, opposed the "Directives," which were seen as an infringement on the privacy of the physician/patient relationship, on the right to refuse treatment, and on the ability of parents to make decisions for their children. Opposition to the "Directives" also came from some conservatives. They feared that the broad interpretation of the law would require the federal government to become involved in investigating other alleged instances of discrimination in other institutions (Russell and Barringer 1983); they also feared further encroachment of the state on the private decision making of its citizens.

The original "Baby Doe Directives" and subsequent revisions were overturned in a series of court cases, and attempts by the federal government to obtain the medical records of Baby Jane Doe were denied. In 1986 the Supreme Court issued a ruling supporting the lower court decisions and affirming parents' rights to make treatment decisions for their children (Bowen v. American Hospital Association et al. 1986). The possibility of the future application of antidiscrimination legislation to treatment decisons about disabled newborns is ambiguous. Legislation has been approved by Congress which recommends the involvement of state child abuse agencies and hospital ethics committees (DHHS 1984b, 1985; Rhoden and Arras 1985; Murray 1985).

The Baby Jane Doe case is a part of larger political issues currently facing U.S. society which are concerned with the role of the government and the role of families and individuals in two major areas: the allocation of resources for social needs, and decision making about medical care.

In reference to Baby Jane Doe, Surgeon General Koop said, "We are not fighting for this baby. We're fighting for the principle of this country that every life is individually and uniquely sacred" (*New York Times* 1983). Although many in this society believe that physiological life should always be maintained, others feel their values may dictate decisions not to prolong life. The issue is whether individuals and families ought to be able to make decisions which reflect divergent values or whether the government is to insure adherence to a value system defined by the state.

There are also questions concerning the allocation of societal resources. The government mandates and finances efforts to save the life of identified individuals through acute care. In the United States today, there is a debate concerning the appropriate role of the government in protecting individuals who are statistically at risk. These "statistical" lives cannot be individually identified but represent individuals who will die withhout the allocation of resources for preventive and primary health services. There is also debate concerning the degree to which individual families should bear or society should share the financial costs and other responsibilities of caring for people with special needs, including children who survive catastrophic illness.

Clinicians making decisions for catastrophically ill newborns usually do not have the choice of giving more preventive and other primary care. Rather, the resources available for different types of care are now determined primarily by public-policy decisions governing the availablity of Medicaid and other third-party payments and, to a lesser extent, by funds for research, training, and social-service programs. It is important to realize that acute interventions and preventive measures need not be conceptualized as mutually exclusive choices. Further reductions in infant mortality would probably result from more investment in each of these areas.

The debate over the Baby Jane Doe issue reflects efforts by various political factions to demonstrate humanitarian concerns and to define societal values and the responsibilities of various sectors of society. In such political discussions, technical, social, and ideological factors are inextricable linked.

NOTES

Support for some of the research presented in this paper came from the Project on Issues of Values and Ethics in Health Care, College of Physicians and Surgeons, Columbia University, which was funded by grants from the National Endowment for the Humanities, the Mallinckrodt Foundation, and the Van Amerigen Foundation and by a Charlotte W. Newcombe, Woodrow Wilson Dissertation Fellowship. I wish to thank John Driscoll, M.D., L. Stanley James, M.D., Zola Golub, R.N., and Katherine Rosasco, R.N. for their aid in conducting research, and Nancy Bonvillain, Arthur Caplan, John Colombotos, Ann Dill, Eva Friedlander, Hannah Lessinger, Jane Bennett Ross, Fran Rothstein, Nina Glick Schiller, Ida Susser, and Bob Zussman for their valuable comments on earlier drafts of this paper.

1. The term "catastrophically ill newborn" is used to refer to babies who are ill and whose illness or condition is socially defined as a catastrophe (a disaster, calamity, or serious misfortunate occurrence) by his or her family and/or professional caretakers.

Although terms such as *anomalous, damaged, deformed, defective,* or *disabled* are sometimes used to refer to such infants, these terms seem to imply that it is the physical state of the child which defines the problem. Catastrophically ill defines a social rather than a physical state, as the term "illness" may be used to refer to a social entity, in contrast to a "disease" which may be defined as a biological entity (Fabrega 1979).

A child may be defined as catastrophically ill because of the presence of a serious illness, prematurity, and/or present or future expected impairment. Not all children with the same physical conditions will be defined as catastrophically ill. Catastrophically ill infants include, but are not limited to, infants who are critically ill.

12

THE FAMILY IN NEWBORN INTENSIVE CARE

Jeanne Harley Guillemin

Although the history of newborn intensive care is relatively brief, the framework for understanding parent-child and parent-staff interaction in this high-technology context is already fixed. This framework is largely psychological, with emphasis on the negative reactions of parents confronted with the serious illness or death of a newborn (Drotar et al. 1975). It has become, in turn, the basis for nursing and social-work approaches to parents of infants in neonatal intensive care units (NICU's). That is, mothers, and often both parents of the newborn, become a second order of patient, the nonmedical, psychological clients of the unit staff.

The social construction of these parents as patients, however, is highly problematic. Acquiring passive or negative roles in the course of an infant's treatment directly diminishes the parents' authority as guardians capable of acting in the child's interest. The loss of a capable guardian, for whatever reasons, puts the infant's welfare in jeopardy. Although hospital staff assume great responsibility in caring for the critically ill infant, they cannot offer adequate substitutes for parental concern and authority. Beyond the NICU staff, the alternatives to parental authority—committees, courts, state agencies—by nature subject the child to impersonal and arbitrary influences.

Why and when does the role of parent become categorically reduced? One answer, strongly implied in the current literature, is that the stress of having a critically ill infant incapacitates parents, rendering them temporarily unfit to make rational decisions. Another answer lies in the institutional imperative of emergency and critical-care medicine that requires complete physician control. The special guardianship relationship of parent to newborn potentially interferes with this requirement. Indeed, a major source of tension within the maximum-care (Level III) nursery revolves around the practical management of potentially disruptive parents (Sherman 1980). In this atmosphere, parents may have no choice but to become some kind of patient: either the good, subservient one who follows directions or the bad one who does not meet expectations (Parsons and Fox 1952).

There can be both psychological and structural reasons why parents of critically ill infants cede their authority to medical professionals. The important question is: What can be done to decrease the likelihood that infants in medical need suffer the loss of parental advocacy? Does the case approach to parental psychology offer the best protection of newborn interests? Or, are there organizational remedies to the serious problem of exposing infants to the depersonalized atmosphere of the central hospital?

THE MOTHER AS PATIENT

Two important factors set newborn intensive care aside from intensive care for adults. First, in the United States nearly all infants are born as hospital patients and are thus already integrated into that institution with an identity and record. And second, the mothers of these infants are also hospital patients and subject to physician authority and institutional rules. Both of these have contributed to the rapid growth of newborn intensive care over the last decade. More than ever in the history of childbirth, skilled personnel and medical resources are prepared for newborn medical trauma, from premature birth to neurological damage or defect. Delivery-room surveillance of problems at birth and access to emergency transport of mothers and/or infants have grown tremendously over the last decade. Pediatricians trained in neonatology at major medical centers now staff lower- and intermediate-level nurseries and are increasingly present in the delivery room to advise about emergency transport (American Academy of Pediatricians 1980). Teams of nurses and physician educators from Level III nurseries train their counterparts in local community hospitals who are unsure of the state of the art in providing resuscitation and post-birth care for distressed newborns. All of these changes make it more likely that a distressed newborn will be admitted to NICU.

As for the patient status of mothers of newborns in intensive care, the general proliferation of childbirth technologies has increased the potential for medicalizing the experience. That is, pregnancy is defined as a pathology and delivery as a crisis, rather than as natural processes of reproduction (Wertz and Wertz 1977). The consequences of treating childbirth as a medical problem are real, whether the medical problems are or not. A woman with a history of diabetes, for example, will find her physician prepared to medically manage the pregnancy. A woman who has had an infant by cesarean delivery may find herself subject to the dictum "once a cesarean, always a cesarean" and therefore an automatic candidate for major surgery in subsequent pregnancies. A woman having her first child while still a teenager or after age thirty-five may also find herself categorically designated for cesarean delivery (Guillemin 1981).

The trend to treat expectant women as patients and, for cautionary reasons, to intensify intervention or overtreat them has a direct effect on the role of parents in the newborn intensive-care unit. If a woman remains hospitalized after childbirth, visiting her infant in the NICU can be difficult or impossible. If she has had her infant in a major medical center, it may be possible to go by wheelchair from one division to another. Indeed, new perinatal centers advertise the convenience of allowing new mothers to be located near the intensive-care nursery. If an infant has been transported to another, distant hospital, the difficulties of visitation are enormous. If the choice is between the infant's proximity to the mother and the infant's need for life-saving emergency treatment, there is no choice.

The hospitalized mother of an NICU infant runs the risk of becoming a psychological client of the unit's nursing and social-psychological staff. This happens, in particular, when physical distance translates into emotional distance and the staff sees the mother as failing to "bond" or establish effective ties with the newborn. In the NICU, the phenomenon of emotional alienation is perceived as a parent's negative reaction to the newborn's illness or defect. Disappointment at not having produced the perfect baby is often strongly felt by mothers, who also tend to blame themselves for their infant's imperfections (Klaus and Kennell 1976). Therapists involved in newborn intensive care have also described both maternal and paternal stages of mourning the lost "perfect" child (Hancock 1976; Holland and Rogich 1980) and eventually accepting their less-than-perfect infant (Benfield, Leib, and Reuter 1976). Grieving for the deceased infant follows the same general patterns observed when adults mourn the death of other adults.

The conclusion drawn from these studies is that parents should be involved with their infants, present at the nursery, and feeling and expressing their emotions. The justification for this involvement lies in the perceived benefits for the parent-child relationship and, in the case of deceased infants, in the eventual emotional stability of the parent. Courses and textbooks in nursing, psychology, and social work, therefore, urge professionals to guide disturbed parents through the appropriate stages of emotional resolution of the crisis generated by the newborn's medical problem. Thus, the parents of a critically ill newborn become patients themselves, subject to the psychologically based interventions of hospital staff.

THE SOCIAL EVALUATION OF PARENTS

In practice, the evaluation of how parents of NICU infants act is more comprehensive than bonding or grieving models. The NICU staff also look to social indicators of how the often-fragile infant patient will be cared for in the future. The ideal situation is one where parents not only accept the newborn's medical problems or anomalies but also are jointly committed to family life.

The example of a single mother confined to her hospital bed for a week or so after childbirth is a case in point. This individual may be at a special disadvantage because she may not have a partner or relative willing and able to assume authority in communicating with physicians and nurses in the NICU. Doubt then arises on the part of the staff (as it does even in the case of a healthy unmarried mother) about the stability of the woman's family life. To what kind of home is this infant going? Will the special care that infant graduates of the NICU often need be guaranteed? Is the single mother emotionally mature enough for the commitment such an infant demands?

Even with married couples, the NICU staff envisions a model of family life with an energetic, dedicated couple devoted to the infant's care and then watches the parents for signs of serious deviation from that model. Emotional outbreaks by one partner are tolerable if the other parent remains calm. When both parents become patients—that is, express hostility, extreme sorrow, or emotional withdrawal—then staff nurses, psychologists, and social workers become worried about the post-discharge care of the infant and, in particular, about child abuse. By the same formula of necessary joint commitment, a woman who has had a difficult birth should have a strong and resolute husband who is accepting of their infant. And, ideally, this mother should regain her strength and appear in the nursery with her husband as soon as possible.

These ideal models, however, are not always obtained. The following three cases, drawn from a series of 103 admissions to a Level III nursery in a major pediatric hospital (Guillemin and Holmstrom 1986), illustrate the dimensions of social and emotional problems encountered by the nursery staff.

In each of these cases, the staff screens out two important sets of facts which have an impact on the parents' ability to respond to their critically ill infant. The first of these is the medical condition and attendant treatment of the infant which affects the reactions of parents. Parents are expected to be strong and to accept, rather than to control, medical decision making. However, the treatment that parents are expected to accept often includes goals that may pertain more to the general aims of progressive medicine than the well-being of the individual child. Neonatology, for instance, is credited with the recognition that very low birthweight newborns (less than 1,500 grams) can survive if given appropriate respirator treatment (Hack et al. 1980; Budetti 1981). The clinical quest for the survival of even smaller infants continues as similar treatment is given to infants born at less than 1,000 grams. The reported results, in terms of both survival and permanent damage, indicate that this is an experimental venture at best. Sixty to 80 percent of such underdeveloped newborns die, and those who survive are likely to have long-term and serious medical needs (Britten, Fitzhardinge and Ashley 1981; Boyle et al. 1983; Kitchen and Murton 1985).

The parents' experience of the hospital referral system and the practical strains of medical care also tend to be screened out by staff. Communication problems abound when an infant is moved from one hospital division to another or from one hospital to another. For some parents, childbirth means negotiating relations with, and multiple billings from, three or more institutional sources. In the worst cases, the charges for newborn treatment can exceed the limits of private insurance or public-health coverage. Sometimes, even in fairly routine cases, parents do not know what their liabilities are.

Moreover, within an intensive-care nursery, the emphasis on staff teamwork can also compound communication problems. Teaching hospitals, where most intensive care units are located, rely heavily on resident physicians working in four-to-eight-week rotations to staff the nurseries. An infant's primary physician can be in the unit one day and, with a change in rotation, gone the next. The strict emphasis on the perceived emotional tenor of the parent-infant relationship denies organizational realities, which are also affecting the parents' emotions and relationships with their children.

For each of these families, the nursing and social work staff took a case approach to the problems that parents were experiencing. The psychological reactions of individuals and couples were either appropriate or inappropriate, with much more benefit of the doubt given to parents who distanced themselves from the unit than those who intruded.

Case One: The Teenage Mother

A fifteen-year-old black woman gives birth by cesarean to twins, each weighing less than 800 grams. The first twin dies in the intensive care unit the day after birth. The second survives but has serious lung, heart, and brain problems. From the beginning, the nurses and social workers are concerned because the father of the infants is not identified. Instead, the grandmother (herself in her early thirties and the mother of four) becomes a regular visitor. The grandmother has already taken responsibility for the mother's first-born child, now about two years old, and is open about her feeling that this newborn should be cared for by the mother. The teenage mother seems emotionally removed. She has dropped out of school, the counselor to whom she was close has left his job, and there are rumors that her current boyfriend has rejected her. Though she lives near the hospital, she visits infrequently and does not hold or touch her infant.

The surviving twin's clinical course is a rocky one, marked by frequent calls to resuscitate in the first week and later by a cardiac operation and brain shunt. After three months in the Level III nursery, the infant is alive but shows signs of severe neurological damage and has endured recurring bouts of infection.

The mother seems incapable of caring for the child, and the grandmother seems unwilling. The alternative of adoption is dismissed by the nursing staff because of the infant's medical condition. Instead, the infant is transferred to a lower-level, mixed pediatric division, where she expires of pneumonia at the age of four months.

Case Two: The Welfare Family

A woman in her mid-thirties gives birth to a large (3,000 gram) infant with severely premature lungs. The infant is given oxygen therapy and subsequently becomes a mystery case: his profusion is poor, he cannot be weaned from the respirator, and he is extremely lethargic, as if asleep. After three weeks, the infant is still on 90 percent oxygen and tests show brain damage. The mother is a frequent visitor, often expressing her guilt about the infant's condition. The father is a department store janitor. They have three other children and a long history of dependence on welfare. One of their children requires monthly out-patient visits at the hospital for a cardiac condition.

The nursing and social-work staff consider this a problem family because they are "high users" of social services. The mother is described as "pushy" because she frequently questions the purpose of tests and treatment. The nurses also feel she is too rough in handling the infant. The father is characterized as aloof. After six weeks the mother consults a fortune teller who predicts the infant will "wake up" soon. The prediction appears to come true, but the infant has chronic lung disease and signs of serious neurological damage. After more than two months in the Level III nursery, this infant is transferred to a neurological division within the same hospital for an additional seven weeks of care before going home with a portable respirator.

Case Three: The Absent Family

A nineteen-year-old mother gives birth to an infant just under 1,000 grams. She is a secretary in a small computer company; her husband, age twenty, is an unemployed mechanic. They live sixty miles from the hospital where their son is being treated for prematurity. The maternal grandmother's telephone is the only way these parents can be reached. They give their consent by phone to having the child included in a cardiac research program, and the infant is operated on for a heart defect (*patent ductus arteriosus*) common among premature infants. After two weeks the parents visit briefly. The infant proves difficult to feed and does not grow. After three weeks he is still on the respirator and intravenous line. The primary nurse describes the mother as having "a low stress tolerance" and as needing encouragement when she telephones to ask about the infant. The parents are difficult to reach and do not visit the nursery. With little information to go on, the staff finds it difficult to assess this family.

After a month, this newborn is also described as a mystery, subject to apnea attacks as well as chronic abdominal distension that could signal bowel infection. The medical staff vacillates between two goals: weaning the infant from the respirator and starting oral feeding. Meanwhile, the infant develops problems from the prolonged use of the endotracheal tube. After five weeks, the condition of the infant stabilizes, and he is moved to a more remote part of the nursery where he is seldom touched or spoken to. At seven weeks, he is transported back to the hospital where he was born, which is close to where his parents live.

ORGANIZATIONAL DETERMINANTS OF THE PARENTAL ROLE

Individual psychologies aside, the participation of parents in newborn hospital care is generally structured by organizational determinants to which all families, normal or deviant, are subject. The first important determinant is the regionalization of neonatal intensive-care services. The second is the development of these services as the basis for progress in fetal and newborn medicine.

The regionalization of newborn intensive care refers to the transport of emergency cases from community or local hospitals to central hospitals that house nurseries capable of giving prolonged maximum diagnosis and treatment to critically ill newborns. The regional structure of the service was developed as an efficiency measure during the 1970s. The rationale was that it was more practical to transport patients to a small number of high-technology centers than to duplicate many of these costly centers in community hospitals (Sugarman 1979).

The result has been widespread availability of transport to newborn intensive care centers, many of which are staffed with specialized personnel and have new technologies and refurbished or expanded space. In the United States, over 250,000 newborns receive intensive care each year.

Most NICU patients, however, spend only a few days in maximum care. The mortality rate in a Level III nursery can range from 10 to 30 percent of admissions, and most of these deaths take place within a week. Many surviving infants have only brief stays as their conditions stabilize and they no longer need maximum care. This does not necessarily mean that their hospital careers are over; for many it is likely to continue in another hospital or hospital division. Commonly, infants are returned from the Level III unit to the hospital nursery from which they were referred. A small minority of newborns, often those with severe congenital anomalies or surgically correctible problems, are sent to other pediatric service divisions. Long-term problem cases, such as those described above, defy the normal admission-discharge pattern. They may be only 10 percent of a unit's admissions, but they can account for as many bed days and charges as the other 90 percent of admitted patients (Guillemin and Holmstrom, 1983).

This skewed pattern in length of stay makes it difficult for the staff to know many parents, except for those whose infants stay for a long time in the nursery. It also makes it difficult for parents to learn about the treatment their infants receive. In fact, as regionalized newborn intensive care has expanded, the role of the parents is one of diminishing influence at the critical junctures when important clinical decisions must be made. Put simply, parents tend to have either a marginal role or become managed as psychological patients.

Additionally, unlike local practitioners and community hospitals, major units in large medical centers have no vested interest in maintaining good relations with patients. This fact is demonstrated in the always secondary and often erratic attention given to parents. Unit nurses are often caught between the heavy technical demands of infant intensive care and their professional concern for families. Psychological and social-work support for families varies greatly from one hospital and unit to the next. The initiation of parent support groups, for example, frequently relies on an individual staff psychologist; if that one professional leaves, such initiatives often cease.

The contribution of neonatologists—the senior physicians in the NICU — to parent-staff relations is also uneven. Many neonatologists are concerned that parents be satisfied with the service. Yet professional rewards go to those physicians and units demonstrating medical competence, which is measured in improved survival rates and active research, not in parent satisfaction. Perhaps as a function of the bureaucratization of newborn care, practitioners now appear to be more willing to call a lawyer if parents disagree with them about treatment then they were a decade ago (Guillemin 1985).

The development of NICUs as the basis for progress in neonatal medicine also structures the participation of parents in their critically ill infant's care. There is a widespread reluctance among pediatricians to acknowledge that the immediate successes with survival rates brought about by effective emergency treatment do not automatically translate into long-term good outcomes. The time frame for treatment in a Level III nursery is so contracted that practitioners usually do not have the leeway to reflect on what happens later to the very premature newborn who survives the first few weeks of crisis. That the infant of less than 1,500 or 1,000 or even 500 grams does survive is interpreted as progress, which, from a purely medical standpoint, it is. Yet, recent national-level comparative research shows that these infants are five times more likely to be rehospitalized in the first year of life than normal weight newborns (Shapiro et al. 1980, 1983). Data on long-term outcomes for critically ill infants and their parents are still scarce. Followup programs that track NICU graduates are more often offered as an optional service to families than supported as essential feedback on the results of treatment decisions. With some exceptions, data on survivors are impressionistically reported to justify continued exploration of the treatment of extremely premature newborns (Budetti et al. 1981). Many neonatologists, therefore, must currently conjecture the outcomes of fundamentally experimental cases. The ability of parents to cope with such problems as cerebral palsy, blindness, and severe mental handicap is considered beyond the medical practitioner's ken.

Yet because of pediatric treatment decisions, parents today have certain new risks attached to bearing children. One is that a very premature infant who might have died in the delivery room ten or even five years ago is likely to be treated aggressively and to survive for ten days or more: that is, death is merely put off. A second risk is that an infant transported to newborn intensive care will survive but with serious iatrogenic problems, such as chronic lung disease from respirator therapy. And a third risk is that the infant who might have died if born a decade ago will survive needing a lifetime of therapy, family support, or institutionalization.

If parents are advised of these risks and are willing to take them in return for the benefits of newborn survival, they have the authority to consent to the full panoply of medical interventions that come with hospital birth. The problem is that many parents are not informed of these risks but are instead reassured by referring obstetricians and pediatricians that "everything possible will be done" in the event of a medical emergency. In addition, since prematurity accounts for most NICU admissions, a certain percentage of mothers at high risk for premature births—teenagers, nonwhites, and the educationally and economically disadvantaged—are unlikely to receive any advance information about hospital options because they often receive no prenatal care (Institute of Medicine 1985). The scenario, then, for many parents is that they are misinformed or uninformed about the risks and benefits attached to newborn intensive care, especially for very low birthweight infants, those with serious multiple anomalies, or even those of normal birthweight with, for example, severe asphyxia.

PSYCHOLOGICAL VERSUS STRUCTURAL CONSTRAINTS

To return to our original question about whether therapy or organizational change will improve the advocate role of parents, it is apparent from the discussion above that the organizational imperatives of regionalization and progressive neonatal medicine are such strong influences on behavior that they risk the misapplication of therapeutic investments aimed at parental psychological distress. They do this by forcing nurses and other staff members to deal with parents as threats to an infant's well-being rather than as co-caretakers of the infant.

If families are traumatized by the birth of a newborn with medical problems, the psychological intervention may be helpful and should be available to them.

Most parents whose infants are transferred to a Level III nursery, however, have only fleeting communications with the staff, who thus are unable to judge the extent of parental trauma. Nurses, psychologists, and social workers invest most of their time and attention in a few difficult, long-term cases, exactly parallel to the enormous medical investment which such difficult, long-term cases receive. Indeed, the parents of such infants inevitably need this psychological support. From one point of view, the deployment of therapists in Level III units is the fulfillment of the NICU's responsibility to address the needs it has created or deepened by aggressively treating such difficult cases.

From a more critical perspective, a conservative function of social-psychological services in NICU is the management of parents as patients to allow physicians a freer hand in making clinical decisions. This may seem a harsh judgment of professionals who are intent on ameliorating the pain of distressed families. Yet, there is in this context a question of advocacy, not unlike that of psychologists working with Vietnam veterans and having to decide the degree to which the patient was deviant or the institutions and goals of that war absurd (Lifton 1979). NICU nurses and consulting therapists answer to physicians. In this subordination, endemic to hospital organization, lies the potential for the instrumental use of the psychological-case approach to promote the aims of medicine, which may not always be in the ultimate best interests of either infants or their families.

SOLUTIONS TO STRUCTURAL PROBLEMS

The rapid development of newborn intensive care testifies to professional and public perception that there is a need for this kind of service. The limits of the system, those related to clinical results, parental authority, and overall cost, are only now beginning to be felt. How is it possible to modify newborn intensive care so that the advantages of regionalization and progressive neonatal medicine are retained and their worst effects eliminated?

There are basically three solutions that, in combination, would continue access to emergency care for newborns in medical need but better sustain the advocacy role of parents. In brief, they are (1) a renewed emphasis on prenatal care so that rates of premature birth decline; (2) the education of community-hospital physicians and nurses in the techniques of intensive care; and (3) a scrupulous evaluation of clinical outcome so as to educate both physicians and parents in the probable risks of treatment decisions.

Although the first of these solutions has been advised by any number of panels and committees, it has had little effect on United States health policy. The segment of our population most likely to be without any health insurance is young people between nineteen and twenty-five, including, of course, many disadvantaged women during their years of maximum childbearing. These are the women who are least likely to obtain adequate prenatal care and most likely to have premature and/or low birthweight infants. Yet, as more than one neonatologist said, "Sharply reduce premature birth, and intensive care for newborns becomes unnecessary." It is clear that the choice in this country has been to attack premature birth after it happens rather than to try to prevent it from happening. This choice reflects a cultural refusal to take a long and comprehensive look at health care. The extent to which federal and state governments can be persuaded to support universal prenatal care will have a beneficial impact on newborn intensive care by reducing premature births and generally improving birthweights.

The second solution, to improve emergency care at the local level may already be taking place, as the current surplus of pediatricians makes them more open to hospital employment as neonatologists. Level III nurseries are equipped to handle a range of cases, from slightly premature infants to infants who should formally be classified as experimental cases. If local hospitals could competently treat a greater proportion of the less severely afflicted infants, neither parents nor their newborns would be subject to the strains of transport and separation. Care would have to be taken to avoid the costly duplication of proliferating technologies that regionalization was intended to avoid, but certainly local and community hospitals could, with properly trained staff, handle less severe cases. Unfortunately, the impetus of the federal "Baby Doe Directive" has been to increase the incentives for local hospitals and nurseries to refer newborns to Level III nurseries. Indeed, to protect infants against medical neglect, the phrasing of the rule virtually required sustained aggressive intervention for all newborns not actually brain dead or dying (Rhoden and Arras 1985). If local practitioners and institutions want to avoid the onus of a difficult decision, while assurring parents that "everything possible is being done," referral to a Level III nursery is an effective short-term strategy. But it may not be a strategy that is in the best interests of either the infant or the family.

The third way to improve newborn intensive care is to extend short-term perspectives on treatment decisions so that the actual outcome, its risks and benefits, can be better predicted. There is some leadership among neonatologists in this direction (Stahlman 1984), but much work needs to be done in following up the records of infants after they are discharged from the NICU. Physicians, obstetricians, and pediatricians who refer infants to intensive care need to be better educated. If physicians were more balanced in their estimates of the value of newborn intensive care, NICUs would be used differently. If parents were advised of the benefits and risks of referral, they would be in a better position to evaluate referral and treatment decisions. The basic problem with the current role of parents in the NICU is that they are less prepared for institutional and professional responses to delivery-room problems than they might be. Thus, information about the benefits and risks of referral must be provided as part of parents' prenatal education.

Ultimately, parents bear the responsibility for their evaluation of and response to referral and treatment possibilities, not simply for a brief period of emotional turmoil, but potentially for a lifetime—their own, the infant's, and those of their other children and family members. The professional urge may be to treat parents as patients, but this approach diverts attention from the larger responsibilities of the parental role and from the larger responsibilities of health institutions and personnel towards newborns and their families.

13

THE ARTIFICIAL WOMB: SOCIAL AND SENSORY ENVIRONMENT OF LOW BIRTHWEIGHT INFANTS

Lucile F. Newman

The term *artificial womb* refers to the technology of intervention in the care of very low birthweight infants. Through the use of the incubator, neonatal intensive care has been successful in enabling the survival of infants previously considered too small to survive. A cultural form itself, this setting provides an opportunity to observe human activities at the very edge of existence. This chapter begins with a description of participant observation in the special-care nursery and views the incubator as a social environment. The social and sensory environment studies are described and findings presented, with special reference to the impact of this environment on the preterm infant.

NEONATAL INTENSIVE CARE AS A SOCIAL ENVIRONMENT

My participant observation in the special-care nursery began in a clinical clerkship in neonatology with fourth-year medical students. A clerkship of this nature is an immersion experience of six weeks duration, with both day and night service. The twelve hour day in the nursery includes: observation of delivery of high risk infants; joining the ambulance team for transport of low birthweight infants from other hospitals; rounds at 8 A.M. and 4 P.M. to monitor the progress of each of the thirty to thirty-five infants in the unit at any time; participation in decision-making meetings on particular problems; and attendance at pathology examinations and autopsies. In addition, I participated in the life of the nursery, a thick social group united by the life-and-death atmosphere as well as the boundedness of the unit within the hospital. The intensity of this experience, the commitment of staff, students, and family to the care of very ill infants, the fragile and constantly changing condition of the infants, and the human histories unfolding daily: all create a bond among those involved that formed the social context for ethnographic observation. Of particular importance are the values and symbols present in this context.

The intensive-care environment is made up of multiple overlapping action patterns—individuals with different roles and different values. The action patterns are visible in the rhythms of the nursery. The most visible and audible is the shift rhythm of the nurses. The nursing staff organize their lives around the twenty-four-hour needs of the nursery by working in shifts. In this nursery, as in most, there are eight-hour shifts beginning at 7 A.M., 3 P.M., and 11 P.M., with a few minutes of overlap around those times when the nurse going off duty transfers instructions and information to the nurse coming on duty. It is a job of constant care. For them, the infants are individuals rather than cases. Their insistence on the individuality of each infant, by sex and by name, and their special loyalties to particular infants seen as attractive or as "fighters" symbolize their daily involvement with the unit as a whole.

A second rhythm is the medical one beginning with rounds at 8 A.M. and 4 P.M., with instructions for care being carried out directly afterward. The coming and going of house doctors other than during their rounds is tied to admissions and the clinical condition of particular infants in the nursery. One of the main values of medicine, in general, and intensive care, in particular, is the value of being "on call." The prime symbol of medical commitment is the subversion of one's own human needs, sleep, food, or social life, to the immediate needs of the patient at risk. The omnipresent "beeper," the instant response to a monitor alarm, the middle-of-the-night call, the proudly bleary-eyed dutiful presence at 8 A..M. rounds, are all indications of the commitment and the willingness to make the care of others one's first obligation. The route of care is scientific. The language is of blood values, hematocrits, oxygen and CO_2 levels, and respiratory requirements. Expected to maintain research productivity, the doctors' interest is often in the new cases, the new problems presented, and the new opportunities for solving them, as well as their own ongoing research.

A third rhythm is the random admission and discharge of infants from the unit. A counterpoint rhythm of visiting parents clusters at mid-afternoon and early evening. Much encouraged by nursing staff involvement with their infant as an individual, parents are often put off by medical staff reference to scientific and objectified risk factors or statistical probabilities. As parents' fear abates, the first acknowledgment of possible survival occurs when they bring siblings in to see the baby. A next level of relief is symbolized on the day of taking the first pictures. Later still, a clear indication of their expectation of survival occurs when they bring clothes (not "hospital clothes") that belong to their baby alone (Newman 1980). In this process, most parents slowly establish personhood for their infant and begin preparation for care at home. During this time, many parents find that support groups are helpful.

The tone of audible rhythms is set by the twenty or so heart-rate monitors and the sounds of respirators and incubators—a mechanical background against which the sounds of human rhythms are set. Physicians, nurses, and parents all respond according to their own roles in the endeavor.

THE INTENSITY OF INTENSIVE CARE

The neonatal intensive care nursery is a workplace and a location for research that can be stressful for those who work there. Jones (1982) has described the work situation through interviews with nursing staff. While their expressed feelings were positive about the value of their work, they were concerned about their feelings of inadequacy when faced with distressed parents and their feelings of anger at the demeanor of some house staff toward them. Marshall and Kasman (1982) have written of nurse "burn-out" in intensive care nurseries resulting from the continual pressure of every action seemingly having a life-or-death significance. Focusing mainly on house staff and fellows, Brody and Klein (1980) describe the intensive care nursery as a small society and concern themselves with the hierarchical structure and competitive nature of research pediatrics. For nursing and medical staff, knowledge that one is performing painful procedures without anesthetic can in itself be a stressful experience. The fact that it is done for the ultimate benefit of the infant necessitates a constant concentration on outcome and a certain degree of denial of present pain.

THE SOCIAL AND SENSORY ENVIRONMENT STUDIES

My acquaintance with the nursery raised questions about the life of preterm infants in such an environment. Decisions about the resuscitation and care of newborns, particularly those on the edge of viability, require speed and certainty of action for the infant's survival (Jonsen and Garland 1976). These functions are accomplished in modern intensive care nurseries not only with the use of incubators and warmers, but with the added assistance of heart-rate and respiration monitoring, intravenous nutrition, and all of the biochemical analyses and technical armamentarium of modern medicine. These interventions, beneficial for survival, intervene also in the establishment of some of the most important relationships in the life of an infant. Moreover, such nurseries are bounded communities with rules for professional staff behavior and sometimes stereotypic relations with the "outside" world of parents.

The origin of the Social and Sensory Environment Study was in the question: What is the life experience of an infant in an incubator? Current studies into the effects of life in an incubator indicate improved survival (Vohr and Hack 1982) and a very specialized environment and perhaps a specializing response (Newman 1981). The studies described in this chapter have focused particularly on the quantity and quality of human interaction available to the infant in intensive care. The method of analysis involves the searching out and analyzing of readily observable environmental and behavioral factors affecting the low birth-weight infant, including both human interaction and other aspects of the incubator environment (Newman 1980, 1981, 1983, 1986).

The life experience of preterm infants in a special care nursery appears to be markedly different from that of infants in a normal nursery. Preterm infants are small, developmentally immature, and at risk. They are isolated in incubators.

Their clinical condition and the therapeutic measures taken to assure their survival take precedence over human interaction; the latter, though regular, may be characterized by invasive procedures and sometimes by impersonal handling. Full-term infants, on the other hand, are not isolated and experience regular interaction, characterized by feeding, holding, talking, and other forms of positive personal communication. It was the objective of the Social and Sensory Environment Studies to observe and describe in detail the surroundings and the behavior of low birthweight infants who live for an extended period of time in the constructed environment of the incubator.

Using direct observation according to precoded behavioral categories, along with tape recording and physiological monitoring, we described in depth the tactile experience and auditory environment for ten very low birthweight infants, that is, those born under 1500 grams, and assessed what kinds of human interaction are experienced under these conditions. We sought an ethnography of the particular natural setting of the nursery, recognizing that a neonatal intensive care unit is a cultural artifact in itself, the incubator an artificial womb, and that we were observing human beings—premature newborns—who were socialized to no other external environment, no other existence.

THE SENSORY ENVIRONMENT OF LOW BIRTHWEIGHT INFANTS

Tactile Stimulation. Individual differences in very low birthweight infants create a fine line between too little handling and too much handling. An example of an often unnoticed response to human interaction can be found in breathing inconsistencies, such as apnea and bradycardia. Heart-rate monitors are usually set to alarm when a reduction of heart rate occurs that is inconsistent with effective breathing. The lowered heart rate and stopped or intermittent breathing compromises circulation, reduces oxygen, and increases carbon dioxide in the blood. Inefficient oxygenation on a continuing basis, or hypoxia, threatens brain function. Studies of handling in the nursery by transcutaneous oxygen monitoring indicate that certain infants are sensitive to handling and suffer an oxygen reduction when handled (Long, Philip, and Lucey 1980). In our first study, individual patterns of apnea after handling were found for two of ten infants. Two different patterns were demonstrated. One is that of Baby A, whose seven apneic episodes in twenty-four hours on Day 3 all occurred within one minute after handling by parents or nurses. A second pattern is exemplified by Baby B. His thirty-six apneic episodes during a twenty-four hour period on Day 3 show peaks during times of most caregiving activity in the nursery—after morning rounds at 8 A.M. and afternoon rounds at 4 P.M.

On the other hand, carefully modulated touching can be beneficial to very low birthweight infants. Stroking and massage are not generally a part of medical attention or nursing routine. This is an activity usually carried out by parents (or researchers). Field (n.d.) has described a study in which light stroking and passive movement of extremities were carried out periodically for ten days.

At the end of this time, the stroked infants weighed more than the controls who had had routine care. They scored better on the Neonatal Behavioral Assessment Scale and required fewer days of hospitalization. Some infants in our studies also engaged in tactile self-stimulation by touching the surfaces available to them within the incubator (Newman 1981). In addition, we found that infants regularly visited by their families regained birth weight faster than nonvisited infants, though there were no differences in interaction time of nursing care for visited or nonvisited infants.

Interaction. Interaction with parents also makes up part of the infant's sensory world. At the present time, most neonatal intensive care nurseries in North America are open and encouraging to parents. Indeed, one of the key criteria for discharge is staff perception that the parents are ready to take charge of the care of their infant. But the environment of the intensive care nursery can be intimidating. As Jerome Bruner once noted, "The degree to which a society elaborates a technology determines the amount of division of labor in the society. The rationale of technology is that its tools are not such that each individual can be equipped with a full set of them. With technological advance more things are possible, but social and technical organization is increasingly necessary to bring them off" (1979:80). In intensive care, this specialization serves to exclude parents from primary knowledge of the techniques of their infant's care.

In our studies, about half of the infants in intensive care were visited by parents. Compared with other studies, this is a comparatively high visitation rate. Whether because of distance, other child-care responsibilities, the sense of having no role in the nursery, or detachment from the possibility of death or disability, parents often feel ill at ease. I have described elsewhere the polarities of "coping through commitment" by those parents who come often, stay long, and impose themselves on their infant's care, and "coping through distance" by those parents who "will get to know him when he comes home" (Newman 1980: 188). Human interaction for these latter infants is often routine, intrusive, and impersonal. Staff time averages from 7-11 minutes per hour. (Much of the care, preparation, paperwork, etc., does not involve interaction.) Our tapes indicate that voices are not audible inside an incubator unless directed inside. Several studies have been concerned with the lack of patterned sensory input for these infants; tactile, aural, and visual stimulation occur separately for them (Newman 1981; Gottfried et al. 1981). If parents do not visit, for the first weeks of life the infant may be isolated from human interaction of a social nature or from the consistent sound of human voices.

CONCLUSION

There is nothing intrinsic to technology that requires the dehumanization of environments. It does, however, require an act of will to create a humane environment under such circumstances. Problems of impersonal care related to therapeutic measures in intensive care have been identified in many studies. They can occur in any area of technical expertise—that is, by concentrating on mechanical and electronic equipment, staff tend to be oblivious to the effects of people in the unit.

The questions posed by the Social and Sensory Environment Studies relate to the life of the infant in an incubator. The auditory environment and handling of low birthweight infants create social experiences that are different from those of the fetus of the same gestational age still *in utero* or from the social and sensory environment of normal-weight infants.

The artificial womb which sustains these infants exists in an environment stressful both to parents and to those who work there. Yet, within that environment there is also a pervasive sense of involvement and of confidence in scientific effectiveness. This ethnography of environmental factors in the special care nursery suggests that attention to the human needs of staff and parents, as well as of the infants, provides a way to relieve some of the intensity of intensive care, at the same time creating an environment conducive to optimum development of infants at risk.

NOTE

The clerkship (1978) and resulting research (1978–86) was supported by the Department of Pediatrics, Brown University, and a grant from the Rhode Island Chapter, March of Dimes Birth Defects Foundation. Grateful acknowledgment is made to Dr. William Oh, Pediatrician-in-Chief, Women and Infants Hospital of Rhode Island, for both support and encouragement, and to the staff and parents of the Special Care Nursery during these years for their good will and continuing help in these studies.

SECTION IV

BECOMING A PARENT

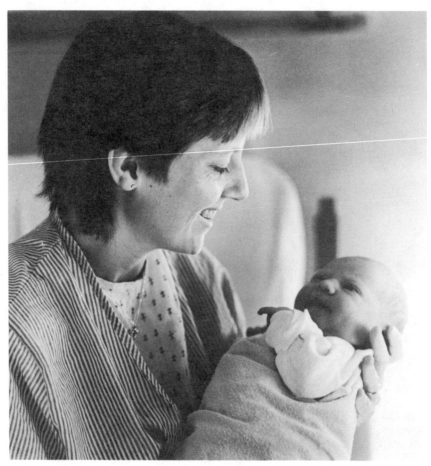

Photograph by LeRoy J. Dierker, Jr., M.D.

BECOMING A PARENT

*Never have I known such exhaustion. Never. I'm too tired
to get out of bed to go to the bathroom. I'm too tired to
ask for soup or tea. I'm too tired to drink it when it's
brought.... Every two and a half hours you're brought in
to me. I walk to the rocking chair. You feed for at least
an hour. I crawl back into bed.... How can I protect you
in my weakened state?.... I need to return to my senses
slowly, properly.... What if I had to do the cooking, and
I felt like this? What if I had another baby tugging at
me, and I felt like this? What if I couldn't afford to pay
someone to help me, and I felt like this? What if I didn't
have your father home with me? What if I did, and it
only meant that I had to cook his dinner too?*
— *Phyllis Chesler, With Child*

*Why isn't more said about the sensuousness between
mother and baby? His waking hours infuse my life with a
steady sensuous pleasure. The growing mutual familiarity,
the sensations I get each time I pick him up, the good
feeling I get of his heft, his smell...and the feel of
him—we merge into one another giving and taking heat,
comfort and love....Love doesn't come from the child's
cooing and smiling....Love comes gradually with our
worry, relief and care—with what we have invested of
ourselves. We must learn the loving of a first child step
by step....*
— *Frances Karlen Santamaria, Joshua Firstborn*

Even for infants not in crisis, the postpartum period is critical for healthy infant
development. Breisemeister and Haines and Trevathan return to the biological
commonalities that characterize newborns and their parents. The human infant,
because of the genetic selection for large brain capacity along with the need to
pass through the narrow birth canal of an upright walking mother, is born at a
point of immaturity and vulnerability uncommon in the animal world. Left on
its own, neglected or abandoned, the newborn infant would not long survive.
Thus, for human beings to survive as a species, that vulnerable infant must be
cared for until it can exist on its own.

The period of relative helplessness extends far beyond the early postpartum
and through the first years of a child's life. The human infant thus must rely on

others to care for it, and, as Breisemeister and Haines point out, the infant has attractive behaviors that make adults—particularly its parents—want to care for it. Parental response to the newborn, however, is culturally determined. In American society, the baby's first cry after delivery is greeted with joy; in other cultures the joy is postponed until delivery of the afterbirth, in recognition that up until this point the woman may still be in danger. In some cultures, the gender of the infant may temper the joy of its birth.

Some postpartum contexts appear to be more conducive to the development of an adequate support system for the newborn. Once again the midwifery model of postpartum care is contrasted with the medical management of that period, as seen in the postpartum experiences described by Trevathan and Briesemeister and Haines. Here, too, socioeconomic differences come into play, for few low-income women have real choices as to where they will give birth and spend the early postpartum period. The infants of such women, often ill or premature, are already more susceptible to potential abuse and neglect than those of economically well-off women, and the lack of opportunity to form a strong bond at birth may further inhibit the development of a strong, positve parent-infant relationship.

It is not only the infant, however, who needs a strong support system during the postpartum period. In contemporary American society, postpartum adjustment is often difficult. Increasingly, women and their infants leave the hospital a short time after birth, often within twenty-four hours. They come home to added responsibilities and to new and redefined social relationships. Particularly for those women who work, the transition to the new maternal role is difficult. Unlike most other societies, in North America there is no clearly defined reintegration of mother and child into society. As Davis-Floyd points out in Chpater 10, hospital ritual alienates women from their own intrabody experience of birth, and when they return home mothers must often recover not only from the physical interventions into the birth process (episiotomy, anesthesia, cesarean section), but also from the assault on their emotions and personal sense of worth. There are no prescribed attendants to help care for the woman during her recovery or provide her with assistance and knowledge on how to care for the new infant. Women with adequate economic resources may be able to hire help for the early postpartum period; others may have mothers, mothers-in-law, or sisters who can come to help. But poor women are often left alone to cope with their new roles and responsibilities. Both Michaelson and Whiteford examine the pressures on women in the process of family formation in this context.

Critical to successful adjustment to motherhood is the presence of a social network of friends and kin who support the new mother in her maternal role. Morse and her coauthors also indicate that support, particularly from the husband, is necessary for a women to successfully breastfeed her infant. The lack of social support among the socioeconomically disadvantaged, noted by the authors in the first section of this book, contributes to the low rate of breastfeeding and high rate of maladaptation to the maternal role among poor women.

Poor adjustment to parent roles is not an exclusive province of the poor, however. The widespread existence of child abuse and neglect crosses class lines and is indicative of the breakdown of support systems in many parts of American society. More active intervention in creating a context for positive parent-child relationships may be necessary. While some changes in medical practice have already taken place, including a concern for early parent-infant contact, rooming-in of baby with mother, and encouragement of breastfeeding, such changes are limited to the early postpartum and are often less available to the poor. The difficult period of adjustment to the infant in the home context, the need to change routines, and perhaps even to change one's self-concept, are largely ignored. Because the human infant remains vulnerable for a prolonged period, long-term parent-infant adjustment is essential. The notion of "successful reproductive outcome" does not end with the delivery of a healthy infant, but continues into the maintenance of the infant's well-being as he or she develops.

14

CHILDBIRTH IN A BICULTURAL COMMUNITY: ATTITUDINAL AND BEHAVIORAL VARIATION

Wenda R. Trevathan

Although a complete study of birth in any culture must consider many factors, we can, for the moment, assume that the phylogenetic and some of the broader ontogenetic factors are more or less the same for all women and infants. Beyond this, however, the variation in experience and attitudes regarding childbirth is wide, both within and between cultures. In order to examine some of the variation, in 1978 I undertook a nine-month study of Hispanic and Anglo women giving birth with lay midwives in a maternity center in El Paso, Texas. The initial impetus for doing the study was a series of papers describing universal or "species specific" behaviors exhibited by human mothers interacting with their newborn babies. Most of the studies had been conducted in hospital settings in the United States and in Western Europe. Although excited about the studies, the anthropologist in me questioned the validity of ascribing universality to a series of behaviors observed in circumstances far from universal and on relatively small and homogeneous samples. I thus selected a study sample that would include women of various ethnic backgrounds who gave birth in a home-like setting under circumstances more typical, perhaps, of those under which women have given birth for generations past and in most parts of the world today.

EL PASO AND THE BIRTH CENTER

El Paso is located in western Texas on the Rio Grande, which at that point forms the border between the United States and Mexico. Across the river from El Paso is Juaréz, Mexico, the largest Mexican border city (population approximately 570,000 in 1980). The entire Juaréz-El Paso metropolitan area has a population of close to one million. The Birth Center (TBC) where this study was conducted is located in downtown El Paso in *Segundo Barrio,* an area of predominantly lower-class Hispanic residents. It is less than a mile from the bridge that leads into Mexico.

According to the director of The Birth Center and most midwives, birth is not a political issue, so their services are offered to anyone, regardless of legal residence status. Potential clients are only required to be committed to breast-feeding their infants. Because of its location and the extremely low cost of maternity care, most of the clients at TBC are Hispanic, and most speak little or no English. Often the women who came here to receive prenatal care crossed the border for exams on "shoppers' passes," and some arrived in labor after having crossed the river border in the middle of the night. After delivering, a number of mothers and infants were never seen again for follow-up care, a fact presumably related to difficulties in crossing the border.

Many of the TBC clients had never received any prenatal care during previous pregnancies. Since it seemed unlikely that they would seek care elsewhere, many women accepted by the midwives would be considered high risk and unacceptable to alternative birth centers elsewhere in the United States. Women with uncontrolled diabetes, pre-eclampsia, active syphillis, and severe pelvic abnormalities were referred to physicians for hospital delivery. Previous cesarean section, abnormal presentation, multiple pregnancy, Rh-negative blood factor, grand multiparity, and age were not reasons to exclude a woman from care at TBC, though these women were monitored more closely during pregnancy and labor for signs that hospitalization was necessary. Women as young as thirteen and as old as fifty-one have delivered at the center, as have fifty-four breech presentations, twenty-eight sets of twins, twenty-four previous cesarean sections, and women with as many as thirteen children. (Recently, however, the midwives in El Paso have experienced more restrictions on their practice. Thus, many of the women who were acceptable as clients at the time this study took place would no longer be allowed to be attended by midwives.)

Between June 1978 and December 1983 (excluding May–December 1982), 3,018 women registered for prenatal care at TBC; 2,885 subsequently delivered there and 163 were referred to hospital care before or during labor (see Table 1). Eighty-one of the women who delivered in the hospital underwent cesarean section, representing less than three percent of the entire sample. Maternal mortality during this period was zero, fourteen infants were stillborn, and eleven died during the neonatal period (i.e., the first twenty-eight days after birth). Most complications during labor and delivery were handled by the midwives, though women were transported to the hospital for a number of reasons, including placenta previa, cephalopelvic disproportion, abruptio placenta, failure to progress, cord prolapse, malpresentation, and premature rupture of the membranes. Twenty-five infants were hospitalized after birth for reasons including respiratory distress syndrome (RDS), prematurity, meconium aspiration, congenital defects, and shock. Delivery outcome was usually much more positive: at five minutes, 80 percent of the infants had Apgar scores greater than 8. Postpartum hemorrhage was somewhat common (12 percent of the

TABLE 1. Summary of TMC Births: June 1978 to December 1983

		Percent
Total number of births	3,018	
Born with midwives	2,855	95
breech	54	
sets of twins	28	
Transport before birth	163	5
C-section	81	2.7
Postpartum transport of mother	16	
Neonatal transport	25	
Maternal Characteristics		
Hispanic	2,742	91
Anglo	253	14
Age		
under 18 years	373	12
19-25 years	1,594	53
26-30 years	667	22
31-40 years	343	11
over 40 years	22	
Marital status		
single	649	22
married	2,295	77
widowed or divorced	56	
Primiparas	1,018	34
More than 4 children	396	13
Fewer than 2 prenatal exams	240	8
More than 6 prenatal exams	2,310	77
No preparation classes	256	8
Complete series of classes	1,556	51
Infant Characteristics		
One minute Apgar greater than 8	1,068	37
Five minute Apgar greater than 8	2,250	79
Weight less than 6 pounds	285	10
Weight between 6 and 9 pounds	2,387	84
Male	1,508	
Female	1,464	

women lost more than four cups of measured blood). Only 119 (4 percent) episiotomies were performed.

MIDWIFERY TRAINING

The midwives associated with The Birth Center refer to themselves variously as "lay," "empirical," or "independent" midwives. In contrast to Certified Nurse Midwives, most of these women did not have medical background or training.

For the first six months of this study there were sixteen women involved in births at the center: eleven students (the director of TBC conducts a midwifery-training program), three interns, and two associate midwives. All were Anglo, and only four spoke Spanish fluently. The remainder had no facility with the language or could speak adequately for simple conversations. All had completed high school, six had completed college, and two had master's degrees. Their experience was variable; students who had never seen a birth enrolled in the program; whereas the director had had primary responsibility for more than 1,000 births. Typical of most lay midwives in this country today and unlike midwives of the past and from other cultures, they were relatively young, most being in their late twenties. Also, many had had no children, a characteristic unusual among midwives of the world.

In September 1978 I enrolled in the one year midwifery-training program at The Birth Center. Although one of my primary reasons for doing so was to gain as much insight into the birth process as possible, it was also a way of gaining access to the women whose deliveries I wanted to observe. Just as anthropologists find that they must become participants in the culture of the people they are observing, I felt that the only way to fully understand what was going on during labor, delivery, and the postpartum period was to immerse myself as thoroughly as possible in the process by training to become a midwife.

As a midwife trainee I took part in prenatal examinations and was able to interview prospective mothers about their willingness to participate in the study. Full participation required completing a personal-history questionnaire, allowing me to be present for labor, delivery, and one full hour after birth, and being available for followup at five days, two weeks, and four months postpartum. During the eight-month period over which the study was conducted, half of all those who delivered agreed to participate. I have little doubt that had I not been a midwife trainee, becoming a familiar figure at the birth center in the process, I would have had far fewer women agree to participate.

Additionally, my ability to make accurate observations at the time of delivery and to complete followup information depended very heavily on the other midwives with whom I worked. I entered the program with ten other women, and over the course of the training period most became supportive of my research. We endured many hardships, including infant deaths, the stress of the daily work schedule, hostility from the medical establishment and other midwives, lack of money, and the intense emotional aspects, both positive and negative, of every delivery.

Most importantly, however, the training enabled me to more accurately perceive and interpret events surrounding each delivery. Knowing what a woman was experiencing physically helped me to determine what was a normal reaction to labor and the range of variation acceptable within that definition. I had also been trained to understand emotional aspects of labor and delivery, and thus I could see that writhing and facial grimaces did not always mean unbearable pain but were part of the normal hard work necessary for delivering a child.

Finally, being trained as a midwife allowed me to witness the birth event not only as a *participant* observer but also as a *contributing* observer (Hazell 1974). Thus, if it became necessary, I could offer assistance to the laboring woman or to the attending midwives. In several instances, when extra hands were needed, I had to abandon my observations. As Hazell (1974) points out, however, becoming a contributing observer carries with it a much higher level of responsibility. Ethical questions that have plagued generations of anthropologists become even more complex when the researcher is a direct contributor to a cultural happening.

THE MOTHERS

Every woman who registered for prenatal care at The Birth Center and whose delivery was expected between October 1978 and May 1979 was informed of the "bonding study," as it was called by the midwives, and invited to participate. Since the initial prenatal examination took up to two hours, the information sheet on the study and the questionnaire requesting background information were given at a subsequent examination. Volunteers were also recruited during childbirth-education classes. In the eight-month period, 152 women agreed to be in the study, approximately 50 percent of all those who delivered during that time period. For various reasons, only 110 women were actually observed for behavior relating to birth and mother-infant interaction.

Eighty-two percent of the 110 women were of Hispanic background; 75.5 percent spoke only Spanish. It was not determined how many were Mexican citizens, naturalized United States citizens, or registered aliens. Many of the addresses on the birth certificates were in Juaréz, and a number of letters sent to El Paso addresses were returned by the post office, suggesting that some of these may have been only temporary or false.

Most of the Hispanic women had annual incomes of less than $3,000 and had fewer than six years of formal education. The Anglo women were typically of a higher socioeconomic class and most had at least a high school education. The demographic and other characteristics of the women who participated in the study are presented in Table 2. A greater percentage of Anglo women were married, though the differences between the two groups were not statistically significant. There were no significant differences between the two groups in parity, number of childbirth-education classes attended, or in attitude toward childbirth (i.e., fear, apprehension, excitement). The mean age for all women in the study was 23.1 (sd=4.7) with a range from 16 to 39, a median of 22.4, and a mode of 21. Mean maternal parity was 2, with a range from 1 to 9.

For most, finances were a primary reason to choose TBC. Clients were asked to make monetary contributions for services according to their incomes. The minimum was $150 based on an income of less than $3,000 per year. The maximum requested was $400 from those who estimated that they earned more than $11,000 per year. This fee covered all prenatal exams, all vitamins, childbirth-preparation classes, the delivery, and postpartum care. Most clients paid the minimum or nothing at all. Total costs at The Birth Center were about 15 percent of costs for prenatal care and delivery with area physicians. Also, most of the women who deliver at TBC have no health and maternity insurance coverage. Since income and occupation had some effect on why the center was chosen for the birth, this decision was not similar in frequency for the Hispanic and Anglo women.

TABLE 2. Characteristics of the Hispanic and Anglo Women, October 1978 to May 1979

	Hispanic(%)	Anglo(%)	X^2	Significance
Income				
<$3,000	*55 (81)	2 (12.5)	24.72	p <.00001
>$3,000	13 (19)	14 (87.5)		
Occupation				
Labor	54 (68)	3 (16)	15.30	p <.0001
Other	25 (32)	16 (84)		
Education				
Primary or less	45 (58)	1 (5)		
Secondary	29 (37)	11 (69)	24.46	p <.00001
Some college	4 (5)	8 (40)		
Reason for delivering with midwives				
Financial	42 (68)	5 (31)	5.63	p <.02
Philosophical	20 (32)	11 (69)		
Marital status				
Single	18 (21)	1 (5)	1.92	ns
Married	68 (79)	19 (95)		
Parity				
Primipara	42 (48)	8 (40)	.14	ns
Multipara	46 (52)	12 (60)		
Childbirth Education				
None	29 (36)	3 (17)	1.67	ns
Most classes	52 (64)	15 (83)		
Attitude toward Childbirth				
Fear	14 (20)	2 (12)		
Apprehensive	36 (52)	6 (35)	4.03	ns
Excitement	19 (28)	9 (53)		
Husband/boyfriend present at birth				
Yes	38 (43)	20 (100)	19.30	p <.00001
No	51 (57)	0		

* The total responses for each category vary because of missing data.

MOTHER-INFANT INTERACTION

Four mother-infant interaction behaviors were examined systematically during the first hour postpartum. These included those that had been previously described as universal to the species: preference for left-side holding of the infant (Salk 1970), orderly progression from fingertip touch of the infant's extremities to palmar massaging of infant's trunk (Rubin 1963; Klaus, Kennell, Plumb, and Zuehlke 1970), intense interest in eye-to-eye contact (Robson 1967; Klaus and Kennell 1976), and use of a high-pitched voice when talking to or toward the infant (Klaus and Kennell 1976).

To gather information to test the hypotheses that these were universal behaviors of human mothers, I observed these women during labor and delivery, plus a minimum of one hour after the birth of the infant. Observations were made behind a one-way mirror situated at the end of the bed on which the women delivered. Time sampling techniques were used to provide a continuous record of maternal touch in one ten-minute segment of the first hour after birth. A ten-second time unit was used as the basis of analysis, with observations beginning as soon after birth as the mother was able to devote most of her attention to the infant, and I could see well enough to make accurate observations. A stop-watch was used to record the number of minutes and seconds that a woman spent looking into the infant's face during the first hour.

A tape recorder was activated the moment the infant's head was born and continued until ten minutes after the actual birth time. The primary purpose of this was to record the mother's voice when talking to or toward her infant, with particular interest in pitch and verbal content. I also noted the side on which the mother first held the infant and any changes in positioning that occurred during the first hour.

Unless a woman requested otherwise, there were usually four midwives, including trainees, present for the actual delivery. Husbands were encouraged to attend the birth as were friends and other family members. Most women gave birth sitting on the bed supported by several pillows. Every infant was placed on the mother's abdomen immediately after birth and remained with her for at least the entire hour. As soon as possible, the family was left alone except for routine checks for uterine bleeding.

Analysis of the data that were gathered to test the hypotheses that these four behaviors are universal indicated that touch may be more variable than previously described. All mothers touched their infants during the first hour postpartum, but there was no evidence of progression from fingertip touch to palmar massaging (Trevathan 1981). The preference for left-side holding of the infant, speaking to the infant in a higher-than-normal pitch, and prolonged maintenance of eye contact during the first hour were confirmed in this study, though there were differences in all except lateral placement when the Hispanic and Anglo women were compared.

For purposes of between-group comparisons, maternal tactile behaviors were divided into three categories: passive holding of the infant; active finger and palmar exploring of the infant's body; and not holding or touching the infant at all, though the infant was still with the mother. Data were collected during a ten-minute period. The Anglo women averaged 38.5 percent of the ten minutes in active finger and palmar exploration and 0.5 percent of the time not touching or holding the infant at all. For the Hispanic women, the figures were 20 percent and 4 percent respectively.

En face orientation was measured for ninety-seven of the women during the entire first hour after birth. Anglo women averaged thirty minutes in the *en face* position, while Hispanic women averaged twenty-two minutes. All but two of the sixty-eight women for whom voice pitch was ascertained during the first hour after birth elevated the pitches of their voices when talking to or toward their infants. Two women, both Hispanic, did not change the voice pitch when the direction of speech switched from adults to infants. Forty-six (54 percent) of the Hispanic women talked actively to their infants during the first hour while sixteen (80 percent) of the Anglo women did so (X^2=4.47, p <.05).

Although audiotapes were obtained for sixty of the mother- infant "conversations" in this study, they have not yet been fully translated and analyzed. However, a few common phrases were noted. If the child was born with a name (i.e., a name had been selected before birth), he or she was usually addressed as such by the mother if she spoke English. Among the Spanish-speaking women, however, the baby would be talked *about* by name, but talked *to* as *"bebé,"* *"niño,"* or *"niña."* Other terms of endearment used by Hispanic women included *"mamacita,"* *"reinita,"* *"reina,"* *"hija,"* *"hijo,"* *"hijito,"* *"mi amor,"* and *"chiquita."* Concern for the infant's health and state was exhibited by Anglo and Hispanic women in such questions or statements as "Are you hungry?" *"Tiene hambre?"* "Don't cry," *"No llores,"* and "What do you want?" *"Qué quiere?"*

In almost all cases where the mother was a fluent speaker of both Spanish and English (N=7), she talked to her infant in Spanish and to the midwives in English, freely moving from one language to the other. The one exception to this was a Hispanic woman whose husband was German. Their common language was English, and she spoke to the infant in that language. During the first hour after this birth, there were phone calls from the father to his parents during which he spoke German and she spoke English, phone calls from the mother to her parents during which she spoke Spanish and he spoke English, and conversations among themselves (mother and father) and speech addressed to the infant, which were in English.

DISCUSSION

As described above, sociocultural background consistently emerged as a factor affecting maternal behavior. Since ethnic status was also correlated with income, occupation, and education, however, it is just as likely that the primary factors influencing behavior were poverty and a lower standard of living as they were differences in cultural background. The majority of Mexican women participating in the study were from a lower socioeconomic class, as indicated by income and occupation, were more likely to have chosen TBC because of its low-cost services, and had fewer years of formal education than the Anglo women who participated in this study. Confirmation of the significance of socioeconomic status in affecting postpartum behavior comes from those women of Mexican background who were also fluent speakers of English. These women had high school or greater education, tended to have incomes higher than $3,000, and most often chose TBC for philosophical, rather than financial, reasons. Their behavior during the immediate postpartum period more closely resembled the behavior of the Anglo mothers (who were largely of similar socioeconomic status) than that of the other Hispanic mothers.

In general, however, there were a number of maternal behaviors that were probably due to Mexican cultural influence rather than socioeconomic and educational factors. In Mexico and other nonindustrial, non-Western cultures, a woman's concept of maternity is largely shaped by her mother and other older women. This was evidenced in the current study by the forty-three mothers (48 percent of all Spanish speakers) who were with their daughters during labor and delivery. The importance of the new member to the extended family was also indicated by the number of other relatives who came to visit during the first hour after birth. In the traditional Mexican culture, childbirth is regarded as a natural event, and medical supervision is not deemed necessary in most circumstances. *Parteras*, or midwives, are called to aid in delivery and a *curandero* (traditional medical practitioner) is rarely consulted. Because of these attitudes, the type of care provided at The Birth Center was not very different from the way birth had been handled in previous generations of Mexican women who participated in the study. Most of the women had themselves been born at home or in a *clinica* with *parteras*. Perhaps the practice that required the most adjustment for these women was the midwives' encouragement of the husband's participation in childbirth-education classes and in the delivery itself. Very rarely did husbands accompany their wives to the classes, and they were present at the deliveries in only 43 percent of the cases.

Women in the dominant United States culture have concepts of maternity that are much more heavily influenced by books, professionals, and peers, than by the advice of their mothers and/or other older women. The tendency is to follow whatever is the current trend, whether it is to be completely pain-free birth, Dr. Spock's advice on child care, or back-to-the-earth, natural, organic, additive-free childbirth and child care. Currently, the trend in childbirth is to have the husband and siblings at the birth, and little emphasis is placed on any social group beyond the nuclear family. Husbands (or boyfriend, in the case of the one unmarried couple) were present at every Anglo birth in this study, and siblings were usually nearby, though they were not necessarily present for the actual birth. At only two of these births was there an older woman: one mother of the parturient and one mother-in-law. One new grandmother visited within an hour of the birth. There was, in addition to these three, a single exception to the nuclear family group: one young primiparous woman was accompanied in labor and delivery by her husband, her parents-in-law, her grandparents, her two brothers, her parents, and several friends. In addition, fifty minutes after birth, the woman's entire childbirth-education class came in for a visit.

Childbirth in the United States is considered to be an illness appropriately handled in the hospital. This accounts, in part, for the lack of visitation by older family members, who are often opposed to or unaware of the fact that their daughters are giving birth in the attendance of lay midwives. The high mobility of the Anglo population also partially explains this, though it is not uncommon for mothers to come from elsewhere to assist their daughters upon return from the hospital after childbirth. Moreover, the border population of Mexicans may also be as mobile as the dominant United States population, so mobility is not as likely an explanation for who attends birth as are attitudinal factors.

The incidence of postpartum depression also differed in the two groups. While the etiology of postpartum depression is uncertain, with physiological, psychological, biochemical and cultural factors implicated under various circumstances, the women who participated in this study lend support to the suggestion that postpartum depression is, to some extent, culturally dependent or defined. Of forty-eight women who answered a questionnaire about postpartum depression two weeks after birth, thirty-six were Spanish speaking and twelve were Anglo. It must be pointed out, however, that the English questions were slightly different from the Spanish questions. The English-speaking women were asked, "Have you been depressed since the baby was born?" The Spanish-speaking women were asked, *"Ha sentido desanimado desde qué nacio su bebé?"* which translates roughly as, "Have you felt discouraged, upset, or listless since the birth of your baby?" This difference may have affected the response. Still, 77 percent of the Spanish-speaking women said they had not been *desanimado*, and 23 percent said they had occasionally felt *desanimado* since the birth of their infant. Of the Anglo women, 17 percent said they had not been depressed, and 83 percent said they had been depressed. Although the numbers are small, the differences between the two language groups are statistically significant.

Other differences of an apparently cultural nature became apparent. Swaddling of the infant is a common practice in Mexican and several other cultures. Anglo women never even mentioned this practice, but Spanish-speaking women almost always wished to swaddle their infants. Approximately two-thirds of the latter group attempted to keep their infants covered during the first hour, compared to fewer than half of the Anglo women. One Mexican woman, in particular, after a midwife uncovered her infant briefly to examine it, got up out of bed, searched for and found a dry towel, and determinedly wrapped her infant tightly in it.

To the constant frustration of the midwives, many of the Mexican infants were brought to the center for follow-up care wrapped in several layers of clothes and blankets, even in the hottest summer months. A scolding by the midwife seemed to have little effect, since the infants would often return two weeks later just as tightly wrapped. This reflects the Mexican tendency to follow the "old ways" rather than seek out the latest trends. The Anglo women were anxious to follow all of the suggestions of the midwives and usually asked many more questions at the followup exam. This is, of course, partly due to the language differences, but it is also suggestive of the Mexicans' inclination to seek advice from relatives and the Anglos' inclination to seek advice from professionals and books. Although most of the books in the TBC lending library were in English, the few that were written in Spanish were rarely checked out by literate Spanish-speaking women. Almost every English- speaking woman had checked out or read one of the popular books on birth and child care.

Another common practice in Mexico is to give the infant *manzanilla* tea (*Matricaria chamomilla*), especially in the three days before the mother's milk comes in. The women who gave birth at The Birth Center were repeatedly advised against any supplemental feeding until breastfeeding was fully established, and they were particularly cautioned against the tea, which tends to make the infants somewhat lethargic. When home visits were made on the day following birth, the midwives often found that the tea was being given despite their admonitions against it. Although stronger negative sanctions were usually applied at that time, these were often ineffective as well, as the tea was often still being given at the five-day visit. Again, this is evidence that cultural norms often outweigh professional advice.

CONCLUSION

Hispanic and Anglo women appear to exhibit systematic differences in visual, verbal, tactile, and other behaviors associated with birth. However, it must be emphasized that, because the two groups of women differed in education and socioeconomic status, it cannot necessarily be concluded that the differences in behavior observed in the immediate postpartum period are attributable to ethnic differences.

The English-speaking women in this sample were probably not representative of the population from which they were derived, whereas the Hispanic women were more representative of the Mexican population. Most of the Anglo women had planned their pregnancies, almost all were married and were accompanied by their husbands/boyfriend, most chose to give birth with midwives for philosophical reasons, and most were highly motivated to bond to their infants and to do all the "right" things in the first few hours and days after birth.

The Hispanic women included those who were highly motivated by philosophical convictions about childbirth and those for whom the pregnancy was unplanned and the child unwanted, at least initially. A factor that undoubtedly contributed to the overall birth experience of the Mexican women was the different cultural background and language of the midwives who attended them. This, plus the presence of many kin right after the birth, probably accounts for the greater ease with which the women were distracted from focusing on their infants during the first hour. It required more concentration for a Spanish-speaking woman to respond to the advice or comments of the English-speaking midwife than it did for English-speaking women to respond to the same advice.

Certainly, many of the behavioral differences observed in these two groups of women can be attributed to growing up in two very different cultures. It is likely, however, that some of the variation is due to differences in education and socioeconomic status that characterize the two groups.

NOTE

Much of the material in this chapter appears in expanded form in Wenda Trevathan, *Human Birth: An Evolutionary Perspective* (Aldine de Gruyter, 1987).

15

THE INTERACTIONS OF FATHERS AND NEWBORNS

Linda H. Briesemeister and Beth A. Haines

Until very recently, the father's role during childbirth was extremely limited in American culture. He was expected to anxiously deliver his wife into the hands of medical practitioners and then to retreat to the fathers' waiting room, pacing continuously until the birth had taken place. He would then get a brief glimpse of baby and mother, rush off to buy cigars with the appropriate label, and announce the birth to all who would listen. Fathers were not allowed into delivery rooms for fear they might faint helplessly away at the supposedly horrifying sight of childbirth.

For the most part, things have changed considerably. Although some hospitals still do not allow fathers in the delivery room, most middle-class parents-to-be take some sort of childbirth courses and expect to experience labor and delivery together. Fathers are given specific tasks during labor and delivery, such as coaching their wife's breathing and lifting her during the pushing phase. The vast majority of childbirth-preparation courses, however, seldom mention any tasks for the father once the birth has been accomplished, and many fathers have an amazingly limited idea of the capacities of the newborn.

The study reported here was designed to address the question of how fathers and newborns behave during their first hour together. Interest in the first hour comes from the recent upsurge of research on early and/or extended contact between mothers and infants. The early work of Klaus and Kennell (1976) was interpreted in the popular press to mean that early mother-infant contact, or "bonding," would make all parents (or mothers, at least) instinctively able to love and care properly for their newborn babies. Before the scientific community had adequately assessed the initial studies, bonding had become the goal of every well-informed parent-to-be. It is not particularly surprising that the response was so great. With changes toward more natural and less medicated births, the idea of spending time with the more alert infant could be seen as a logical development. Thus, in some ways the time was ripe for change in the realm of newborn care. In addition, with the promise of a more successful parent-infant relationship, the value of bonding seemed unquestionable to many parents and childbirth educators.

The scientific community took a much more critical look at the concept of bonding. Some studies of bonding have shown what appear to be differences between groups who have or have not experienced early or extended contact, while other studies have shown no differences (Goldberg 1983; Lamb 1982). A number of researchers have pointed out that the studies address different aspects of the question. For example, does bonding mean early contact or extended contact, or both (Goldberg 1983)? Others have criticized the methodology of many of the studies and the lack of demonstrated long-term effects of early or extended contact (Lamb 1982). It also has been suggested that the observed effects may vary depending on the level of social support the mother receives as well as on the time together (Anisfeld and Lipper 1983).

One aspect of the problem that has received surprisingly little attention is the question of what actually happens during the time that the infant and the parents are together. Usually, scientific method dictates that a phenomenon be thoroughly described before any manipulations are tried or hypotheses tested. No such description exists for the mother-infant data. Moreover, only a small number of studies have considered the father's role postpartum (Jones 1981; Palkovitz 1982; Toney 1983; Pannabecker, et al. 1982). Most of these studies do not report the actual behaviors the fathers produced, and one that does report behaviors (Toney 1983) included an investigator who seemed to be coaching the fathers during their interactions. The study here describes the behaviors fathers and newborns produced with as little interference as was possible in a hospital setting.

METHODS

A one-hour modified narrative recording was made for each of thirty families. All mothers were primiparous and primigravida and experienced normal vaginal deliveries. The ages of mothers ranged from twenty to thirty years, and fathers ranged from nineteen to thirty-six years. Using the Hollingshead Index (1965), all families had an SES Quotient of IV or above (most were III or II)—in ordinary terms, this means they were mostly middle class. All but one couple had attended childbirth classes, and all fathers but one attended the birth (this father watched from outside the delivery room).

Names of possible participants were obtained from one group of obstetricians to insure uniform prenatal care. Families were contacted before the delivery in order to obtain consent. Only mothers who remained conscious and alert during labor and delivery were kept in the study.

All infants were normal and healthy according to the hospital pediatrician's evaluation. Only infants with an Apgar of 8 or above at five minutes were included. All mothers had elected to room in, and, except for the early treatment differences, they received the same care. All deliveries took place in fully equipped delivery rooms on standard horizontal delivery tables. Some deliveries were assisted by forceps. After birth, all infants were placed on their mother's abdomen while the placenta was expelled. The infant was then held up for the mother to see and then placed under a radiant warmer. Standard procedures during this time included a brief examination, silver nitrate eye drops, and the placement of identification bracelets on one ankle and one wrist.

Families were randomly assigned to either the routine-care or the early-contact group. Differential treatment began with the departure from the delivery room. The routine-care group mothers and fathers went to a recovery room for one hour. Some infants went directly to the triage nursery for at least four hours. Some infants went first to the recovery room with their parents. No infant stayed longer than one hour, and most stayed less than a half hour. Mothers eventually went to a room and were reunited with the infants after their release from the nursery.

Early-contact group families went directly from delivery to a private room. A private nurse, who stayed with the family for six hours, was responsible for the usual nursery procedures for the infant and recovery-room procedures for the mother. The only separation occurred when the infant was weighed. The parents were allowed to hold the infant as much as they wanted as long as all necessary procedures were accomplished.

The observation consisted of the first full hour the fathers, infants, and mothers were together. For early-contact families this was the hour following birth beginning with the entrance into the private room. For routine-care families the hour began whenever the infant was released from the nursery and the father was present. Therefore, the time for routine-care families varied from four to fourteen hours after birth (mean 8.46 hours).

The observation technique was based on Clarke-Stewart (1973). A stenographic pad was used to record behaviors as they occurred. Father behaviors were recorded on the left side of the page, and the right side was used for infant behaviors and states. States were defined according to Brazelton's method (1973). The center of the page was reserved for the behaviors of mothers and any other person who interacted with the family. Behaviors occurring simultaneously were recorded on the same line. Behaviors occurring sequentially were recorded one below the other down the page (in their respective columns). If a behavior continued, a vertical line was drawn down the page until it stopped. Infant state was recorded at the beginning of the observation and again whenever it changed. The position of the father, mother, and infant was noted at the start of the hour and continuously for the rest of the time. The observer had a small electronic beeper with an earphone. Every thirty seconds it would sound a tone and the observer would make a horizontal slash on the paper so that the continuous recording was divided into thirty-second intervals. A stopwatch timed the observation hour.

The definitions of most behaviors had previously been agreed upon during a reliability study. The two observers used in the study established an average reliability of r=.88 (Pearson Product-Moment Coefficient was used to calculate correlations). Of the fifty-three scores obtained, only five were below .75, and thirty-six scores were above .90.

The observer tried to be as inconspicuous as possible. Before the observation, she answered any questions and reminded the parents that she would not talk during the observation. After the hour, she talked to the parents, admired the baby, and generally tried to create a comfortable environment.

Since father-infant interaction was the focus of this study, the mother's behavior (other than her position in the room) was only recorded when it involved both the father and the infant. The behavior of other individuals such as nurses was noted.

The Statistical Package for Social Sciences was used to obtain frequency distributions. Because some behaviors occurred rather infrequently and because in many cases the distributions were not normal, the nonparametric Mann-Whitney U-Test (Sokal and Rohlf 1969) was chosen to compare the distributions. Significance was set at the .05 level.

RESULTS

Infants. Human infants, while capable of a wide range of behaviors, are the most vulnerable of newborn creatures and thus require intense caregiving from the moment of birth. Selection for large cranial capacity and the need for that large-brained infant to pass through a birth canal designed for bipedal locomotion resulted in the need to have the infant emerge more immature than most other animals. Selection has also provided the infant with a number of features that help the infant attract a caregiver. These features are reflected in the frequencies of infant behaviors seen in Table 1.

It is important to note that the two groups of infants exhibited different behav-iors more frequently. Desmond et al. (1966) showed that newborns tend to have a period of alertness following birth that lasts for about an hour. The early-contact group infants demonstrated this alertness along with many other attractive behaviors. They spent some of the time doing quiet alert looking. They also were more likely to make noises (fuss, vocalize) and cry, and were very responsive to their parents' attention. In contrast, the routine-care group infants were more likely to be asleep, and when they were awake it was for significantly less time than the early-contact group. This does not suggest that the routine-care group was incapable of the behaviors seen in the early-contact group, but rather only that the parents did not experience that first period of alertness with the infant. These infants most likely produced attractive behaviors

TABLE 1. Infant Behaviors Significantly More Frequent by Group

Early Contact	Routine Care
State 4 (alert)	State 1 (deep sleep)
State 5 (crying)	State 2 (light sleep)
Variable State	State 3 (fluttering eyes)
Root	Yawn
Fuss	
Vocalize	
Quiet	

in the nursery right after birth until they fell into the deep-sleep period that usually follows the first hour or so of alertness.

For the early-contact group, the first hour involved extensive interaction with the parents. These infants spent very little time in their cribs. When they were in the alert state, they were usually face-to-face with one of their parents. When they cried or vocalized the parents usually responded verbally; when they rooted they were fed (except for the bottle-fed babies, who were not fed at this time). Thus, the environment these infants experienced was contingently responsive to their needs. This is the beginning of learning and perhaps the root of Emde's "basic trust" (1980). The parents, by responding to the infant, essentially begin to teach the infant that his or her needs will be met.

The routine-care group, on the other hand, did not experience a contingent environment for the entire first alert period. Some had a short time with their parents before the nursery, but most of this time was usually disrupted by the usual medical procedures following birth. While in the nursery the babies' needs are certainly attended to, but generally certain tasks are of primary importance, such as measuring, weighing, and bathing. For the most part the nurses do not have the time to hold and talk to the infants under their care. Although the nursery is not an unsympathetic place, the infants still do not receive the kind of attention that parents provide.

The behaviors displayed by the routine-care group in their first hour of contact reflect the tendency for newborns to sleep a fair amount. The first hour with their fathers seldom included more than a short period of alertness. It has been documented elsewhere (Brazelton 1961) that the periods of alertness tend to be shorter after the initial hour and perhaps are less predictable.

Fathers. Just as infants are genetically programmed to produce attractive behaviors, some evidence exists that adults are also keyed to respond to these behaviors and to the physical features of infants. Men and women respond to reflex smiles, eye contact, and finger grasping and perceive them to be attempts at interaction (Greenberg and Morris 1974; Pryor 1973); and exaggerated infant features are preferred over actual proportions (Gardner and Wallach 1965; Huckstedt 1965). While there seems to be a gender-specific developmental pattern in the establishment of preferences for infants (Fullard and Reiling 1976), other studies have shown that males are interested in infants (Parke et al. 1972; Parke and O'Leary 1976; Parke and Sawin 1976). Some evidence suggests that the time following birth may be an important time for organizing paternal behavior. Rodholm and Larson (1982) showed that unrelated males and fathers showed the same pattern of touching newborns as new mothers. Peterson et al. (1979) suggest that the birth environment may facilitate the assumption of the paternal role.

In this study, the combined totals showed the most frequent father behaviors to be talking with mother, looking at the infant, holding the infant, and talking to the infant (in descending order of frequency). Table 2 shows the behaviors each group exhibited more frequently than the other. The early-contact group fathers participated in the culturally expected behavior of telephoning to announce the birth, doing so significantly more frequently in the first fifteen minutes of their hour. Invariably the fathers placed the calls and gave the news. Most of the mothers also talked, but only after the father had made the announcement. The fathers seemed to feel this was their first priority and began interactions with the infant after the calls were completed.

The other father behaviors more frequent in the early-contact group show the fathers' interest in the mothers. Immediately following birth, the fathers tended to continue their roles of coaches. They continued to stay close to their wives and look after their needs. In most cases the mothers were holding the infants. Thus, the fathers were in close proximity to both mother and infant. (The measure of this "triadic interaction" was higher in this group, but not significantly so.) The parents tended to do infant care together. For example, many fathers actually helped the mother breastfeed by transferring the infant from side to side or by actually holding the baby to the breast. This sort of intense triadic interaction was not common in the routine-care group.

TABLE 2. Father Behaviors Significantly More Frequent by Group

Early Contact	Routine Care
Kiss mother	Converse with mother
Stroke mother	Stroke infant's head
Next to mother	Stroke infant's foot
Talk on phone**	Put finger in infant's hand
	Adjust clothing
	Dyadic interaction
	Caress infant*
	Feed infant *
	Hold infant *
	Stroke infant's hand or arm**

* Indicates behaviors derived by combining similar behaviors; for example, all the feeding behaviors together equal "feed infant."

**First 15 minutes only

The early-contact parents were still in the rather elated state that generally follows the birth of a healthy infant. They continued to work as a team to accomplish whatever tasks were necessary and included the infant in their intense interactions. They experienced the first hour of infant alertness together and tended to marvel continuously at each new behavior the infant displayed. In a few cases, the mothers whose labor was slightly more difficult spent more time resting. In these cases, the fathers alone would hold and talk to the infants. The hour showed the organization of the fathers' attention to the infant increasing. Toward the end of the hour, the fathers who were somewhat apprehensive about handling the infant seemed much more confident and assured as they held or carried the baby.

The routine-care group fathers had a very different kind of experience with their infants. The time of this observation varied from four to fourteen hours after the birth, depending on when the father was back for the first time after the infant had spent four hours in the nursery. Even after four hours, the initial elation of the birth had somewhat worn off. Many fathers in this situation were very tired after the labor and the waiting. In other cases, the fathers had returned home to sleep, and some had even been at work all day. In many cases, the mothers had already been reunited with the infant; in most cases the mothers were feeling very much recovered.

An interesting pattern was significantly more frequent in the routine-care group for the first fifteen minutes only. As the infant was wheeled in or upon entering the room, fathers tended to approach the infant, vocalize, and stroke the infants hand. This pattern is remniscent of our cultural pattern of approach and handshaking and may demonstrate early enculturation. Fathers in the routine-care group showed more frequent dyadic (father-infant) interaction. They held the infants more, did more stroking, and were more likely to feed the infants. They appeared to be more involved, but in actuality, since many of the babies were asleep, their behaviors may be interpreted differently.

Much of the behavior directed at the infant was intended to wake the infant. Although holding a sleeping newborn may be considered by some to be a pleasurable experience, these fathers really seemed to want to wake up and make contact with their offspring. When they failed to make eye contact, they proceeded to a tactile sort of connection and they often resorted to eliciting the hand grasp reflex. Although this usually succeeded, it did not seem to be as satisfying to them as eye-to-eye or vocal contact. It is interesting to note that Caudill and Weinstein (1969) reported that American mothers were less likely to manipulate sleeping infants and more likely to use visual and verbal stimulation than were Japanese mothers The fathers in this study may have been trying to establish the sort of interaction appropriate to our culture. When that did not succeeed, they settled for a different style, perhaps one less valued in American culture. In any case, the fathers were obviously frustrated by the sleeping.

The routine-care group fathers also exhibited more infant-feeding behavior. It should be noted that early-contact group fathers could not feed the infants because of hospital policy. No formula or water (for breastfeeding infants) was given at the first feeding. Routine-care group fathers were very interested in feeding their infants (either formula or water) and were very active feeders. Much of the head-stroking behavior (see Table 2) is actually the fathers' attempting to get the infants to suck.

Routine-care group fathers held the infants more than fathers in the early-contact group. This reflects the contact the mothers had usually experienced before the fathers' arrivals. Having had their first hour or more alone with their infants, many mothers actively encouraged the fathers to hold the infants. Many fathers picked up sleeping infants from their cribs and sat on a chair across the room from the mothers. In general, the mothers were more active in the routine-care group. They were significantly more likely to leave the room (to ask the nurses a question, for instance) and were often involved in self-grooming or other non-infant-related activities. The fathers were not involved in mother care, and the coaching role seemed to have totally disapppeared among fathers who had left the hospital after the birth. The parents functioned as independent units— mothers reporting their activities and fathers bringing messages from the outside world.

Mothers. Since mother behaviors were reported during triadic interaction only, they do not reflect the full range of mothers' activities but rather those things that the mothers did while in close contact with both father and infant. For the entire sample, the most frequent triadic behaviors were looking at infant, holding infant (cradled left), vocalizing to infant, and stroking infant's head.

For the early-contact group, more frequent behaviors were holding the infant and feeding the infant. This demonstrates again the close triadic interaction taking place as the mother laid in bed and the father stayed close, helping even with breastfeeding. The only triadic activity more frequently displayed by the routine-care group was cleaning the infant. All cases of diapering during the routine-care group's hour were triadic interactions. Usually the mother diapered and the father assisted. In general, however, diapering was very infrequent during the observation hour.

TABLE 3. Mother Behaviors Most Frequent by Group

Early Contact	Routine Care
Puts nipple in	Cleans infant
Adjusts nipple	Leaves room (non-triadic activity)
Holds cradled right	
Lays in bed	
Feeds infant*	
Holds infant*	

*Indicates behaviors derived by combining similar behaviors; for example all the feeding behaviors together equal "feed infant

Father's Questionnaire

TABLE 4. Results of the Father's Questionnaire

	Early Group	Routine Group
Attitude toward pregnancy	4.335	4.353
Feelings about the baby	4.462	4.474
Feeling about infant care	4.188	4.212
Past experience with children	3.600	3.980
Change in life style	4.493	4.445

The fathers in both groups were also asked to fill out a questionnaire on their attitudes about birth-related issues (based on Leonard 1976). Their answers were evaluated using a scale of 1 to 5 (1 being negative and 5 positive). ANOVA revealed no statistically significant differences between the group means on any of the questions (Table 4).

In general, these fathers seemed to have very positive attitudes about infants and about how fatherhood would affect them. Since the questionnaires were filled out at a very early stage in parenthood, they may only reflect the feelings of the early postpartum period. It is interesting to note that the lowest means were in the area of past experience with children. This may reflect American culture's tendency to have female babysitters and a general decrease in family size which decreases the exposure most people have to younger siblings.

DISCUSSION

The interactions of infants and caregivers can be viewed on several levels. The ultimate level, certainly, is species survival. Infants provide attractive behaviors, and adults respond to the activity and the appearance of the child. The interactions are mutually beneficial. The infant gains food, warmth, locomotion, and stimulation, and the adult gets satisfaction from the alert-looking infant's reaction to soothing (Emde 1980) and from many physical features of the infant, such as soft skin (natal coat), grasp reflex, and vocalizing.

How an infant is cared for, however, is not a totally biological question. The interaction also takes place in a specific culture. The culture values certain behaviors over others and defines the norms of parental behavior. From the beginning, the infant is surrounded by culture. Language encodes culture, and thus the infant is being patterned from the time it can record experience (perhaps beginning in utero). Condon and Sander (1974) showed that infants move in synchrony with spoken language. The culture defines the normal birthing situation and the roles of all the people involved.

Since fathers are experiencing labor and delivery more frequently, it is important to consider the impact of this change on our culture. It is unlikely that anything magical or irreversible happens during the first hour after birth, but it is a time that provides a context for focusing certain behaviors that may be culturally relevant. During that time infants tend to be visually and vocally active, behaviors that fathers find very attractive. Although most fathers in this study perceived visual orientation to be a voluntary activity, they considered most other behaviors to be involuntary. Fathers seemed to view their infants as capable of interaction after the infant had looked at them for a length of time. Since this behavior is maximized in the first hour, it may lead fathers to view their infants as more competent and better able to communicate than if this behavior is missed.

Fathers also tended to respond verbally to their infants' vocalizations, which may set up a communication style for the newborn. As Caudill and Weinstein pointed out (1969), ours is a visual and vocal culture. Our patterns are not as tactile as those of many other groups. For example, Brazelton (1972) has noted that Mayan mothers experience breast milk "let down" in response to infant movement; mothers in the United States experience it in response to infant cries. Americans also tend to care for infants at a distance—cribs, strollers, infant seats—rather than through continuous carrying. By doing this, we need to see and hear our infants' needs rather than feel them. Perhaps it is important to encourage first-hour contact for fathers (and mothers) to enhance their learning of visual and vocal cues.

This time of alertness begins the learning of contingent interaction— infant produces behavior, parent responds. Fathers seem to learn the patterns just as easily as mothers. What differs, perhaps, is the cultural expectation that the mother will be primary caretaker. As more mothers return to work and share caretaking with fathers, the fathers need to establish a caregiving relationship with their child. Even though some evidence suggests that fathers and mothers have different interaction styles (Clarke-Stewart 1980; Lamb et al. 1982), any caretaker has to be attuned to the infant's needs.

The more time a parent spends with an infant, the more able that parent is to predict that child's behavior. The better able a parent is at predicting what will interest, distract, or comfort an infant, the more success the parent will experience in taking care of the infant. Success leads to self-confidence. As a parent gains confidence in his or her abilities in caregiving, the task becomes more pleasurable and, therefore, more likely to be willingly continued. Due to a variety of cultural reasons, such as the general lack of paternity leaves in this country, it is often the mother who experiences early successes with the newborn. Success with a newborn usually requires a great deal of work and patience. It is easy to see how the father who immediately goes back to work may find it difficult to commit the time and energy required really to get to know the newborn. He probably feels genuine love and affection for the child, but abhors the thought of spending long hours alone with what to him is a very unpredictable little creature.

Early success experienced in the neonatal period may encourage the father to continue to interact with the infant. As he invests more time he will become more attuned to the infant's needs and develop the skills appropriate to the child's developmental level.

One area of continuing discussion in the literature on bonding is the concept of developing affection or love for the infant. Often the attempt is made to demonstrate the strength of this emotion by measuring caregiving or interaction style. Some authors have pointed out that measures of attachment are inappropriate for the newborn period, because that is a feature of a much older child. Perhaps assessing affection or love is equally inappropriate at this age. It is very easy to love a newborn or the idea of a newborn. Parents who, for whatever reason, are removed from their child still express love and affection for that child. A father who has never seen or held his child may feel he sincerely loves that child. It might be more significant to view the amount of time and energy a parent is willing to invest in the child not as a measure of love but as a measure of involvement. How well does the parent know the infant? Knowing an infant comes with time, actual caregiving, and interaction. Perhaps a better question of the "bonding" studies would be, "Has it increased involvement with the child?"

CONCLUSION

This study shows that fathers interact with their newborns and that the period immediately following birth enhances certain father-infant behaviors important in American culture. The experience benefits both father and infant and may begin a contingently responsive relationship. The behaviors demonstrated by these fathers might help medical practitioners to facilitate interactions between fathers and infants who were separated at birth.

16

DELAYED ACCOMPLISHMENTS: FAMILY FORMATION AMONG OLDER FIRST-TIME PARENTS

Linda M. Whiteford and Michael W. Sharinus

The transition to parenthood has been called a time of crisis, anxiety and stress (Richmond-Abbot 1983; Feldman and Rollins 1970; Curtis-Boles 1983, among others). It is a time of profound emotional, physical, and familial change. The ways in which couples make that transition to parenthood may predict the quality of their marital relationship for the first decade following the birth of their child (Dyer 1963).

This research focuses on a small sample of first-time parents over the age of thirty and measures how they perceive the quality of their marital relationship for the first decade after the birth of their child. It analyzes these self-descriptions in the light of sociodemographic variables, such as educational level and occupation. The couples were asked to evaluate their relationships using a series of standardized instruments designed to measure communication skills, marital adjustment, perception of happiness and idealized self. The research draws on two conceptual orientations: (1) parenthood as a period of adaptive transition and (2) life phase as an influence on adaptation.

Older first-time parents are conceptually interesting because they start to have their children at a time when the majority of their age mates are already raising adolescent children. Few studies have focused explicitly on this group, and no study has attempted to measure objectively their marital adjustment to parenthood. The major reason for this is that until recently the group was too small either to arouse much interest or to provide adequate samples. For a variety of reasons—not the least of which is the availability of relatively safe, legal, effective, socially acceptable birth control—this situation has changed over the past twenty years. From the 1960s to the 1980s, the proportion of women in our society who wait until they were past twenty-five before having children has grown by about 30 percent, now accounting for about a third of the mothers in the country. Although this may be a transitional group, its size has become significant.

HYPOTHESES

In the present study of older first-time parents, we have chosen to focus on how individuals adapt to their new life situation after becoming parents. At the beginning of this exploratory work, we developed four hypotheses about what we would find: (1) life phase would have an influence on marital adjustment to parenthood; (2) older couples would perceive themselves as happier than other couples; (3) educational level would be directly related to communication skills among older parents; and (4) mothers employed outside the home would be happier than mothers who did not work outside the home.

Our research findings supported the first and second of our hypotheses but did not support the third and fourth. Life phase (which was operationalized as "being involved in activities that were appropriate to that time of the respondents' lives") does appear to influence marital adjustment to parenthood, and the older couples of our sample did perceive themselves to be happier than other couples. However, education was not positively associated with greater interpersonal communication skills, nor was maternal employment outside of the home associated with more successful marital adjustment and maternal happiness. Although level of education was associated with better communication skills for men, women in our sample were striking in that they shared an inverse relationship between educational level and interpersonal communication skills. The women who were most successful with interpersonal communication—both according to their own self-ratings and those of their partners—were women who had the least amount of formal education. Similarly, our research indicated the obverse of our fourth hypothesis. That is, women in this sample who worked outside the home reported that they were less happy than women who were not employed outside the home. Working women did, however, have higher "idealized-self" scores than women who remained at home. To account for the results requires a reconceptualization of the issues and a more detailed examination of the data.

Parenthood and Marital Satisfaction

Alpert and Richardson (1978) indicate that parenthood may negatively affect marital satisfaction, lead to conflict, and reduce self-esteem. For some couples, the loss is offset by a later rise in parental satisfaction (Glenn and Weaver 1978; Spanier, Lewis, and Cole 1975; Rossi 1968). Wilkie (1981) shows that women who delay childbearing may experience increased stress because of their own inexperience and the unavailability of their own parents to provide support with crucial child-rearing functions. There are also numerous studies examining self-esteem and mental health in relation to overall marital satisfaction and, more recently, in relation to changes in family structure such as the transition to parenthood. Specifically, a decrease in overall self-esteem with relation to childbearing was examined by Rossi (1968) and LeMasters (1957).

Marital satisfaction has been seen to be affected by self-esteem, communication, social roles, and self-image (Cowan and Cowan 1983). There is often a decline in marital satisfaction for the first decade after the birth of a child. Not surprisingly, longitudinal research indicates that the type of relationship the couple has before the birth of the child is highly predictive of the level of marital satisfaction following the birth of a child (Cowan and Cowan 1983; Grossman et al. 1980; Boles 1981). The amount and quality of communication between partners have been positively correlated with marital satisfaction (Navran 1967; Honeycutt, Wilson, and Parker 1982; Boles 1983). Schafer and Braito (1979) examined the correlation between marital satisfaction and self-image. Social roles or task-sharing arrangements have been correlated with marital satisfaction by Frank, Anderson, and Rubinstein (1980) and by Chadwick, Albrecht, and Kunz (1976). More recently, investigators have studied the father's role in parenting and marital satisfaction (Radin 1983; Russell 1982; Sagi 1982; Coysh 1983). The variables discussed in the literature on parenthood and family formation provided the variables used in the present research. They are communication, marital adjustment, perception of happiness, perception of self, and self-esteem.

Parenthood and Life Phase

Although studies have examined the functioning of marriages before and after the birth of a child in an effort to predict positive adjustment to birth and new parenthood, none have looked directly at the effect of life phase on the couples' adaptation to parenthood or the amount of parental stress involved in this transition (Grossman et al. 1981; Shereshefsky and Yarrow 1973; Cowan and Cowan 1983). The concept of life phase is being used here not to refer to any specific pyschological theory, but rather to a perspective shared by developmental psychology, sociology and anthropology. It is used here to refer to the age-differentiated, socially-structured role domains of life. An underlying assumption of the present research is that the type of adaptation made to parenthood is predicated upon the individual's being able to utilize the skills he or she has developed and the individual's feeling that those skills are appropriate for his or her activities and sequence (and timing) of life events.

Research in the area of life phase focuses on age as a determinant of social patterns in the ordering, spacing, and timing of major life events (Rossi 1980; Gutmann 1965; Neugarten 1979; Erikson 1959; Vaillaint 1977; Levinson 1978). Such research suggests that people between thirty and forty are frequently involved in a variety of activities that differentiates them from both younger and older groups. For some members of this age cohort, this is a period of self-evaluation and recognition of where they are in their careers and a time of choice about whether to stay in that career or change. For others, it is a time to examine their vulnerability to aging and the inevitability of death.

The perception of invulnerability, which typifies people in their early twenties, changes as people reach the ages of thirty to forty and see their own parents age. In many cases, couples in their thirties and forties are preparing for their own children to leave home as the children reach adolescence and young adulthood. Some individuals feel a sense of urgency at this time as they recognize that they have not accomplished all they thought they would by the time they were thirty or thirty-five. Major changes occur during this period—divorce, remarriage, a new job, a return to school to complete an interrupted education or retrain for a new vocation. Some people speak of their "biological clock"—not just in terms of their potential for motherhood, but also in terms of their own need to strive and to accomplish. A fear of diminished opportunity may also mark this time period.

Erikson (1959) identifies the middle-adult years as those which are built around the task of developing the "capacity for intimacy." Vaillant (1977) and Levinson (1978) describe changes the men they studied experienced during this period of their lives between the early thirties and early forties. "Men leave the compulsive, unreflective busywork of their occupational apprenticeships and once more become explorers of the world within" (Vaillant 1977:220). Rossi describes this time as "a watershed during which both outer life structure and inner concept of self undergo profound change" (1980:10). Rossi, analyzing Levinson's research, describes how men incrementally increase their involvement with their work as a central priority until at some time in their middle-adult years when, a shift occurs from this high centrality of work to a greater emphasis on the family and private life. Most importantly, Rossi adds the concept of intimacy mentors to Levinson's concept of career mentor.

Levinson makes much of the role of "career mentors" in the work histories of his male subjects; my impression is that women played the role "intimacy mentors" to their husbands. If so, this makes the developmental task in early adulthood in the Levinson men consistent with Erikson's life cycle but inconsistent in the case of women in early adulthood. It implies that women, typically younger than their husbands, have already resolved the intimacy issue by their twenties, while men are still engaged in this task well into their thirties (Rossi 1980:11).

This inconsistency by sex with Erikson's model helps to explain the findings of the present research. Further, it may be that as women increasingly assume less gender-specific roles they mirror the developmental plateaus previously described for men.

If the research on life phase is accurate, then one would expect that the experience of parenting would be different for older parents as they simultaneously experience the crisis of first birth and the "watershed" of profound personal change. Older first-time parents provide a provocative example of what

Neugarten (1979) has termed "asynchrony of life events." According to Neugarten, synchrony of phases with the life cycle is influenced by gradual, normal changes in time perspective. As people move from their twenties to their thirties, "life is restructured in terms of time left-to-live rather than time-since-birth" This change is accompanied by heightened introspection, stocktaking, and interiority. The concept of synchrony is complicated, however, by the cognizance of the multiple contexts within which one may seek syn-chrony. For example, Neugarten suggests that chronological age no longer serves as the kind of marker it once did. This stems from the fact that the phasing of different contexts of life is not always synchronous: a man may be "on time" in terms of his work or career but "off time" by being a father of an infant born of a late or second marriage. Equally interesting is the situation of the older first-time mother who may be "on time" with her career but "off time" as a new mother.

METHODOLOGY

Design. The present research was designed to explore some of the changes occurring among older first-time parents. The concept of life phase is used to help explain the findings and to provide a context by which to understand better the dynamics of adjustment to new parenthood occurring for couples in their thirties and forties. The methodology was developed with two primary concerns: (1) to include male partners in the research design and (2) to use standardized, closed-ended instruments to elicit quantifiable data on marital adjustment, marital satisfaction, and interpersonal skills. Including the male partner in such research has become a valuable aspect of the analysis of response to birth and family formation (Whiteford 1983; Bing 1970; Eldridge 1970; Roberts 1969; Richman and Goldthorp 1978).

Following Cowan and Cowan's significant recent work on family formation and parental adaptation (1983), we focused on marital communication (Hill, Stycos, and Black, Marital Communication Test, 1970) and marital adjustment (Locke-Wallace Short Marital Adjustment Test, 1959) as indicative of the flexibility of the marital relationship. Two individual measures were included to provide a general sense of idealized self-concept (adapted from Pearson's Self-Concept) and a perception- of-happiness index.

Subjects and Procedures. In the spring of 1984, childbirth educators in Tampa, Florida, were asked to review their client records and provide the researchers with the names and addresses of couples in which both partners were over thirty years old, were expecting their first child, and had completed childbirth-education classes during the first three months of that year. We obtained the names of forty couples who fit the research requirements and to whom we mailed the research instruments. Eight couples had moved, and we were not able to find them for the research. Of the remaining thirty-two couples, fifteen responded fully with both partners returning completed questionnaires (thirty completed questionnaires).

Measures. Interpersonal communication skills were measured using an instrument that each partner completed independently of the other. The same instrument was used for men and women. From the raw data we generated a communication-skills index for each couple. This index was computed by squaring the differences between the responses of the male and female partners, summing these squared differences, and taking the square root of this sum. Lower values of this index indicated that the couple had good communication skills and higher scores indicated less than optimal skills. This instrument consisted of thirteen individual items which explored areas such as handling of family finances, caring for children, and sharing of household tasks. The index scores ranged from a low of 2.65 to a high of 8.85, with a mean of 5.13 and a standard deviation of 1.35.

Marital adjustment was also measured for each couple. The partners completed identical instruments independently of each other. Due to the nature of this instrument, it was broken into two parts for analysis. For the first eight items, an index score was computed for each couple with lower scores indicating good marital adjustment skills, and higher scores indicating poorer marital adjustment skills. Indices for the marital- adjustment instrument were computed in the same way the indices for the communication skills were computed. Scores on this instrument ranged from a low of 0.00 to a high of 3.61, with a mean of 2.09 and a standard deviation of 0.94. The remainder of the items on this instrument were open-ended and therefore this part did not lend itself to easily quantifiable scoring. In this section we looked for relatively large differences in response between the spouses.

The same happiness-scale instrument was provided for each partner. The instrument was a line with areas marked for very unhappy (indicated with a score of 0) to perfectly happy (indicated by a score of 35). All respondents were asked to indicate where on the line they felt they belonged. When the instrument was designed, the midpoint was to represent the amount of happiness from marriage for an "average" couple. From this measurement we were able to obtain both individual and combined happiness scores (Table 1). Individual scores ranged from a high of 35 to a low of 15. Couple scores ranged from a high of 70 to a low of 35 with a mean of 52.67 and a standard deviation of 10.63. Most people in this sample indicated that they thought they were happier than the average person.

Only women were asked to complete the ideal-self instrument. They were to indicate how their perception of themselves now corresponded to the person they would like to be. For this instrument there was a raw-score range of 0 to 25. For the fourteen women who completed this instrument, the scores ranged from a high of 24 to a low of 7, with a mean of 14.60 and a standard deviation of 6.48.

TABLE 1. Happiness Scores for Each Partner of Each Couple

Couple #	Female	Male	Male Plus Female
1	20	15	35
2	35	25	60
3	20	20	40
4	35	35	70
5	25	25	50
6	35	32	67
7	35	25	60
8	20	23	43
9	25	25	50
10	25	20	45
11	25	35	60
12	35	25	60
13	20	20	40
14	35	25	60
15	25	25	50
X	27.67	25.00	52.67

*Individual scores can range from a low of 0 to a high of 35, with 15 representing the average amount of happiness people get from marriage.

RESULTS

Demographic Variables. In a comparison of the scores for the women only, two demographic variables were included—employment and education. For the employment variable an effort was made to distinguish between employment within or outside the home. Though the sample was too small for generalization, women not employed outside the home tended to show better communication skills than women who were employed outside of the home. They also seemed to have better marital-adjustment skills and to report themselves as happier than women working outside the home. Women employed outside the home, however, scored higher on ideal-self than did women who worked fulltime in the home.

When the variable, "highest educational level," was examined, three categories emerged. Those individuals who had graduated from high school and had attended college were put into the first group; college graduates were placed in another; and those with a postgraduate education were placed in a third category. Women with a high school education only showed remarkably higher interpersonal communication skills than did women with postgraduate education or those with college degrees (Table 3). Women with a postgraduate education showed the poorest marital-adjustment skills, while women with the least amount of education showed the best skills in this category. The happiest women were those with the least education, while the least happy women were those with the most years of formal education (Table 4). Women with college educations and those with postgraduate training were more likely to have lower self-images than women whose formal education ended after high school.

TABLE 2. Happiness Scores for Women

Employed Outside The Home	Not Employed Outside The Home
35	35
25	35
25	35
35	20
25	25
25	35
20	
0	
20	
X 25.56	30.83

*Individual scores can range from a low of 0 to a high of 35, with 15 representing the average amount of happiness people get from marriage.

TABLE 3. Marital Adjustment and Communication Skills of Women

Employed Outside the Home

High School/Some College		College Graduate		Postgraduate	
CS	MA	CS	MA	CS	MA
4.90	2.00	5.48	1.00	6.33	2.24
5.92	3.61	5.83	2.00	8.49	3.46
4.12	2.00	4.80	1.00	5.29	2.83
X= 4.98	2.54	5.35	1.71	7.41	2.85

Not Employed Outside the Home

3.74	0.00	2.65	2.24	4.58	2.00
6.00	1.73	4.24	2.65	4.58	2.65
X= 4.87	0.87	3.82	2.51	NA	NA

CS=Communications Skills; MA=Marital Adjustment
*Communication skills and marital adjustment index scores of women are separated by nature of employment and highest level of education attained. For both instruments, the lower index scores indicate better marital adjustment and communication skills.

TABLE 4. Happiness Scores of Women by Level of Education

High School/Some College	College Graduate	Postgraduate
35	20	20
25	35	35
35	20	20
25	25	
35	25	
	35	
	25	
X 31.00	26.43	25.00

X for all females= 27.67; pHo = .153846

*The scores can range from a low of 0 to a high of 35, with 15 representing the average amount of happiness people get from marriage.

When scores of the instruments were examined with respect to employment and education, women who had postgraduate education and worked outside the home were least happy and had the worst scores for communications skills, marital adjustment, and ideal self. The group of women who were happiest and had the best scores for communications skills and marital adjustment were those with least education and who were not employed outside the home. These two groups were the extremes. The other four categories arranged by educational level and employment had score differences that were fairly evenly distributed (Table 4)

All of the men worked in businesses outside the home or were self-employed (except one who was temporarily unemployed and looking for a job); for our analysis we grouped men by the educational level they had attained. The scores for the happiness instrument were very evenly distributed over this variable (Table 5).

TABLE 5. Male Communication Skills and Marital Adjustment

High School/Some College		College Graduate		Postgraduate	
CS	MA	CS	MA	CS	MA
8.49	3.46	5.29	2.83	4.80	1.00
4.90	2.00	4.12	2.00	2.65	2.24
5.77	1.00	4.58	2.00	5.83	2.00
3.74	0.00	4.58	2.65		
4.24	2.65	5.92	3.61		
		6.00	1.73		
		6.33	2.24		
X= 5.43	1.82	5.30	2.44	4.42	1.75

*Communication-skills and marital-adjustment index scores for men are separated by highest level of education attained. For both instruments, lower index scores indicate better communication skills and marital adjustment.

When happiness scores were compared within each couple, in seven cases the women was the happier partner, in two cases the male was happier, and in six cases no difference was reported. Although the people in this sample seem to indicate a greater degree of happiness than the overall population, women indicated a greater degree of happiness than did men. When the female partner had the higher educational level, the couple showed relatively poor marital-adjustment skills.

DISCUSSION

The results of this research are intriguing precisely because they fail to satisfy our third and fourth working hypotheses: that education would be directly related to greater communication skills among older parents and that mothers employed outside the home would be happier than mothers who did not work outside the home.

The first hypothesis was based on earlier research that showed a strong relationship between education and communication skills. Nevertheless, in our sample of older first-time parents there was no association between communication skills and level of education. Despite the small sample, we tested the relationship of communication-skills score above and below the mean and presence or absence of a college degree. A Fisher's Exact Test of the probability of a distribution like that of our sample occurring by chance yielded a probability of .573 (Table 6). While it is presumed that better-educated people in our sample have gained skills in other kinds of communication, there is no evidence that they have gained skill in interpersonal communication within marriage. Similar testing failed to reveal a relationship between education and marital adjustment, or education and self-reported happiness, though on average our sample reported their happiness being at a relatively high level.

Our second surprise came with the discovery that the mothers in our sample who worked outside the home did not rate themselves as happier than those who remained at home. In fact, again using the Fisher's Exact Test, we found some indication of the reverse. Dividing the sample by those who did and did not remain at home and by those who rated their happiness at 35 (the highest score) and those who rated themselves at less than 35, we obtained a probability of .119 (Table 7). This suggests that close attention should be paid to this relationship in any future retest.

Our reasoning was that women who were working outside the home, having delayed childbearing until later in life, would likely be women satisfactorily pursuing careers that they find rewarding. With the birth of a child, their tasks and perhaps their rewards become doubled both in their careers and in their family life. While the first premise of this argument might legitimately by questioned, one further statistic, though falling just short of the .05 level of confidence, provides support to that premise.

TABLE 6. Communication Skills by Education

| | | Has a College Degree | |
		Yes	No
Scored above mean for comunications skills	Yes	5	3
	No	5	2
		pHo = 0.573	

TABLE 7. Happiness by Workplace

| | | Works Outside Home | |
		Yes	No
Self-reported level of happiness	35	2	4
	<35	7	2
		pHo=.119	

TABLE 8. Communication Skills by Work Place

| | | Works Outside Home | |
		Yes	No
Scored at or above mean for	Yes	3	5
communcations skills	No	6	1
		pHo = .084	

We compared the interpersonal communications skills of women who did and did not work outside the home, again using the Fisher's Exact Test because of low N, and dividing the sample by those scoring at or above the mean for communications skills from those below the mean. The result, with a probability of .084 that the distribution occurred by chance, was that the women who stayed home had better interpersonal communication skills (Table 8).

Before returning to the concepts of intimacy mentor and life phase, it is worth summing up that women in the sample who stayed home showed some tendency toward greater self-reported happiness and better interpersonal communication skills, regardless of level of education, which is not associated with either. At the same time, whether or not by chance, women in our sample with the most formal education and who worked outside the home constituted extreme cases of poor marital adjustment, poor communications scores, low self-image, and unhappiness.

LIFE PHASE AND INTIMACY MENTORS

If the ten years between thirty and forty in an individual's life are marked by a move away from the "compulsive, unreflective busywork of...occupational apprenticeships" and toward personal, empathetic, and introspective relationships, then the family, and particularly the new infant provide the perfect context for that expression. The Rossi and Levinson concepts of career mentors and intimacy mentors as explanations of variation in adjustment to parenthood suggests that women whose primary identification is based on their role as wife and mother provide an easier and more adaptable environment for adjustment to parenthood. Such women may act as intimacy mentors to their husbands during the period in which the husbands are developing their career opportunities through contacts outside of marriage. According to Rossi, such women may have resolved the task of developing intimacy by their twenties. It may be that those individuals who in their twenties focused their lives on career development, be they men or women, delay learning the skills of intimacy, sharing, and self-revelation—the very skills required for successful marriage and parenting.

Working women with postgraduate educations who are married to men who are also working may, like their husbands, fail to learn the skills of nurturing and intimacy. The result may be a couple in which neither member is structurally specified as the caretaker or intimacy mentor. Couples with no member in a caretaker role undergo a radical transformation with the addition of a dependent infant. Structurally the couple may remain without a caretaker, but the family unit is no longer composed of self-sufficient individuals.

The structural constraints that until recently have required women to provide the family environment with its flexibility, intimacy, and emotional base are changing. Women who select career paths through postgraduate education and combine childrearing with employment may find it very difficult to create such a family environment. Their own personal development may mirror the developmental path traditionally taken by men—delayed personal gratification in exchange for career advancement. In such couples, no one may be the intimacy mentor.

In contrast to the group of women described above, those who were full-time caregivers consistently showed the highest scores for happiness, best marital adjustment, and best communications skills. This can be explained in part by the fact that they are immersed in an environment which stresses and rewards intimacy. This provides them with time and a context in which to develop those very skills that facilitate marital adjustment and communication. It is important to note that these women, while they may only have high school educations, are not recent high school graduates. These are women who have delayed having children, but not necessarily for reasons of career advancement. They may, thus, have mastered Erikson's "capacity for intimacy" before they became mothers thereby providing their partners with intimacy mentors.

Men in the present sample had happiness scores that were evenly distributed across all levels of education. However, men with postgraduate levels of education showed the best communication skills and highest marital-adjustment scores. These scores contrast with the scores attained by women with the same educational characteristics. This inverse relationship is associated with life phase:

men with postgraduate educations were actively involved in career development using skills appropriate to that phase of their lives. During their thirties and forties they begin to develop the intimacy that marks their next life phase. In this, the men were consistent with Neugarten's "synchrony of life events." Women in this population who have postgraduate educations were "out of phase" for the life phase traditionally held by females in this society, for they had not mastered the intimacy skills that other women may have mastered by their thirties and forties.

The present research is provocative. Of the four issues raised at the beginning of our research, two held true: (1) life phase appears to have an influence on marital adjustment to parenthood, and (2) older first-time parents perceive themselves as happier than the general population. But two issues had results inverse to those we expected. The research showed (1) education was not associated with greater communication skills among older women, and (2) mothers working outside the home were not happier than those who did not work outside the home. Examining the small sample studied here illustrates the interplay between social roles, timing and sequencing of life events, and the development of interpersonal skills in the transition to parenthood.

The issues raised here should help focus future research on a rapidly growing population. According to Monthly Vital Statistics, "Between 1972 and 1982, the first birth-rate for women in their early 30s more than doubled, increasing from 7.0 first births per 1,000 women aged 30–34 to 14.6, while the rate for women aged 35–39 years rose 83 percent from 1.8 to 3.3" per 1,000 women (1982). Clearly, this population is increasing at a rapid rate. We know very little about how they are adapting to parenthood or what variables may make that transition more or less traumatic. Based on our exploratory research, it appears that life phase and the development of interpersonal skills strongly influence the process of adjustment. Future research needs to elicit information concerning the roles played by intimacy mentors and how and when members of couples acquire those interpersonal skills. The issues raised in the present research are significant not only because they are important to an increasing population, but also because they offer insight into the pan-human problem of adaptation to parenthood.

NOTE

This research was made possible by a grant from the College of Social and Behavioral Sciences of the University of South Florida, 1982–83. I would like to thank Virginia Kiefert for her assistance with this research.

17

BRINGING UP BABY: EXPECTATION AND REALITY IN THE EARLY POSTPARTUM

Karen L. Michaelson

All known cultures pattern reproductive behavior—the proper behaviors for the soon-to-be parents during pregnancy, the appropriate attendants at and expectations for childbirth, and the expected roles of the parents to the infant and to others in their society (Mead and Newton 1967). Women do not just give birth physically to a child, they give birth within a specific set of social relations and cultural definitions of the maternal role and its expected behavior (Whiteford 1983). In most societies, women learn the behaviors appropriate to childbirth and infant care from other women. When a woman's labor begins, she is supported by other women through the birthing; her sisters. mother, grandmother, cousins, and friends might be with her to share the joys and burdens of the early postpartum weeks.

Yet, in American society there is presently a lack of a clearly demarcated reintegration of the mother into society after the birth of a child. In many other societies there is a specific waiting period after birth during which the women is catered to by her kin or by childbirth specialists, after which she reenters society in a structured way to take on a clearly defined new role. The birth of an infant climaxes nine months of waiting, which for many women in the United States includes adequate physical prenatal and intrapartum care. "But during the first month at home with a new baby, when the family's needs for support and guidance may be acute, relatively few have contact with any health professionals" (Gruis 1977:182). Nor are there culturally prescribed individuals who remain with the mother and baby to assist in the transition. Increasingly, women are leaving the hospital twenty-four to forty-eight hours after the baby is born and have no followup to see how well they are doing once they return home. The current pattern of returning for a maternal postpartum exam at four to six weeks after birth means that a woman is left without professional support during a potentially difficult period in her life. This is particularly true of those women who have had normal uncomplicated births and those who have had children previously and are presumed to "know the ropes." At the same time, the support of kin and friends for the maternal role may be inadequate for the major changes that occur in a woman's life during the postpartum period.

THE STUDY

In the summer of 1983, I conducted a pilot study that examined new mothers' preparation for childbirth, their concerns during pregnancy, experience of birth, and postpartum adjustment. Twenty women from rural eastern Washington and twenty women from urban Spokane were interviewed within the first six weeks postpartum. The urban women were selected by a random sample of births announced in the local newspapers; the rural population consisted of all births taking place in a rural northeastern Washington county during a six-week period in May-June 1983. In each population there were two home births and one birth in a free-standing birthing center. Most of the rural women gave birth in a small community hospital and were attended by family practice physicians. Most of the urban women gave birth in one of Spokane's large tertiary-care hospitals, and were attended by either obstetricians or family practice physicians. The women were all married, had from high school diplomas to postgraduate degrees, and were between twenty and their mid-thirties. Twenty-one of the women were giving birth to their first child; nineteen had had prior children, ranging from one other child to seven other children. Nine of the women had cesarean deliveries, and the remainder were delivered vaginally, with interventions ranging from none to epidural anesthesia and forceps. The women were interviewed with an open-ended questionnaire.

Preparation for Childbirth

Although there were differences in the type of birth experience each mother had, depending on whether she delivered at home, in a community hospital, or in a larger hospital, there was remarkably little difference in the women's preparation for childbirth or in their postpartum concerns. All but one of the women had taken some form of childbirth-education class, either during this pregnancy or a previous pregnancy. Several women had taken multiple classes, with the additional class usually being an exercise class; some had taken refresher classes (usually Lamaze) for the birth of a second or third child.

By their own report, most women felt well prepared for their childbirth experience. There were of course, gaps between the expectation and reality of childbirth even for those who had taken childbirth classes. Women who had cesarean deliveries or who had unexpected interventions, such as anesthesia or forceps, found that their careful reading and preparatory classes were sometimes less than adequate for their experience.

Preparation for Parenthood

For all women, preparation for the postpartum period was woefully lacking. One midwife, who had herself recently given birth, commented, "Right now, when parents take the baby home, it's kind of like at the end of a movie where every one walks off into the sunset. But when you take the baby home, this is just the beginning of everything....People need to be told what the realities are. When you have a new baby, life does not just go on like it did before. You're not going to get the house cleaned as often, or you might have pancakes for dinner three nights in a row" (Massenda 1984).

During the first few weeks and months after becoming a mother, substantial changes take place in a woman's life. There is a need for a new concept of time, a different organization of self, and a changed coordination of routine (Shereshefsky et al, 1973: 173). Women whose lives have been primarily oriented toward work and the public sphere now find themselves confined largely to home and the domestic sphere. Although in other cultures the new mother can count on kin to assist in child care or perhaps on worksite daycare, for many women in the United States, birth can be the beginning of an oppressive trap (Seiden 1978:99) in which the dependent child is her burden alone. These demands are exacerbated by fatigue and frequently by the need for physical healing. The cultural assumptions are that these women chose motherhood (they could, after all, have used birth control or gotten an abortion) and that they knew what they were getting into.

Yet, there is ample evidence that women—or indeed parents—do not know what they are getting into, even those who have had children before. Evidence of maladaptation to parenthood exists in the appalling figures on child neglect and gross child abuse and in the statistics which indicate that married couples without children are happier than married couples with children (Seiden 1978: 88).

One reason that it is difficult for parents, and particularly mothers, to know what they are getting into when they bring home the new baby is that there is little information available to new parents about the early postpartum period and the real trials, tribulations, and joys of bringing up baby.

During pregnancy, women fantasize about their upcoming maternal role (Mercer 1981: 234). As their attachment to the developing infant grows through their pregnancy, they try on a variety of roles, searching for the one that suits their values and lifestyles. They study other mothers for cues and perhaps recall their own childhood experiences or their experiences with babysitting or caring for siblings. Yet, despite the fact that much of the psychological literature on pregnancy stresses the need for a woman's coming to grips with her relationship with her own mother prior to the birth of her child and cites the benefit of having a positive experience of having been mothered as being essential to developing adequate mothering skills, being a daughter simply is not adequate preparation for being a mother. For many women, prior experience with mothering consists of playing with dolls and occasionally babysitting—both rather inadequate sources of parent-role information.

The women in this study found few formal sources of information about mothering and their early postpartum role. None reported attending parenting classes, though they are available through the local hospitals. Several cited books as a source of information about childrearing and had read extensively about labor and delivery. But these books focused mainly on babycare and not on maternal adjustment. It appears that prior to the birth of their child, most women focus on the events of the birth itself and are not ready to prepare for the postpartum period until they have cleared that dramatic hurdle. Discussions with local childbirth educators and midwives support this view. Once the infant is born, most women find that they have little time to read, particularly in the early postpartum weeks.

Thus, most women did what women have always done: sought out someone older and wiser. Fifty-seven percent of the women giving birth for the first time said they got most of their child-care advice from their mothers; slightly fewer multiparous women specified their mother as a source of advice, primarily because they cited their own prior experience. The second most common source of advice was the doctor—usually a pediatrician or family practitioner—or other medical personnel. Mothers-in-law also were significant sources of advice. Primiparous women tended to have more sources of advice on childrearing, largely because they reported a greater need for information for this first-time experience.

But the information sought from these older and presumably wiser sources had mostly to do with the infants' well-being and less with parental adjustment to their new role. If a woman actively seeks help during the postpartum period, it is for the baby, not for herself. Yet there is evidence that the primary problems women experience in the early postpartum are not ones of lack of child-care knowledge but of adjustment to a new role, with new responsibilities and restrictions. Several studies have indicated that the first few months of parenthood are not a period of unmitigated joy in the growth of the new family but are a period of crisis, characterized by loss of sleep, worry over appearance, social isolation, and lack of preparation for parenthood (Dyer 1963; Lemasters 1957). Indeed, the child-development specialist Brazleton refers to the first few months of new parenthood as "paradise lost."

ADJUSTMENT TASKS OF THE EARLY POSTPARTUM

A variety of research indicates that the tasks of the first few months postpartum are fourfold:[1]

Physical Restoration. This may include healing from the episiotomy, sore breasts, and fatigue, among other physical aspects of recovery. There are cultural aspects to this healing as well. In a society that values slimness and youth, the return of a woman's prepregnancy figure is not a minor concern. The need to fit into one's old clothes may not merely be vanity but an expression of a pressing need to regain self-esteem and control over one's presentation of self (Gruis 1977: 182–4).

In the group of new mothers in this study, concern for physical healing took place primarily in the first week postpartum. At that time, 42.8 percent of the first-time mothers reported concern for healing of the episiotomy, though only 10 percent of the multiparous women had that concern. In part, this was because fewer multiparous women had episiotomies—for example among that group there were four home births that did not involve episiotomies—but also it is not surprising that primiparous women were concerned with the healing of an incision in a very sensitive and private part of their body. In this early period, cesarean-sectioned mothers were universally focused on healing and on pain and were also concerned about their inability to care for their child properly because of the pain. In the first week, only two of the multiparous women were concerned with the return of their figures, but seven of the first time mothers already expressed concern with their weight and shape. By the fourth through sixth week postpartum, there was a dramatic increase in the number of mothers expressing concern for regaining their prepregnancy figure. Fifty-eight percent of multiparous women and 67 percent of primiparous women reported this as a major concern, and most had begun active exercise and dietary restraint to achieve their desired weight goal. By this time, those women with other children at home also reported an increase in problems with "nerves" or control of the emotions, especially in relation to familial stress increased by the burden of the new infant. For mothers who had cesarean deliveries, physical healing was still a concern for two-thirds of them at four to six weeks.

Learning infant needs. Because modern society provides little opportunity for learning about infant care through experience, new mothers must adjust to their infants' demands and learn how to care for them "on the job." Most women, however, are confident in their skills as mothers by six weeks. Even in the first week postpartum, few mothers expressed concern over their ability to care for their infant, and by the sixth week postpartum this concern had virtually vanished. The only mothers expressing concern over their inability to mother their infants adequately were those who had delivered by cesarean section; they were still often concerned that they were doing an inadequate job because of their physical condition. Infant care is easier than most expect it to be, even for first time mothers (Gruis 1977:185). It is apparent, however, that though the skills of babycare can be more or less easily acquired, satisfaction with the parental role is substantially harder to come by (Lederman, Weingarten, and Lederman 1981).

Relationship with the newborn. Parents need to know what is normal for their own baby and to become accustomed to its routines and patterns. First time mothers in this study, for example, reported a concern for "baby noises" and the sound that the infant made while sleeping. These concerns were most pronounced in the earliest weeks of the postpartum period, and by six weeks the mother had adjusted to the infant's patterns. Other concerns during the first week, for all of the mothers, concerned feeding the child adequately. First-time mothers had more general concerns and worries, such as Sudden Infant Death Syndrome (SIDS) and the infants' overall health, while those who had had babies before expressed concern only for specific medical problems such as jaundice. By four to six weeks, most of these concerns had vanished for both groups.

Accommodating a new family. Parents are seldom prepared for the changes and realignment of relationships that a new baby brings. The new family member cannot be simply added on; he or she must somehow be integrated into an existing set of relationships that the parents already have with each other, with siblings, if they exist, and with family and friends. This integration is not always easy. Inglis (1971) reports that in a study of couples three months after the birth of their first child, two-thirds of them reported having marital problems. The quality of the relationship with the husband is often contingent on the active interest and involvement of the father as a parent (Lederman, Weingarten, and Lederman 1981: 208). At the same time, fathers often feel prepared for birth but not for parenthood, and the husband-wife problems that develop in the early postpartum often increase when the child is older (Wente and Crockenberg 1976:353). Multiparous women, in particular, often have a deep concern for relationships and family integration.

The new mothers I studied, in fact, reported a variety of changes in their relationships after the birth of a child. Within their immediate family, 26.3 percent of the multiparous women and 33.3 percent of the primiparous women reported that they now spent less time with their husbands. At the same time, 47.4 percent of the multiparous women and 62 percent of the primiparous women reported that they were closer to their husbands. Interestingly, the same women often reported both phenomena, which indicates, presumably, a decrease in the quantity but an increase in the quality of time spent together. Mothers who had delivered by cesarean section frequently said they were closer to their husbands and that their husbands had taken on a nurturing role during their convalescence. These mothers were often focused more on physical healing and on the evolution of the relationship with their spouses than on their new infant in the early postpartum. Despite a sense of growing closeness with their husbands, new mothers also expressed concern over their spouses' demands on them versus the new demands placed on them by the infant. Many women were apologetic for the added burden they felt they were placing on their spouses, for their crabbiness, and for other perceived faults. Several also expressed a concern for future problems that they thought might occur in their relationship if existing tensions did not diminish.

Changes also occurred in the new mothers' other relationships. Multiparous women reported fewer changes in their extended-family relationships, possibly because they had worked out these relationships with the birth of a previous child. First-time mothers, however, reported marked changes in their extended-family relationships: 71.4 percent reported an increase in closeness to their own family, specifically an increase in closeness to their own mother. A few women reported that after the baby's birth they underwent a reconciliation of a relationship with the husband's family and/or mother-in-law, and sometimes the new closeness to the woman's own family was seen as a reconciliation.

It must be noted that most of the women in the study had extended families living in close proximity to them at the time of their infant's birth. Both the Colville area and the Spokane area have relatively stable populations with generations remaining in the area. Many women reported that their parents and/or their husbands' parents lived in the same town or county and that they socialized with them at least once a week. Several women, in fact, lived in the same neighborhood as their kin and saw them on a daily basis. More than weekly visits were very common.

Changes in friendship patterns were harder to analyze. About one-third of each group reported no change in their friendships. Of those who did note changes, most reported becoming closer to those friends who also had children. Primiparous women frequently reported that they saw their friends less. It appears that changes in household routine eliminated much time for social interaction and that what time remained was devoted to socializing with the family. It would be interesting to correlate changes in friendship patterns with proximity of kin.

Overall, social life for all of these mothers was characterized by going out less frequently, staying home, and other modifications of lifestyle, all of which indicate a restriction of the woman to the domestic sphere and to some degree an isolation from the larger society, mitigated fortunately by the close presence of kin for many of the women. The addition of an infant to the household routine complicates things, whether or not it is the first baby. Primiparous women, for example, frequently noted that it was simply harder to go out, that the time it took to prepare the baby's things for a simple trip was rather like deploying a major troop movement, which sometimes made it too difficult to simply go out for casual purposes. About 38 percent of the first-time mothers also expressed deep concern for lack of time for themselves. Presumably those who already had children had given up on having time for themselves or had learned how to make time for themselves out of their busy days. Interestingly, while virtually all of the multiparous women said they expected the changes in their life-styles or relationships that occurred with the addition of another child, at the same time, at least one-fourth of that group cited severely negative changes in their lives. They also reported that the extra child was "more work" or "took up more time" than expected. About half of the first- time mothers said that motherhood was not what they expected it to be (though this was not always negative: many said that, despite the problems, there was more joy than they ever thought possible). The primiparous women who felt motherhood to be what they expected it to be felt that they had anticipated many of the changes but had not expected them to be so extreme.

MATERNAL ADJUSTMENT AND SOCIAL SUPPORT

The primary concerns of new mothers tend not to be the handling of the infant—the physical aspects of bringing up baby—but the need to incorporate the new member into one's social world and the need to regain one's figure and control over self-presentation. And, while most classes aimed at the postpartum period focus on childcare—such as hospital films on infant safety, bathing, etc—little attention is paid to the fatigue, emotional tension, isolation, and feeling of being tied down that new mothers feel in the early postpartum period. It has become more apparent in the past several years that a critical factor in postpartum adjustment and the development of adequate mothering is not knowledge of the various methods of childcare but the support system available to the new mother that positively backs up her new role. Couples with childrearing friends, for example, report fewer postpartum adjustment problems than others (Lederman, Weingarten, and Lederman 1981: 207).

The geographical proximity of support-network members has a significant effect on how important they will be postpartum (Bryant 1982:1760). A woman with no nearby support system often must take care of her infant while she is still physically uncomfortable and is undergoing the profound changes that occur at a social and emotional level after childbirth. Satisfaction with motherhood, not simply the learning of childcare tasks, appears to be directly related to the support of family and friends for the maternal role. The women in this pilot study perhaps had fewer postpartum conflicts than others might have had because most of them lived near and could call upon the resources of a support network of kin. All were married, and the new infants were by and large welcome additions to the family circle. Support for the maternal role within the larger family was high.

MOTHERHOOD MYTHS AND POSTPARTUM ADJUSTMENT

Society's popular view of motherhood also provides a yardstick by which many women measure their performance as mothers in the early postpartum period. Prior to 1960, "not only did women spend most of their adult energies raising a family rather than pursuing employment; this pattern was thought to be congruent with and supportive of a set of intrinsically female skills and preferences" (Luker 1984: 113). Even for those women who worked, a paying job was an adjunct to a woman's primary role as mother. Particularly in the 1950s, women were idealized as enjoying total involvement with their children, and the popular media portrayed mother at home baking cookies and rocking the cradle, happy in her domestic role. In reality, during this period there was an increasing contradiction between the growing number of women entering the workforce and the ideology of mother at home (Margolis 1984). Still, for many women giving birth today, this idealized view of motherhood is the one they have learned from their own mothers and carried to their expectations of the maternal role in the postpartum period.

As more women entered the workforce after 1960 there was a basic philosophical change in the idea of motherhood. The increased opportunity for a woman to have status outside the home and family has meant that a woman's primary place is no longer solely in the home, but that the role of mother is one of many that a woman may choose (Luker 1984). Yet, the increase in role options has not demythologized the maternal role. The new mother, who may herself have only recently left the workforce to have her baby, is faced with the myth of the 'supermom,' which implies that a woman can do it all, and if she cannot she must be less of a woman. Supermoms love the baby automatically, and, despite physical discomfort, they provide optimum care, stimulation, and love to the infant while maintaining a superior relationship with husband and other family members. In a society that romanticizes motherhood in this way, the woman who resents her infant's demands, who wishes only to sleep for more than two hours at a time, and who feels hostile when she cannot cope with the multiple demands of her family feels guilty.

Culturally, the postnatal period is depicted in the misty tones of baby-product commercials, a madonna-like mother smiling down at her newborn, full in her contentment. Yet the reality of early postpartum does not resemble the image projected. The complexity of the adjustment to the demands of infant and family creates a contradiction for the new mother between the culturally acceptable image of motherhood and the realities of becoming a mother. In truth, beyond mythology, motherhood and childrearing are not seen as crucial and valued roles. And, despite the ability to choose other roles along with motherhood, once a woman gives birth to a child, her life changes substantially. She is no longer free; she is not just superwoman, she is supermom! "And, tragically, that lack of freedom is reinforced and institutionalized by the very nature of society....Whatever her situation, every woman who has a child is punished for having done the very thing which society tells her is her womanly goal" (Chicago 1985:224).

Women react to the demands of motherhood with a varying capacity for flexibility and a varying readiness to find satisfaction in these new rythms in their life (Shereshefsky et al, 1974: 173). It appears that the women who adjust most easily to the birth of a new child are those who are less enslaved by the experience because they have adequate support from others, do not aspire to be the perfect selfless mother, can call on a good mothering image, and are not passively feminine, but actively seek to control their circumstances (Breen 1975).

CONCLUSIONS

Overall, it is apparent that positive postpartum adjustment is a continuum through pregnancy and childbirth which requires support to enhance the mother's self-esteem and create realistic, rather than romanticized, notions of the rewards and problems of new motherhood. It is clear, also, that the roles that a woman takes on after the birth of her child are not developed in isolation. For one, the infant provides cues with its unique personality—a baby with colic certainly poses different problems of adjustment from the rare baby who immediately sleeps through the night. Social-group approval or sanctions and a variety of environmental or situational circumstances restrict or enhance the options a given woman may have in defining her mothering role. The new mother needs flexibility, and cognitive, communication, and social skills which the society provides altogether few opportunities for learning. The large number of neglected, abused, and abandoned children indicates that too many mothers have difficulty in adjusting to that role.

NOTES

Research for the pilot study of rural and urban childbirth presented in this chapter was supported by a grant from the Northwest Institute for Advanced Study. An earlier version of this paper was presented at the meetings of the American Anthropological Association, Denver, 1984.

1. The four tasks of postpartum recovery are taken from the analysis of Gruis (1977).

18

WHAT DETERMINES
THE DURATION OF BREASTFEEDING?

Janice M. Morse, Margaret J. Harrison, and Karen M. Williams

Since the 1950s, health professionals have made a concerted effort to increase the rate and duration of breastfeeding. Numerous studies showing the advantages of breastfeeding in Third World countries have been used to develop a "breast-is-best" policy that has also influenced policy for Western nations, including the United States and Canada (American Academy of Pediatrics 1982; Canadian Pediatric Nutrition Committee 1979). In response to this trend, an enormous amount of research has been conducted to determine the factors associated with the initiation, maintenance, and early termination of breastfeeding. The assumption underlying this research is: if factors that facilitate breastfeeding (or inhibit bottle feeding) can be identified, then breastfeeding rates can be further increased. The most recent goal set in the United States is to have 75 percent of all new mothers breastfeeding their infants by the year 1990 (Smith 1984).

The debate concerning the advantages of breast or bottle feeding is beyond the scope of this discussion. Rather, in this chapter the factors associated with the duration and termination of breastfeeding will be reviewed, and suggestions for alternate directions for research will be presented. The authors argue that present research, focusing primarily on maternal factors rather than on a holistic approach, over-simplifies the problem. The tendency of researchers to attribute past events, such as delivery-room variables, to the length of time that breastfeeding is maintained is simplistic. Patterns of breastfeeding are societally structured rather than a function solely of a single mother's experiences with birth. For example, breastfeeding is often terminated prematurely due to a lack of "fit" between the mothers' and infants' lives. Therefore, the most fruitful method of extending breastfeeding might be to explore new patterns of breastfeeding that will fit contemporary women's lives rather than to demand that women's lives fit a breastfeeding schedule. Furthermore, societal norms not only suggest that there is a right place and method of feeding for infants at various developmental

261

stages, but also an appropriate time for weaning. The onset of weaning is often due to external social pressure on the mother when the infant reaches the age at which society deems him or her to be "too old to breastfeed." It is paradoxical, therefore, that efforts to promote breastfeeding are targeted at the mother rather than at society in general.

HISTORICAL TRENDS

Changing patterns of infant feeding have been documented over the past fifty years. In 1933, 87.8 percent of infants in the United States were breastfed; by 1936, this incidence was reduced to 74.6 percent (Eastman et al. 1976). There had been an even more dramatic decline to 38 percent by 1946; to 32 percent by 1952, and down to 18 percent by 1966 (Meyer 1968). By 1977, however, the rate of breastfeeding had been restored to 33 percent (Cummingham 1977), and by 1979, it had increased to 49.7 percent (Martinez and Nalezienski 1979).

Surveys have also shown a consistent correlation between breastfeeding and socioeconomic status and level of maternal education. The lowest rates of breast-feeding are associated with economically and educationally disadvantaged mothers (Hirscham and Sweet 1974; Sauls 1979; Sjolin, Hofvander, and Hillervick 1977). Ironically, because nutritional and hygiene standards are lower in these groups, bottle-fed infants are considered by health professionals to be at increased health risk (Mata 1978).

RECENT RESEARCH

Despite the tremendous amount of research and money spent on educational programs, many mothers choose not to breastfeed. The reasons for the high rate of bottle feeding are still being debated in the literature. Influences on the mother's decision to breastfeed or not have been cited as occurring before, during, and after the birth of her baby.

Prenatal Influences. Several studies have shown that the woman's choice of infant feeding is made prenatally, sometimes as early as during the woman's adolescence (Guthrie and Kan 1977). Hally et al. (1984) note that 75 percent of their sample of primigravidae had made a firm decision regarding method of infant feeding by the thirty-fourth week of pregnancy. These studies indicate that, while prenatal teaching may be of value for some mothers (Wiles 1984), discussions of breastfeeding should be included in the health curricula at high schools or earlier (Berger and Winter 1980).

There has been an extensive debate over the influence of advertising on women's decisions to purchase and use infant formula (Jelliffe 1975). Although this has primarily been an issue for Third World countries, some hospitals and public-health clinics in North America have refused to allow the formula companies to advertise on their premises or to distribute literature and formula samples. Yet, a comparison of the duration of breastfeeding in a sample of mothers who received gift packages of infant formula and those who did not indicated no statistically significant differences between the two groups (Bergeuni, Dougherty, and Kramer 1983)

Perinatal Influences. The immediate postnatal environment is considered to play a vital role in the success of breastfeeding. Researchers have noted that the mother's experience during labor is related to whether or not the mother breastfeeds: mothers who have experienced complications during labor, such as forceps delivery or a cesarean section, are less likely to breastfeed (Whichelow 1982).

The work of Klaus and Kennell (1976) on the concept of maternal-child bonding showed that mothers who had prolonged contact with their infants were more likely to breastfeed and also exhibited increased attachment behaviors (Carlsson, Larsson, and Schaller 1980; Klaus et al. 1972). This research has contributed to relatively recent changes in delivery-room procedure to provide parents with time with their new infant immediately after birth.

Rigid hospital scheduling of infant-feeding times and the promotion of complementary and supplementary bottle feeding has also been noted as interfering with lactation (de Chateau, Holmberg, and Wineberg 1977). Over the past fifteen years, hospitals have made a greater effort to permit rooming in and feeding on demand (Verronen et al. 1980). Furthermore, the attitudes of health professionals, particularly nurses, toward breastfeeding have been extensively examined. Nurses who have negative attitudes about breastfeeding are considered to hinder breastfeeding attempts by postpartum mothers (Ellis and Hewat 1983, 1984; Hood et al. 1978).

Postpartum Factors. The concept of a *doula*, or a person to support the mother during lactation, was first described by Raphael (1973). Studies have repeatedly shown that mothers cannot successfully breastfeed without support (Houston 1984; Rousseau et al. 1982). The person who assumes the role of the *doula* differs among cultures; for example, it will be the mother's mother in Mexican-American families, a close friend in black-American families, and the woman's husband in Anglo-American families (Baranowski et al. 1983).

Surveys investigating why mothers have not continued to breastfeed reveal two predominant reasons. The first is insufficient milk. Breast milk does not resemble cows' milk or formula, and many mothers think that the slightly blue color of human milk indicates that it is "weak." Mothers also attribute infant fussiness to "not enough milk," and, rather than stimulate the milk supply, they interpret this as a cue to switch to bottle feeding (Sjolin, Hofvander, and Hillevik 1977; Whichlow 1982).

The second reason is convenience (Goodine and Fried 1984; Yeung 1983) or returning to work (Riordan 1983; Yeung 1983). Eighteen percent of the women who weaned within four months of delivery cited this as the primary reason for ceasing to breastfeed (Rousseau et al. 1982). Other reasons frequently cited, such as tiredness (Gunn 1984), insufficient milk (Gunn, 1984; Gussler and Briesemeister 1980), and a difficult baby, may also be directly associated with the stress of women's workload. Only recently have researchers noted that breastfeeding may simply be time-consuming and hard work (McCaffery 1984).

Limitations of Research. From the preceding discussion, it is evident that breastfeeding is complex and multivariate. Yet the research methods used to determine the duration of breastfeeding and the variables included are delineated according to the paradigmatic preferences of the researcher rather than reflecting the multivariate reality. Even the choice of a dependent variable to measure "success" in breastfeeding differs according to the perspective of the researcher (Harrison, Morse, and Prowse 1985). However, in spite of the complexity of the issue, researchers continue to use univariate statistical methods to analyze continuation of breastfeeding. Such an approach may produce invalid results and spurious correlations (Morse 1982).

A second limitation is that researchers focus on antecedent events (either prenatally or in the early postnatal period) and correlate factors from this time with the subsequent duration of breastfeeding. A more fruitful approach is to examine ongoing events, such as changing attitudes towards the infant during the rapid developmental stages of the first few months of life.

A third problem with research that has examined mother's choice of infant feeding or the mother's reasons for weaning is that it is based on forced-choice questionnaires rather than on observational data and open-ended interviews. The deductive nature of such survey research frequently loses validity as mothers check the socially acceptable responses and the real reasons are left unexplored. With the exception of the research on maternal-child bonding, there is a dearth of observational research on the nursing couple and the interaction of the dyad within the family. This may be due to the inconvenience and the perceived invasion of privacy associated with conducting such longitudinal research in the home.

The Present Study. During the past two years, with the use of telephone interviews, we have conducted longitudinal research on innovative patterns of breastfeeding (Morse, Harrison, and Prowse 1986) and have examined the assumptions and beliefs underlying breastfeeding research (Harrison, Morse, and Prowse 1985). Two major areas that have a profound impact on the duration of breastfeeding have been identified from this research: (1) the incompatibility of present breastfeeding patterns with the life-style of many North American women and (2) the degree of social coercion toward weaning.

BREASTFEEDING PATTERNS

As previously noted, one of the major reasons for ceasing to breastfeed is convenience or returning to work or school. Mothers may wean from the breast because of economic necessity and limited maternity leave or simply because of the desire to return to work. Others may feel constrained by the infant's schedule and/or wish to allow their husband and others more involvement in infant feeding.

For mothers who wish to work or to otherwise spend time away from the infant each day and still continue to breastfeed their infant, the advice given by health-care professionals for maintaining lactation is that breasts must be emptied three or four times per day. Without this regular emptying, lactation will cease (see, for example, La Cerva 1981). As milk supply is a matter of supply and demand, Goldfarb and Tibbets (1980:180–1) suggest that cessation of lactation will occur within one month due to the "dwindling supply of milk and the preference for some babies for the bottle." According to this advice, if the mother wishes to continue to breastfeed, it is necessary to express the breasts every four hours to ensure that the milk supply is maintained.

Although this recommendation appears reasonable, in practice it may not be feasible. Rarely is there a private place in the work setting for the women to express. Bathrooms are not private, and there is usually nowhere to sit. Few women have private offices, and professional women report that their positions do not allow for predictable breaks. The final part of the recommendation, that the expressed milk be refrigerated and fed to the infant the next day, is also not always feasible, though some women have solved this problem with plastic bags, ice, and Thermos flasks.

The medical belief that lactation will diminish without regular stimulation cannot be substantiated in the literature. Reports from the Third World contradict this position: anthropologists report mothers nursing once or twice per day without expressing and continuing to do so for long periods of time (Gussler and Mock 1983; Morse 1984). In clinical practice, we also observed this method of infant feeding, termed *minimal breastfeeding*, to be practiced by Canadian women (Morse, Harrison, and Prowse, 1986).

Thirty women who were using minimal breastfeeding (MBF) were interviewed monthly by telephone until the infant was weaned. This study provided extensive data on the management of lactation (Morse, Harrison, and Prowse 1986). Women in this study used MBF for three reasons: as a method for slow weaning, for convenience while working, and as a "comfort" nursing strategy for nursing older infants. Although the sample in this study was small, none of the mothers experienced problems with their breasts (engorgement, leaking, or infections), nor did any report problems with a reduction of their milk supply.

They reported that their breasts "adjusted" to the new schedule. All of the infants were fed formula from a cup, bottle, or spoon in their mother's absence. Apparently, mothers were able to continue breastfeeding as long as they or their infant desired. For the mothers who were weaning, MBF was maintained for a mean of six weeks (s=1.77 weeks). Working mothers used MBF for a mean of 19.77 weeks (s=12.55), and mothers who were comfort nursing used it for a mean of 39.4 weeks (s=19.69).

Despite advice from health professionals that frequent expression of milk was necessary for continued lactation, these women had discovered MBF during the slow weaning process or had learned of it from a friend. Others tried this pattern of nursing as a last resort, rather than cease breastfeeding their infant. One mother, a lawyer, said, "I cannot express! What would I do if I'm in court? Do I say 'Excuse me Judge... '?"

Although there is a lack of research on the actual need for expressing, health professionals teach that it is always essential for the management of lactation. The possibility of nursing the infant fewer times a day, supplemented with formula when the mother is away, is never offered as an alternative. Only the most resourceful mothers discover, through necessity, that it is not always required:

> If you read anything, they always say to express milk while you are at work... and it is such a hassle! I think it turns people off. *And you don't have to do that!*

Medical knowledge and recommendations for maintaining breastfeeding are replete with assumptions rather than knowledge based on science. Medical advice to the breastfeeding mother on the necessity for expressing milk may paradoxically produce demands that result in a decision to wean from the breast rather than to continue lactation. In these instances, the clinician's perceptions of reality regarding breastfeeding restrict maternal options and decrease, rather than increase, the duration of breastfeeding.

SOCIAL COERCION FOR WEANING

Anthropologists have long noted that the method of infant feeding selected by parents is a reflection of cultural norms. Work by Raphael (1973) has called attention to the role of the *doula* in the mother's efforts at breastfeeding. The support may be in the form of psychological support for the mother, the provision of knowledge on the techniques of breastfeeding, or assistance with household duties and with the care of other children while the mother is nursing. Significantly, Raphael noted that without the support of a *doula*, breastfeeding was not likely to be successful. Cross-culturally, in the extended family situation the *doula* was most likely to be the mother's mother or mother-in-law. In North American society, the *doula* might also be a female friend, the husband, a formal support group, such as La Leche League, a health professional, or even a book on breastfeeding.

In our longitudinal study of breastfeeding patterns, we asked mothers, "Who is most supportive of your breastfeeding?" and, "Who is least supportive of your breastfeeding?" With few exceptions, mothers identified their husbands or their mothers and mothers-in-law as the *doula* during the first few months. All reported that their families, friends, and acquaintances, as well as their physician and nurse, supported their breastfeeding. However, this pattern changed in the course of the study. Between the fifth and the tenth month, friends and acquaintances became quiet about the mother's breastfeeding. Mothers reported that their friends "didn't say anything." Then, from approximately the eighth month, friends began to suggest that the infant should be weaned. Mothers reported that friends questioned "Why are you *still* breastfeeding?" and one mother said, "One friend jokes about it—'Oh, you haven't weaned him yet'—not *really* joking, you know!"

Mothers reported that this feedback made them feel nervous and anxious about breastfeeding. They became quiet about the fact that they "were *still* breastfeeding"" and concealed this from those who they thought would not understand. They no longer nursed their infant in public. Mothers stated this in a number of ways: "I'm getting comments on his age. I refuse to nurse him in public when he asks. He fusses, but I just refuse." "Only close friends know—that means others can't comment." "We were grocery shopping yesterday and it was Kelley's usual naptime and he began to fuss and started pulling my blouse. My neighbor looked at me and asked 'Are you *still* nursing?' It was so obvious I couldn't say no!" At this time, several mothers deliberately sought out a friend who was also breastfeeding or made contact with La Leche League and made new friendships within that group.

Family members followed a similar pattern of withdrawal of support for breastfeeding. Between the tenth and thirteenth month they refrained from commenting about breastfeeding and then began suggesting that the infant should be weaned. Even in situations where the mother or the mother-in-law previously served as *doula*, she began to encourage weaning. Various reasons were presented for encouraging weaning, such as the belief that prolonged breastfeeding is a drain on the mother's body. A more subtle reason given was the wish of the grandparents to care for their grandchild: "My mother says I would be freer and Jenny could stay with her more if I weaned her."

As the child becomes older, family members increasingly view breastfeeding as a sexual activity. Repeatedly mothers reported that their families "dropped hints" or told the child rather than the mother that they were "too old to nurse." The implication was that the child was becoming too aware to nurse, and thus such behavior was inappropriate. One mother stated directly: "She [the mother-in-law] is afraid that I'm turning her grandson into a sexual pervert!"

With the exception of one case, the last person to withdraw support for breastfeeding was the husband. This occurred between the thirteenth and twentieth month. The sexual implications of the child sucking and the violation of the norms of modesty appeared to underlie the withdrawal of support: "He doesn't really say [if he supports breastfeeding or not]. But he wasn't impressed when she was pulling up my blouse and trying to nurse" "My husband wants me to wean, but he lets me do my own thing. At times he says 'What is a big boy like that doing *there*.'"

Mothers, sensing societal disapproval as the infant became older, reduced the number of places they would nurse the infant. Initially, mothers felt it acceptable to nurse the infant in public, such as in church or in front of family or friends. But as the baby learned to speak, to crawl, and then to walk, the number of places that the child could be nursed became more limited until all mothers nursed at home in a special chair. This pattern of "closet nursing" has been previously described by Avery (1977). Often the mother and infant have a special term for the chair used for nursing, or for breastfeeding per se, so that if the infant requests to nurse in a public place, others listening will not understand the request. This prevents embarrassment to the mother.

With the exception of two cases, weaning occurred within one month of the withdrawal of all support, and in the remaining two cases within three months. One of these mothers continued to nurse, concealing this fact from her husband, who thought the child was weaned!

The attitudes of health professionals appeared to resemble the norms of the larger society. Thus, the personal attitudes of the physician or nurse towards breastfeeding may be in conflict with the official policy of encouraging breastfeeding. Observing this implicit message, mothers observed that physicians were a little too quick to suggest that the infant be placed on a bottle when breastfeeding problems occurred, and mothers who practiced breastfeeding for more than six months may even withhold this information from health professionals. Of the thirty mothers in this sample, only eleven reported that their doctors knew they were still breastfeeding when they were first interviewed. One mother reported, "I haven't talked to him about it. He asked me at six weeks whether the babe was breast or bottle fed, and that's all."

Although all doctors knew that their patients were breastfeeding initially, when the infant was twelve months of age, only four of the sixteen doctors knew that nursing was continuing. None were informed after the infant's sixteenth month. Mothers said, "He doesn't ask, so I don't tell."

Although physicians were "officially" supportive, they were not considered the main source of support in any instance. None were identified by mothers as serving in the role of the *doula*. The mothers explained: "Well, he supports it on paper, but he is inclined to suggest the bottle when there are any problems"; or "The doctor's quite supportive, but not a great source of information." One mother felt that she needed to conceal the fact that she was nursing a twenty-six month old toddler from her dentist, when he prescribed penicillin for dental problems:

I sort of misled the dentist to believe that Lisbeth was about
one-year old. A week later I ran into him at a restaurant. There
I was with a two-year old, and I felt awful. But it's hard to
know if the dentist remembered me as a patient. I'd done most
of the research on penicillin myself and found it to be harmless
[in breast milk].

The attitudes of nurses were similar. One infant was admitted to a hospital at
twenty-one months. Although recently weaned, the child wanted to nurse, and
breast milk soon became the only food the child would take. The mother noted
that while the nurses did not openly oppose her nursing the infant they "didn't
say anything."

The duration of breastfeeding is thus a reflection of societal norms. When
the baby is perceived to be past the appropriate age for breastfeeding, the decision
to wean is facilitated by the *doula* and significant others. There is some evidence
that this mechanism—social coercion for weaning—is operational and effective
even when the mother herself wishes to continue to breastfeed. One mother who
called reported that, though she "loved to nurse" and thought it the best thing she
could do for her baby, she felt pressured by her neighbors to wean the baby onto
formula.

CONCLUSION

The determinants of the duration of breastfeeding have been examined extensively
by researchers, but the present trend of this research has serious limitations in
both the paradigmatic assumptions underlying the research and the research
methods used. Our preliminary research, despite the small number of subjects,
suggests that concurrent sociocultural factors rather than (or perhaps as well as)
antecedent events are important considerations for understanding the course of
breastfeeding.

Presently, all of the efforts of health professionals are targeted toward
educating the mother and, to a lesser extent, the father on the importance of
breastfeeding. However, the research discussed in this chapter suggests that
health education should not be specifically aimed at the mother but at society in
general, particularly Anglo-American grandparents. Moreover, a variety of
patterns of breastfeeding, such as minimal breastfeeding, needs to be encouraged
so that mothers who wish to continue nursing their infant may have the option
to do so.

NOTE

This chapter was prepared with the assistance of a National Health Development
Program Research Scholar Award to Dr. J. Morse.

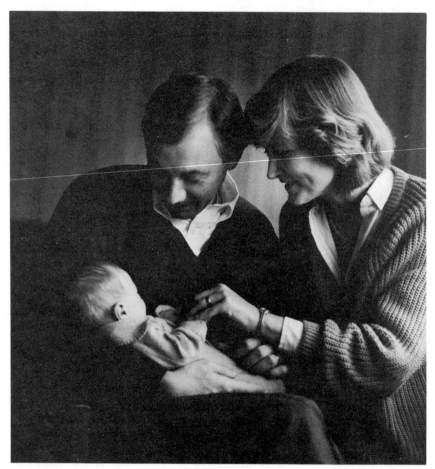

Photograph by LeRoy J. Dierker, Jr., M.D.

CONTRIBUTORS

Barbara Alvin received her Ph.D. in biostatistics from the University of Washington. She currently is an assistant professor of mathematics at Eastern Washington University.

Margaret S. Boone received her Ph.D. in cultural anthropology from the Ohio State University. She is a social science analyst with the U.S. General Accounting Office, Program Evaluation and Methodology Division.

Linda Haines Briesemeister received her Ph.D. in anthropology from the Ohio State University. She is currently a visiting assistant professor at the University of Wisconsin-Parkside.

Robbie Davis-Floyd received her Ph.D. in anthropology and folklore from the University of Texas at Austin. She is a frequent speaker at academic and childbirth education conferences.

Jeanne Harley Guillemin received her Ph.D. in sociology from Brandeis University. She is a professor of sociology at Boston College.

Beth A. Haines is a doctoral candidate in developmental psychology at the University of Wisconsin-Madison, where she serves as a lecturer in the Department of Psychology.

Margaret J. Harrison received her master of science in nursing degree from the University of Rhode Island. She is now an assistant professor of nursing at the University of Alberta, where she is a doctoral candidate in the Department of Family Studies.

Ellen S. Lazarus received her Ph.D. in anthropology at Case Western Reserve University. She is a visiting assistant professor at Oberlin College and a research associate in the Department of Reproductive Biology at Case Western Reserve School of Medicine.

Betty Wolder Levin earned the Ph.D. in sociomedical sciences from Columbia University. She is currently an associate in the Division of Sociomedical Sciences at Columbia University and an assistant professor in the Department of Health and Nutrition Sciences at Brooklyn College of the City University of New York. She is a member of the Hastings Center Research Group on the Care of the Newborn.

Ronnie Lichtman received her master's degree in maternity nursing and nurse-midwifery at Columbia University, where she is currently pursuing doctoral studies in sociomedical sciences with a specialization in anthropology. She teaches midwifery at Columbia University, and is a partner is a private practice.

John Marcucci received his Ph.D. in anthropology from Southern Methodist University. He is currently director of the Multicultural Community Center in Dallas.

Karen L. Michaelson received her Ph.D. in anthropology from the University of Wisconsin-Madison. She is an associate professor of anthropology and health sciences at Eastern Washington University where she holds an administrative position.

Janice M. Morse received both a Ph.D. in nursing and a Ph.D. in anthropology from the University of Utah. She is currently a professor of nursing on the Faculty of Nursing at the University of Alberta, where she also is a research associate in the Department of Anthropology.

Lucile F. Newman received her Ph.D. in anthropology from the University of California-Berkeley. She is currently an associate professor of community health at Brown University.

Marilyn L. Poland has a master's degree in maternal child health nursing from Boston University and a Ph.D. in physical anthropology from Wayne State University. She is currently an associate professor in the Department of Obstetrics and Gynecology at the Wayne State University School of Medicine where she serves as co-director of the Institute for Maternal and Child Health.

Caroline Park has a bachelor's degree in nursing from the University of Manitoba and an M. Ed. from the University of Alberta. She is an assistant professor of nursing at the University of Alberta.

Rayna Rapp received her Ph.D. in anthropology at the University of Michigan. She is currently an associate professor in the Department of Anthropology, the Graduate Faculty, at the New School for Social Research where she serves as chair of the department.

Barbara Katz Rothman holds the Ph.D. in sociology from New York University. She is currently an associate professor of sociology at Baruch College and the Graduate Center, City University of New York.

Carolyn Sargent received her Ph.D. in anthropology from Michigan State University. She is currently an associate professor of anthropology at Southern Methodist University.

Michael Sharinus is a doctoral candidate in the Ph.D. program in applied anthropology at the University of South Florida.

Wenda R. Trevathan received her Ph.D. in anthropology from the University of Colorado, and now holds a position as assistant professor of anthropology at New Mexico State University.

Linda M. Whiteford received her Ph.D. in anthropology from the University of Wisconsin, Milwaukee, and a masters degree in public health from the University of Texas. She is currently an associate professor of anthropology at the University of South Florida where she is the leader of the Medical Track in Applied Anthropology.

Karen M. Williams is a candidate for the master's degree in nursing at the University of Alberta.

BIBLIOGRAPHY

Abrahams, Roger D. 1973. Ritual for Fun and Profit (or the Ends and Outs of Celebration). Paper presented at the Wenner-Foundation Symposium # 59, "Ritual: Reconciliation in Change." Burg Wartenstein.

Adams, Jeffrey L. 1983. The Use of Obstetrical Procedures in the Care of Low Risk Women. *Women and Health* 8(1):25–34.

Affonso, D.D. 1976. The Newborn's Potential for Interaction. *Journal of Obstetric, Gynecological, and Neonatal Nursing* 5(6):9–14

————. 1973. Assessment of Pain During Labor. In *Current Concepts in Clinical Nursing*. E.H. Anderson, ed. St. Louis: C.V. Mosby.

Alpert, J., and M. Richardson. 1978. Conflict, Outcome, and Perception of Women's Roles. *Educational Gerontology* 3:79–87.

Amarasingham, Loran R. 1980. Movement among Healers in Sri Lanka: A Case Study of a Sinhalese Patient. *Culture, Medicine, and Psychiatry* 4:71–92.

American Academy of Pediatrics. 1982. Policy Statement Based on Task Force Report: The Promotion of Breast Feeding. *Pediatrics* 69:654–61.

————. 1980. Estimates of Neeed and Recommendation for Personnel in Neonatal Pediatrics. *Pediatrics* 65:850–53.

Anderson, Barbara G., J. Rafael Toledo, and Nancy Hazam. 1982. An Approach to the Resolution of Mexican-American Resistance to Diagnostic and Remedial Pediatric Heart Care. In *Clinically Applied Anthropology*. Noel Chrisman and Thomas Maretzki, eds. Dordrecht, Holland: D. Reidel.

Angelini, D.J. 1978. Nonverbal Communication in Labor. *American Journal of Nursing* 78:1220–22.

Anisfeld, Elizabeth and Evelyn Lipper. 1983. Early Contact, Social Support, and Mother-Infant Bonding. *Pediatrics* 72(1):79–83.

Anspach, Renee R. Forthcoming. *Life and Death Decisions in Neonatal Intensive Care: A Study in the Sociology of Knowledge.* Berkeley: University of California Press.

Antonovsky, Aaron, and Judith Bernstein. 1977. Social Class and Infant Mortality. *Social Science and Medicine* 11:453–70.

Arms, Suzanne. 1975. *Immaculate Deception.* Boston: Houghton Mifflin.

Arras, John D. 1985. Toward an Ethic of Ambiguity. *Hastings Center Report* 14(2):25–33.

Asbury, J. 1980. Labor Pain: The Role of Childbirth Education, Information, and Expectations. In *Problems in Pain*. C. Peck and M. Wallace, eds. London: Pergamon.

273

Asch, Adrienne, and Michelle Fine. 1984. Shared Dreams: A Left Perspective on Disability Rights and Reproductive Rights. *Radical America* 18(4):51–58.

Auletta, Ken. 1982. *The Underclass.* New York: Random House.

Avery, Jimmie. 1977. Closet Nursing: A Symptom of Intolerance or a Forerunner of Social Change? *Keeping Abreast Journal.* July-September:212–27.

Babcock, Barbara, ed. 1978. *The Reversible World: Symbolic Inversion in Art and Society.* Ithaca: Cornell Unversity Press.

Badinter, Elisabeth. 1981. *Mother Love: Myth and Reality—Motherhood in Modern History.* New York: Macmillan. (Translated from the French).

Baranowski, Tom, et al. 1983. Social Support, Social Influences, Ethnicity, and the Breastfeeding Decision. *Social Science and Medicine* 17:1599–1611.

Barber, Bernard, ed. 1978. Medical Ethics and Social Change. *Annals of the American Academy of Political and Social Science* 437:1–141.

Barnard, Kathryn E. 1980. *Psychosocial Aspects of Pregnancy.* Report for the Surgeon General's Task Force on Improving Pregnancy Outcomes and Infant Health. Washington, D.C.: U.S. Government Printing Office.

Barton, John J., et al. 1980. Alternative Birthing Center: Experience in a Teaching Obstetric Service. *American Journal of Obstetrics and Gynecology* 137:377–84.

Bauwens, E.E., and S. Anderson. 1978. Home Birth: A Reaction to Hospital Environmental Stressors. In *The Anthropology of Health.* E.E. Bauwens, ed. St. Louis: C.V. Mosby.

Beck, Neils C., and Lawrence J. Siegel. 1980. Preparation for Childbirth and Contemporary Research on Pain, Anxiety, and Stress Reduction: A Review and Critique. *Psychosomatic Medicine* 42(4):429–47.

Bee, H.L., et al. 1982. Prediction of IQ and Language Skill from Perinatal Status, Child Performance, Family Characteristics, and Mother-Infant Interaction. *Child Development* 53:1134–56.

Bell, David. 1975. *A Time to Be Born.* New York: Morrow.

Benfield, D. Gary, Susan A. Leib, and Jeanette Reuter. 1976. Grief Responses of Parents after Referral of the Critically Ill Newborn to a Regional Center. *New England Journal of Medicine* 294:975–78.

Berger, Anna, and S.T.Winter. 1980. Attitudes and Knowledge of Secondary School Girls Concerning Breast Feeding. *Clinical Pediatrics* 19:825–26.

Bergeuni, V., C. Dougherty, and M.S. Kramer. 1983. Do Infant Feeding Formula Samples Shorten the Duration of Breastfeeding? *Lancet* 1:1148–56.

Bing, E. 1970. *The Adventure of Birth.* New York: Simon and Schuster.

Blackwell, A., et al. 1983. An Administrative Petition to the United States Department of Health and Human Services. June 29. San Francisco: Public Advocates.

Boles, A.J. 1983. Marital Satisfaction During the Transition to Parenthood. Paper presented at the meeting of the American Psychological Association, Anaheim, California.

———. 1981. Multivariate Analysis of Marital Satisfaction. Paper presented at the meeting of the American Psychological Association, Los Angeles.

Boone, Margaret. 1985. Social and Cultural Factors in the Etiology of Low Birthweight among Disadvantaged Blacks. *Social Science and Medicine*

20(10):1001–11.

———. 1982. A Socio-Medical Study of Infant Mortality among Disadvantaged Blacks. *Human Organization* 41(3):227–36.

Boston Women's Health Book Collective. 1985. *Our Bodies, Ourselves: A Book by and for Women.* New York: Simon and Schuster.

Bowen *vs.* American Hospital Association et al. 1986. Supreme Court of the United States. No. 84-1529. Argued January 15, 1986. Decided June 9, 1986

Boyle, M.H., et al. 1983. Economic Evaluation of Neonatal Intensive Care of Very-Low-Birthweight Infants. *New England Journal of Medicine* 308:1330–37.

Brackbill, Yvonne, J., and Diony Young. 1984. *Birth Trap: The Legal Low-Down on High-Tech Obstetrics.* St. Louis: C.V. Mosby.

Brazleton, T.B. 1973. *Neonatal Behavioral Assessment Scale.* London: Spastic International.

———. 1972. Implications of Infant Development among the Mayan Indians of Mexico. *Human Development* 15:90–111.

———. 1961. Effect of Maternal Medicine on the Neonate and His Behavior. *Journal of Pediatrics* 58:513–18.

Breen, Dana. 1975. *The Birth of a First Child.* London: Tavistock.

Brenner, Harvey. 1973. Fetal, Infant, and Maternal Mortality During Periods of Economic Instability. *International Journal of Health Services* 3:145–59.

Brewster, Arlene. 1984. A Patient's Reaction to Amniocentesis. *Obstetrics and Gynecology* 64:443–44.

Britton, S.P., S. Fitzhardinge and S. Ashley. 1981. Is Intensive Care Justified for Infants Weighing Less than 801 Grams at Birth? *Journal of Pediatrics* 99:937–47.

Brody, E.B., and H. Klein. 1980. The Intensive Care Nursery as a Small Society: Contribution to the Socialization and Learning of the Pediatric Intern. *Paediatrician* 90:169–81.

Brody, Howard, and James R. Thompson. 1981. The Maximin Strategy in Modern Obstetrics. *The Journal of Family Practice* 12(6):977–86.

Bromwich, Rose M. 1985. "Vulnerable Infants" and "Risky Environments." *Zero to Three* 6(2):7–12.

Brooks, C. 1980. Social, Economic, and Biological Correlates of Infant Mortality in City Neighborhoods. *Journal of Health and Social Behavior* 21:2–11.

Brown, E. Richard. 1979. *Rockefeller Medicine Men: Medicine and Capitalism in America.* Berkeley: University of California Press.

Brozan, Nadine. 1979. Two Fundamentalists Crusade Against Abortion in 20 Cities. *New York Times.* September 29.

Bruner, Jerome S. 1979. *On Knowing: Essays for the Left Hand.* Cambridge, Mass.: The Belknap Press of Harvard University Press.

Bryant, Carol Anne. 1982. The Impact of Kin, Friend, and Neighbor Networks on Infant Feeding. *Social Science and Medicine* 16:1757–65.

Budetti, Peter, et al. 1981.*The Costs and Effectiveness of Neonatal Intensive Care.* Background Paper #2: Case Studies of Medical Technologies. Office of Technology Assessment. Washington D. C., U.S. Government Printing

Office.

Burke, Meredith B., and Aliza Kolker. 1982. Amniocentesis and the Social Construction of Pregnancy. Paper presented at the meetings of the District of Columbia Sociological Society, Washington, DC.

Burnett, C., et al. 1980. Home Delivery and Neonatal Mortality in North Carolina. *Journal of the American Medical Association* 244(24):2741–45.

Burns, Tom, and Charles D. Laughlin. 1979. Ritual and Social Power. In *The Spectrum of Ritual: Bio-Genetic Structural Analysis*. E.G. Aquili et al., eds. New York: Columbia University Press.

Burst, Helen V. 1983. The Influence of Consumers on the Birthing Business. *Topics in Clinical Nursing* 5(3):42–54.

Canadian Pediatric Committee Nutrition Committee. 1979. Infant Feeding. *Canadian Journal of Public Health* 70:376–85.

Carlsson, S.G., K. Larsson, and J. Schaller. 1980. Early Mother-Child Contact and Nursing. *Reproduction, Nutrition, and Development* 20:881–89.

Carver, Cynthia. 1981. The Deliverers: A Woman Doctor's Reflections on Medical Socialization. In *Childbirth: Alternatives to Medical Control*. S. Romalis, ed. Austin: University of Texas Press.

Cassidy, Claire Monod. In press. Worldview Conflict and Child Malnutrition: Change Agent Dilemmas. In *Child Survival, Culture, and the Value of Children*. Nancy Scheper-Hughes, ed. Dordrecht, The Netherlands: D. Reidel.

Caudill, W., and H. Weinstein. 1969. Maternal Care and Infant Behavior in Japan and America. *Psychiatry* 32(1):12–43.

Chadwick, B., S. Albrecht, and P. Kunz. 1976. Marital and Role Satisfaction. *Journal of Marriage and the Family* 38:431–40.

Charles, Allen G., et al. 1978. Obstetric and Psychological Effects of Psychoprophylactic Preparation for Childbirth. *American Journal of Obstetrics and Gynecology* 131:44–52.

Chase, Helen. 1977. Infant Mortality and Its Concomitants, 1960–1972. *Medical Care* 15:622–74.

Chesler, Phyllis. 1979. *With Child, A Diary of Motherhood*. New York: Berkley Books.

Chess, Stella, and Alexander Thomas. 1982. Infant Bonding: Mystique and Reality. *American Journal of Orthopsychiatry* 52(2):213–22.

Chicago, Judy. 1985. *The Birth Project*. New York: Doubleday.

Clarke-Stewart, A. 1980. The Father's Contribution to Children's Cognitive and Social Development in Early Childhood. In *The Father-Infant Relationship*. F.A. Pederson, ed. New York: Praeger.

———. 1973. Interactions between Mothers and Their Children. *Monograph of the Society for Research on Child Development* 38(6–7).

Clausen, Joy P. 1985. A Transcultural Perspective on the Delivery of Perinatal Health Care. In *Bioethical Frontiers in Perinatal Intensive Care*. C. Harris and F. Snowden, eds. Natchitoches: Northwestern State University Press.

Cleveland Vital Statistics. 1984. *Annual Report*. City of Cleveland. Division of Health.

Cohen, Richard L. 1981. Factors Influencing Maternal Choice of Childbirth Alternatives. *Journal of the American Academy of Child Psychiatry* 20:1–15.

Cohen, S.E., M. Sigman, A.H. Parmalee, and L. Beckwith. 1982. Perinatal Risk and Developmental Outcome in Preterm Infants. *Seminars in Perinatology* 6:334–39.

Colon, D.D. 1981. *Born at Risk.* New York: St. Martin's Press.

Committee on Perinatal Health. 1976. *Toward Improving the Outcome of Pregnancy: Recommendations for the Regional Development of Maternal and Perinatal Health Services.* White Plains, N.Y.: March of Dimes National Foundation.

Condon, W.S., and L.W. Sander. 1974. Neonate Movement Is Synchronized with Adult Speech: Interactional Participation and Language Acquisition. *Science* 183:99–101.

Converse, Thomas A., Richard S. Buker, and Richard V. Lee. 1973. Hutterite Midwifery. *American Journal of Obstetrics and Gynecology* 116(5):719–25.

Corea, Gena. 1985. *The Mother Machine.* New York: Harper and Row.

Corwin, E.H.L. 1952. *Infant and Maternal Care in New York City: A Study of Hospital Facilities.* Committee on Public Health Relations. New York Academy of Medicine. New York: Columbia University Press.

Cowan, P., and C. Cowan. 1983. Quality of Couple Relationships and Parenting Stress in Beginning Families. Paper presented at the meeting of the Society for Research in Child Development, Detroit.

Cox, Bonnie, E., and Elaine C. Smith. 1982. The Mother's Self-Esteem After a Cesarean Delivery. *Maternal and Child Nursing* 7:309–14.

Coysh, W.S. 1983. Predictive and Concurrent Factors Relating to Father's Involvement in Childrearing. Paper presented at the meeting of the American Psychological Association, Anaheim, Calif.

Craig, Kenneth D. 1978. Social Modeling Influences on Pain. In *The Psychology of Pain.* R.A. Sternbach, ed. New York: Raven Press.

Craig, Kenneth D., and J. Allen Best. 1977. Perceived Control over Pain: Individual Differences and Situational Determinants. *Pain* 3(2):127–35.

Crane, Diana. 1975. *The Sanctity of Social Life: Physicians' Treatment of Critically Ill Patients.* New York: Russell Sage Foundation.

Cranley, Mecca S. 1981. The Roots of Attachment: The Relationship of Parents with Their Unborn. In *Perinatal Parent Behavior: Nursing Research and Implications for Newborn Health.* Birth Defects Original Article Series 17(6). R.F. Lederman et al. New York: Alan Liss.

Cunningham, Allan S. 1977. Morbidity in Breast-fed and Artificially Fed Infants. *Journal of Pediatrics* 90:726–29.

Curtis-Bowles. H. 1983. Self Changes in Early Stages of Parenting. Paper presented at the meeting of the American Psychological Association, Anaheim, Calif.

Danziger, Sandra Klein. 1979. Treatment of Women in Childbirth: Implications for Family Beginnings. *American Journal of Public Health* 69(9):895–901.

d'Aquili, Eugene G., and Charles D. Laughlin. 1979. The Neurobiology of Myth and Ritual. In *The Spectrum of Ritual: A Bio-Genetic Structural Analysis.* E.G. d'Aquili et al., eds. New York: Columbia University Press.

David, R., and E. Siegel. 1983. Decline in Neonatal Mortality, 1968–1977: Better Babies or Better Care? *Pediatrics* 71:531–40.

Davis, Karen. 1978. *Health and the War on Poverty: A Ten Year Appraisal.*

Washington, D.C. The Brookings Institute.

Davis-Floyd, Robbie E. 1987a. Obstetric Training as a Rite of Passage. *Medical Anthropology Quarterly* 1(3):288–318.

———. 1987b. The Technological Model of Birth. *Journal of American Folklore* (in press).

———.1986a. Afterward: The Cultural Context of Changing Childbirth. In *The Healing Power of Birth*. Rima Star. Austin Texas: Star Publishing.

———. 1986b. Birth as an American Rite of Passage. Ph.D. dissertation, University of Texas.

———. 1986c. *Routines and Rituals: A New View*. NAACOG Update Series. Princeton, N. J.: NAACOG Continuing Professional Education Center.

Davitz. Lois J., Joel R. Davitz, and Yasuko Higuchi. 1977a. Cross-Cultural Inferences of Physical Pain and Psychological Distress. Part 1. *Nursing Times* 73(16):512–23.

———. 1977b. Cross-Cultural Inferences of Physical Pain and Psychological Distress. Part 2. *Nursing Times* 73(16):556–58.

Davitz, Lois J., Yasko Sameshima, and Joel Davitz. 1976. Suffering as Viewed in Six Cultures. *American Journal of Nursing* 76(8):1296–97.

de Beauvoir, Simone. 1953. *The Second Sex*. New York: Bantam.

de Chateau, Peter, H. Holmberg, K. Jakobsson, and J. Winberg. 1977. A Study of Factors Promoting and Inhibiting Lactation. *Developmental Medcine and Child Neurology* 19:575–84.

Department of Health, New York City. 1984. *Summary of Vital Statistics*.

———. 1982. *Summary of Vital Statistics*.

———.n.d. *Infant Mortality Rates by Birthweight Group* 1950–1981.

Department of Health and Human Services. 1985. *Federal Register* 50 (April 15): 14878.

———. 1984a. *Federal Register* 49 (January 12): 1622.

———. 1984b. *Federal Register* 49 (December 10): 48160.

———. 1983a. *Federal Register* 48 (March 7): 9630.

———. 1983b. *Federal Register* 48 (July 5): 30848.

———. 1982. *Federal Register* 47 (June 16): 26027.

Desmond, M.M., A.J. Rudolph, and P. Phitaksphrawan. 1966. Transitional Care Nursery: A Mechanism of a Preventive Medicine. *Pediatric Clinics of North America* 13:651–55.

DeVitt, Neal. 1977. The Transition from Home to Hospital Birth, 1930–1960. *Birth and the Family Journal* 4(2):47–58.

DeVries, Raymond G. 1983. Image and Reality: The Evolution of Hospital Alternative Birth Centers. *Journal of Nurse-Midwifery* 28(3):3–9.

Dick-Read, Grantly. 1970. *Childbirth Without Fear: The Principles and Practice of Natural Childbirth*. New York: Harper and Row.

Dobbs, Kathe B., and Kirkwood K. Shy. 1981. Alternative Birth Rooms and Birth Options. *Obstetrics and Gynecology*. 58:626–30.

Douglas, Mary. 1973. *Natural Symbols: Explorations in Cosmology*. New York: Vintage Books.

———. 1966. *Purity and Danger*. London: Routledge and Kegan Paul.

Driscoll, John, Jr. n.d. Personal communication, based on unpublished statistics from Columbia-Presbyterian Medical Center NICU and other NICUs.

Driscoll, John, et al. 1982. Mortality and Morbidity in Infants Less than 1001 Grams Birth Weight. *Pediatrics* 69:21–22.

Drotar, Dennis, et al. 1975. The Adaptation of Parents to the Birth of Infants with Congenital Malformations: A Hypothetical Model. *Pediatrics* 1975:710–17.

Dubowitz, L.M.S., V. Dubowitz, and C. Goldberg. 1970. Clinical Assessment of Gestational Age in the Newborn Infant. *Journal of Pediatrics* 77:1–7.

Duff, Raymond S., and A.G.M. Campbell. 1973. Moral and Ethical Dilemmas in the Special Care Nursery. *New England Journal of Medicine* 289:890–94.

Duignan, N.M., J.W. Studd, and A.D. Hughes. 1975. Characteristics of Normal Labor in Different Racial Groups. *British Journal of Obstetrics and Gynecology* 82:593–601.

Dyer, E.D. 1963. Parenthood as Crisis: A Restudy. *Journal of Marriage and Family Living* 25:196–201.

Earhardt, C., H. Abramson, J. Pakter, and F. Nelson. 1970. An Epidemiological Approach to Infant Mortality. *Archives of Environmental Health* 20:743–57.

Eastman, E., D. et al. 1976. Further Decline in Breastfeeding. *British Medical Journal* 1(6005):305–7.

Egeland, Byron, and Brian Vaughn. 1981. Failure of "Bond Formation" as a Cause of Abuse, Neglect and Maltreatment. *American Journal of Orthopsychiatry* 51(1):78–84.

Ehrenreich, Barbara, and Dierdre English. 1973. *Witches, Midwives, and Nurses: A History of Women Healers.* Old Westbury, N.Y.: Feminist Press.

Eisner, V.,et al. 1979. The Risk of Low Birthweight. *American Journal of Public Health* 69:887–93.

Eldridge, R. 1970. How to Give Birth to a Daughter. *Redbook* 135(May): 81ff.

Ellis, Donelda J., and Roberta Hewat. 1984. Factors Related to Breastfeeding Duration. *Canadian Family Physician* 30:1479–84.

———. 1983. Do Nurses Help or Hinder Mothers Who Breastfeed? *Journal of Advanced Nursing* 8:281–88.

Emde, R.N. 1980. Emotional Availability: A Reciprocal Reward System for Infants and Parents with Implications for the Prevention of Psychosocial Disorders. In *Parent-Infant Relationships.* P.M. Taylor, ed. New York: Grune and Stratton.

Enkin, Murray, and Iain Chalmers, eds. 1982. *Effectiveness and Satisfaction in Antenatal Care.* Philadelphia: J.B. Lippincott.

Erb, Lois, Gail Hill, and Doreen Houston. 1983. A Survey of Parents' Attitudes Towards Their Cesarean Births in Manitoba Hospitals. *Birth: Issues in Perinatal Care and Education* 10(2):85–91.

Erickson, E.H. 1959. *Identity and the Life Cycle: Selected Papers.* Psychological Issues, Volume 1.

Erickson, J. David, and Tor Bjenkedal. 1982. Fetal and Infant Mortality in Norway and the United States. *Journal of the American Medical Association* 247(7):987–91.

Ettner, Frederic. 1977. Hospital Obstetrics: Do the Benefits Outweigh the Risks? In *21st Century Obstetrics Now.* David Stewart and Lee Stewart, eds. Marble Hill, Mo: NAPSAC.

————. 1976. Comparative Study of Obstetrics, with Data and Details of a Working Physician's Home O.B. Service. In *Safe Alternatives in Childbirth*. David Stewart and Lee Stewart, eds. Marble Hll, Mo: NAPSAC

Fabrega, Horacio. 1979. The Scientific Usefulness of the Idea of Illness. *Perspectives in Biology and Medicine* 22:545–58.

————. 1972. Concepts of Disease: Logical Features and Social Implications. *Perspectives in Biology and Medicine* 15(4):538–617.

Feeley-Harnik, Gillian. 1981. *The Lord's Table: Euchrist and Passover in Early Christianity*. Philapdelphia: University of Pennsylvania Press.

Feldman, G., and A. May Freiman. 1985. Prophylactic Cesarean Section at Term? *New England Journal of Medicine* 312(19):1264–67.

Feldman, H., and B. Rollins. 1970. Marital Satisfaction over the Family Life Cycle. *Journal of Marriage and the Family* 32:2–28.

Feldman, Sylvia. 1980. *Choices in Childbirth*. New York: Bantam.

Field, T.S., et al. n.d. Effects of Tactile-Kinesthetic Stimulation on Preterm Neonates. unpublished manuscript.

Filkens, K., and J.F. Ruso, eds. 1985. *Human Prenatal Diagnosis*. New York: Marcel Dekker.

Flynn, A. M., et al. 1978. Ambulation in Labor. *British Medical Journal* 2:591–93.

Fogel, Catherine Ingram. 1981. High Risk Pregnancy. In *Health Care of Women: A Nursing Perspective*. Catherine Ingram Fogel and Nancy Fugate Woods, eds. St. Louis: C.V. Mosby.

Folkenberg, Judy. 1984. Illness, Poverty, and Infants: Preventing Early Damage. *Grantsmanship Center News*. January/February:4–6.

Ford, C.S. 1964. *A Comparative Study of Human Reproduction*. New Haven: Human Relations Area Files Press.

Foster, George and Barbara G. Anderson. 1978. *Medical Anthropology*. New York: John Wiley and Sons.

Fox, Daniel M., et al. 1986. Special Section on the Treatment of Handicapped Newborns. Daniel M. Fox, guest editor. *Journal of Health Politics, Policy, and Law* 11(2):195–303.

Fox, Renee. 1980. Evolution of Medical Uncertainty. *Health and Society* 58(1):1–49.

————. 1976. Advanced Medical Technology—Social and Ethical Implications. *Annual Review in Sociology* 2:231–68.

Frank, E., C. Anderson and D. Rubinstein. 1980. Marital Role Ideals and Perception of Marital Role Behavior in Distressed and Non-distressed Couples. *Journal of Marital and Family Therapy* 6: 269–82.

Frohock, F.M. 1986. *Special Care: Medical Decisions at the Beginning of Life*. Chicago: University of Chicago Press.

Fullard, W., and A.M. Reiling. 1976. An Investigation of Lorenz's Babyness. *Child Development* 47:1191–93.

Fullerton, Judith D. Townsend. 1982. The Choice of In-Hospital or Alternative Birth Environment as Related to the Concept of Control. *Journal of Nurse-Midwifery* 27(2):17–22.

Gardner, B.T., and L. Wallach. 1965. Shapes of Heads Identified as a Baby's Head. *Perceptual and Motor Skills* 20:135–42.

Garland, Corine, et al., eds. 1981. *Early Intervention for Children with Special Needs and Their Families.* WESTAR Series Paper #11. Chapel Hill: Frank Porter Graham Child Development Center, University of North Carolina.

Gaskin, Ina May. 1978. *Spiritual Midwifery.* revised edition. Summertown, Tenn.: Book Publishing Co.

Geertz, Clifford. 1973. *The Interpretation of Cultures.* New York: Basic Books.

Gendlin, Eugene. 1978. *Focusing.* New York: Dodd, Mead.

Gilligan, Carol. 1982. *In a Different Voice.* Cambridge, Mass: Harvard University Press.

Glenn, N., and C. Weaver. 1978. A Multivariate Multisurvey Study of Marital Happiness. *Journal of Marraiage and the Family* 40:269–82.

Gliedman, John, and William Roth. 1980. *The Unexpected Minority: Handicapped Children in America.* Carnegie Council on Children. New York: Harcourt Brace Jovanovich.

Goffman, Erving. 1963. *Stigma: Notes on the Management of a Spoiled Identity.* Englewood Cliffs, N.J.: Prentice-Hall.

Goldberg, Susan. 1983. *Parent-Infant Bonding: Another Look.* Child Development 54:1355–82.

Goldfarb, J., and E. Tibbets. 1980. *Breastfeeding Handbook: A Practical Reference for Physicians, Nurses, and Other Health Professionals.* New Jersey: Enslow Publishers.

Goodine, L.A., and P.A. Fried. 1984. Infant Feeding Practices: Pre- and Postnatal Factors Affecting Choice of Method and Duration of Breastfeeding.*Canadian Journal of Public Health* 75:439–44.

Goodlin, Robert C. 1980. Low Risk Obstetric Care for Low Risk Mothers. *Lancet* 10(May):1017–19.

Goodman, Ellen. 1979. *Turning Points.* New York: Fawcett Columbine.

Gortmaker, S. 1979. The Effects of Prenatal Care Upon the Health of the Newborn. *American Journal of Public Health* 69:653–60.

Gottfried, A.W., et al. 1981. Physical and Social Environments of Newborn Infants in Special Care Units. *Science* 214:673–75.

Gottlieb, B.H. 1981. Social Networks and Social Support in Community Mental Health. In *Social Networks and Social Support.* B.H. Gottlieb, ed. Beverly Hills: Sage.

Gral, R., et al. 1981. *The Father Book: Pregnancy and Beyond.* Washington, D.C.: Acropolis Books.

Greenberg, M., and N. Morris. 1974. Engrossment: The Newborn's Impact upon the Father. *American Journal of Orthopsychiatry* 44(4):520–31.

Greenberg. R. 1983. The Impact of Prenatal Care in Different Social Groups. *American Journal of Obstetrics and Gynecology* 145:797–801.

Grossman, F., et al. 1980. *Pregnancy, Birth, and Parenthood.* San Francisco: Jossey-Bass.

Gruis, Marcia. 1977. Beyond Maternity: Post Partum Concerns of Mothers. *American Journal of Maternal Child Nursing* May/June:182–88.

Guillemin, Jeanne. 1985. Physician Attitudes Towards Critically Ill Newborns. unpublished survey data.

———. 1981. Babies by Cesarean: Who Chooses, Who Controls? *Hastings Center Report* 11:15–18.

Guillemin, Jeanne, and L.L. Holmstrom. 1986. *Mixed Blessings: Intensive Care for the Newborn*. New York: Oxford University Press.

————. 1983. Legal Cases, Government Regulations, and Clinical Realities in Newborn Intensive Care. *American Journal of Perinatology* 1(1):89–97.

Gunn, Tania. 1984. The Incidence of Breast Feeding and Reasons for Weaning. *New Zealand Medical Journal* 97:360–63.

Gussler, Judith D., and Linda H. Briesemeister. 1980. The Insufficient Milk Syndrome: A Biocultural Explanation. *Medical Anthropology* 4(2):3–24.

Gussler, Judith D., and Nancy Mock. 1983. A Comparative Description of Feeding Practices in Zaire, the Phillipines, and St. Kitts-Nevis. *Ecology of Food and Nutrition* 13:75–85.

Gustaitis, Rasa, and Ernle W.D. Young. 1986. *A Time To Be Born, A Time To Die: Conflicts and Ethics in an Intensive Care Nursery*. Reading, Mass: Addison Wesley

Guthrie, Helen A., and Eva Kan. 1977. Infant Feeding Decisions—Timing and Rationale. *Journal of Tropical Pediatrics/Environmental Child Health* 23:264–66.

Gutmann, D. 1965. Women and the Conception of Ego Strength. *Merrill-Palmer Quarterly* 11:229–40.

Hack, Maureen, et al. 1980. Changing Trends of Neonatal and Postneonatal Deaths in Very Low Birthweight Infants. *American Journal of Obstetrics and Gynecology* 137:797–800.

Hahn, Robert A., and Arthur Kleiman. 1983. Biomedical Practice and Anthropological Theory:Frameworks and Directions. *Annual Review of Anthropology* 12:305–333.

Haire, D.B. 1972. *The Cultural Warping of Childbirth*. ICEA News.

Hall, D.G.E. 1968. *A History of South-East Asia*. Fourth edition. New York: St. Martin's Press.

Hally, Margaret R., et al. 1984. Factors Influencing the Feeding of First-Born Infants. *Acta Paediatrica Scandinavica* 73:33–39.

Hancock, Emily. 1976. Crisis Intervention in a Newborn Nursery Intensive Care Unit. *Social Work in Health Care* 1:421–33.

Hanmer, Jalna. 1981. Sex Predetermination, Artificial Insemination, and the Maintenance of Male-Dominated Culture. In *Women, Health, and Reproduction*. Helen Roberts, ed. London: Routledge and Kegan Paul.

Haraway, Donna. 1985. Manifesto for Cyborgs: Science, Technology, and Socialist Feminism in the 1980's. *Socialist Review* 80:65-107.

Harris, Harry. 1974. *Prenatal Diagnosis and Selective Abortion*. Cambridge, Mass.: Harvard University Press.

Harrison, Margaret J., Janice M. Morse, and Margaret Prowse. 1985. Successful Breastfeeding: The Mother's Dilemma. *Advanced Journal of Nursing*. 10:261–69.

Harrison, Michelle. 1982. *A Woman in Residence*. New York: Random House.

Harwood, Alan. 1971. The Hot-Cold Theory of Disease: Implications for Treatment of Puerto Rican Patients. *Journal of the American Medical Association* 216(7):1153–58.

Hazell, Lester. 1974. *Birth Goes Home*. Seattle: Catalyst Press.

Heckler, Margaret. 1983. *Healthy Mothers, Healthy Babies: A Goal We Can All*

Help Attain. Editorial. Public Health Reports 98(6) 529.

Hein, Herman. 1982. Secrets from Sweden. *Journal of the American Medical Association* 247(7):987–91.

Helper, Malcolm M, et al. 1968. Life-Events and the Acceptance of Pregnancy. *Journal of Psychosomatic Research* 12:183–88.

Henshaw, Stanley, and Greg Martire. 1982. Abortion and the Public Opinion Polls. *Family Planning Perspectives* 14:53–62.

Hern, Warren. 1975. The Illness Parameters of Pregnancy. *Social Science and Medicine* 9:365–72.

Hilberman, Mark. 1975. The Evolution of Intensive Care Units. *Critical Care Medicine* 3(4):159–65.

Hill, R.L., J.M. Stycos, and K.W. Black. 1970. *Family Development in Three Generations.* Cambridge, Mass.: Schenkman Publishing.

Hilton, Bruce, et al., eds. 1973. *Ethical Issues in Human Genetics.* New York: Plenum.

Himmerstein, D., et al. 1984. Patient Transfers: Medical Practices as Social Triage. *American Journal of Public Health* 74:494–96.

Hinds, M., G. Bergeisien, and D. Allen. 1985. Neonatal Outcome in Planned *vs.* Unplanned Out-of-Hospital Births in Kentucky. *Journal of the American Medical Association* 253(11):1578–82.

Hirsham, C., and J.A. Sweet. 1974. Social Background and Breastfeeding among American Mothers. *Social Biology* 21:39–47.

Hobel, Calvin, et al. 1973. Prenatal and Intrapartum High-Risk Screening: Prediction of the High Risk Neonate. *American Journal of Obstetrics and Gynecology* 117:1–9.

Holland, Lin, and Lee Ellen Rogich. 1980. Dealing with Grief in the Emergency Room. *Health and Social Work* 5:12–17.

Hollingshead, A.B. 1965. *Two Factor Index of Social Position.* New Haven, Conn.: Yale Station.

Homans, H. 1982. Pregnancy and Birth as Rites of Passage for Two Groups of Women in Britain. In *Ethnography of Fertility and Birth.* C. MacCormack, ed. New York: Academic Press.

Honeycutt, J., C. Wilson, and C. Parker. 1982. Effect of Sex and Degrees of Happiness on Perceived Styles of Communicating In and Out of the Marital Relationship. *Journal of Marriage and the Family* 44:395—406

Hood, Lynley J., et al. 1978. Breastfeeding and Some Reasons for Electing to Wean the Infant: A Report from the Dunedin Multidisciplinary Child Development Study. *The New Zealand Medical Journal* 624:273–76.

Hook, Ernest B. 1981. Rates of Chromosome Abnormalities at Different Maternal Ages. *Obstetrics and Gynecology* 58:282–85.

———. 1973. Behavior Implications of the Human XXY Genotype. *Science* 179 (January 12):139–49.

Hook, Ernest B., Philip K. Cross, and Dina M. Schreinemachers. 1983. Chromosomal Abnormality Rates at Amniocentesis and in Live-born Infants. *Journal of the American Medical Association* (April 15):2034–38

Hostetler, John A. 1974. *Hutterite Society.* Baltimore: Johns Hopkins University Press.

Houston, Mary J. 1984. Supporting Breast Feeding at Home. *Midwives*

Chronicle and Nursing Notes 97:42–44.

Hsu, Lillian. 1982. *Keeping Genetic Service Accessible: Report from a Conference on the Continuing Role of the Prenatal Diagnosis Laboratory of New York City.* June.

Huckstedt, B. 1965. Experimentelle Untersuchungen zum "Kindchinscheme." *Zeitschrift für Experimentelle und Angewandte Psychologie* 12:421–50.

Hutchins, Vince, Samuel S. Kessel, and P. J. Placek. 1984. Trends in Maternal and Infant Health Factors Associated with Low Infant Birth Weight, United States, 1972 and 1980. *Public Health Reports* 99(2):162–71.

In the Matter of Claire C. Conroy. 1985. Supreme Court of New Jersey A-108. September term, 1983. Argued March 19, 1984. Decided January 17, 1985.

Inch, Sally. 1984. *Birth-Rights: What Every Parent Should Know About Childbirth in Hospitals.* New York: Pantheon Books.

Infants. 1978. *The Encyclopedia of Bioethics.* W.T. Reich, ed. New York: The Free Press 2: 717–51.

Inglis, S.M. 1971. An Exploratory Study Concerning Emotional Tensions of the Post Partum Period. Master's thesis, University of Washington.

Institute of Medicine. 1985. *Preventing Low Birthweight.* Washington, D.C.: National Academy Press.

————. 1983. *Research Issues in the Assessment of Birth Settings.* Washington, D.C.: National Academy Press.

Jelliffe, Derrick B. 1975. Advertising and Infant Feeding. Editorial. *Journal of Tropical Pediatrics and Environmental Child Health* 21: 161-62.

Jenness, D. 1935. *The Ojibwa Indians of Parry Island: Their Social and Religious Life.* Bulletin 78. Ottowa: Canada Department of Mines.

Joans, Barbara. 1980. Dilemmas and Decisions of Prenatal Diagnosis. Symposium at the New York City Technical College. April.

Johnson, Jean E. 1973. Effects of Accurate Expectations about Sensations on the Sensory and Distress Components of Pain. *Journal of Personality and Social Psychology* 27(2):261–75.

Johnson, S. M., and L. F. Snow. 1982. Assessment of Reproductive Knowledge in an Inner-City Clinic. *Social Science and Medicine* 16:1657–62.

Jones, C.L. 1982. Environmental Analysis of Neonatal Intensive Care. *Journal of Nervous and Mental Disease* 179(April):130–42.

Jones, Collette. 1981. Father to Infant Attachment: Effects of Early Contact and Characteristics of the Infant. *Research in Nursing and Health* 4:193–450.

Jonsen, A.R., and M. Garland, eds. 1976. *Ethics of Newborn Intensive Care.* San Francisco: Health Policy Program, University of California.

Jordan, Brigitte. 1986. The Hut and the Hospital: Information, Power, and Symbolism in the Artifacts of Birth. To appear in *Birth: Issues in Perinatal Care and Education* 13 (2).

————. 1985. Biology and Culture: Some Thoughts on Universals in Childbirth. Paper presented at the meeting of the American Anthropological Association, Washington, D.C.

————. 1983. On the Social Distribution of Authoritative Knowledge in Childbirth. Paper presented at the meeting of the American Anthropological Association.

————. 1978. *Birth in Four Cultures: A Cross-Cultural Investigatioon of*

Childbirth in Yucatan, Holland, Sweden, and the United States. Vermont: Eden Press Women's Publications.

———. 1976. The Cultural Production of Childbirth. In *Women and Children in Contemporary Society.* N. Harmond, ed. Lansing: Michigan Women's Commission.

Kay, Margarita Artschwager, ed. 1982. *The Anthropology of Human Birth.* Philadelphia: F.A. Davis Co.

Kelley, Gerald, S.J. 1979. Quoted in *Principles of Biomedical Ethics.* Tom L. Beauchamp and James R. Childress. New York: Oxford University Press.

Kennell, John H., and Marshall H. Klaus. 1984. Mother-Infant Bonding: Weighing the Evidence. *Developmental Review* 4(3):275–82.

Kitchen, William H., and Laurence J. Murton. 1985. Survival Rates of Infants with Birth Weights between 501 and 1,000 g. *American Journal of Diseases of Children* 139:470–71.

Kitzinger, Sheila. 1980. *Women as Mothers: How They See Themselves in Different Cultures.* New York: Vintage Books.

Klaus, Marshall H., and John H. Kennell. 1982. *Parent-Infant Bonding.* St. Louis: C.V. Mosby.

———. 1976. *Maternal-Infant Bonding: The Impact of Early Separation or Loss in Family Development.* St. Louis: C.V. Mosby.

Klaus, Marshall, et al. 1972. Maternal Attachment: Importance of the First Postpartum Days. *New England Journal of Medicine* 288:460–63.

Klaus, Marshall H., et al. 1970. Human Maternal Behavior at the First Contact with Her Young. *Pediatrics* 46:187–92.

Kleinman, Arthur. 1975. Explanatory Models in Health Care Relationships. In *Health of the Family.* Washington, D.C.: National Council for International Health.

Konner, M.J. 1976. Maternal Care, Infant Behavior, and Development Among the !Kung. In *Kalahari Hunter-Gatherers: Studies of the !Kung San and Their Neighbors.* R. B. Lee and I. DeVore, eds. Cambridge, England: Cambridge University Press.

Koontz, Ann M. 1984. Pregnancy and Infant Health: Progress Toward the 1990 Objectives. *Public Health Reports* 99(2):184–92.

Kubler Ross, Elisabeth. 1969. *On Death and Dying.* New York: Macmillan.

Kuhse, Helga, and Peter Singer. 1985. *Should the Baby Live? The Problem of Handicapped Infants.* New York: Oxford University Press.

La Cerva. V. 1981. *Breastfeeding: A Manual for Professionals.* New York: Medical Examination Publication Co.

Laderman, Carol. 1983. *Wives and Midwives: Childbirth in Rural Malaysia.* Berkeley: University of California Press.

Lamb, M.E. 1982. Early Contact and Maternal-Infant Bonding: One Decade Later. *Pediatrics* 70 (5):763–68.

Lamb, M.E., et al. 1982. Mother- and Father-Infant Interaction Involving Play and Holding in Traditional and Non-Traditional Swedish Families. *Developmental Psychology* 18(20):215–21.

Lazarus, Ellen S. 1984. Pregnancy and Clinical Care: An Ethnographic Investigation of Perinatal Management for Puerto Rican and Low Income Women in the United States. Phd diss. Case Western Reserve University.

Leach, Edmund. 1979. Ritualization in Man in Relation to Conceptual and Social Development. In *Readings in Comparative Religion.* Fourth edition. Willam A. Lessa and Evon Vogt, eds. New York: Harper and Row.

Leavitt, J. W. 1983. Science Enters the Birthing Room: Obstetrics in America Since the Eighteenth Century. *Journal of American History* 70 (2):281-304.

Leavitt, Judith Walzer, and Whitney Walton. 1982. Down to Death's Door: Women's Perceptions of Childbirth. In *Childbirth: The Beginning of Motherhood. Proceedings of the Second Motherhood Symposium.* Madison, Wisconsin.

Lederman, Regina Placzek, C.G. Weingarten, and E. Lederman. 1981. Post-Partum Evaluation Questionnaire: Measurements of Maternal Adaptation. In *Perinatal Parental Behavior: Nursing Research and Implications for Newborn Health.* R. Lederman et al. New York: Alan R. Liss.

Lee, Kwang-Sun, et al. 1980. The Very Low-Birthweight Rate: Principle Predictor of Neonatal Mortality in Industrialized Populations. *Journal of Pediatrics* 97:759-64.

Lee, Kwang-sun, et al. 1976. Determinants of the Neonatal Mortality. *American Journal of Diseases of Children* 130:842-45.

LeMasters, E.E. 1957. Parenthood as Crisis. *Marriage and Family Living* 19:352-55.

Leonard, S.W. 1976. How First-Time Fathers Felt Toward Their Newborns. *Maternal Child Nursing.* November/December: 361-65.

Leslie, Charles, ed. 1976. *Asian Medical Systems: A Comparative Study.* Berkeley: University of California Press.

Letters. 1958. *Ladies Home Journal.* May.

Letters. 1968. Response to Zachary. *The Lancet.* (August 3): 7562.

Levin, Betty Wolder. 1985. Consensus and Controversy in the Treatment of Catastrophically Ill Newborns: Report of a Survey. In *Which Babies Shall Live: Medicine, Ethics, and the Imperiled Newborn.* Thomas H. Murray and Arthur L. Caplan, eds. Clifton, N.J.: Humana Press.

———. 1982. Cultural factors in the Choice of Medical Treatment: A Study of Decision-Making in Neonatology. Paper presented at the meeting of the American Anthropological Association, Washington, D.C..

Levinson, D.J. 1979. *The Season's of a Man's Life.* New York: Ballantine Books.

Lex, Barbara. 1979. The Neurobiology of Ritual Trance. In *The Spectrum of Ritual: A Bio-Genetic Structural Analysis.* E.G. d'Aquili et al., eds. New York: Columbia University Press.

Lifton, Robert Jay. 1979. Advocacy and Corruption in the Healing Professions. In *Nourishing the Humanistic in Medicine.* W.R. Rogers and D. Bernard, eds. Pittsburgh: University of Pittsburgh Press.

Lim, M.A., W.P. Wong, and T.A. Sinnathuray. 1977. Characteristics of Normal Labor among Different Racial Groups of Malaysia. *British Journal of Obstetrics and Gynecology* 84:600-4.

Lipkin, M., and P.. Rowley, eds. 1974. *Genetic Responsibility.* New York: Plenum.

Locke, H., and K. Wallace. 1959. Short Marital Adjustment and Prediction Tests: Their Reliability and Validity. *Marriage and Family Living* 21:251-55.

Long, J.G., A.G.S. Philip, and J. Lucey. 1980. Burnout in the Neonatal Intensive Care Unit. *Pediatrics* 65:182–90.

Lorber, 1971. Results of Treatment of Myelomeningocele: An Analysis of 524 Unselected Cases, with Special Reference to Possible Selection for Treatment. *Developmental Medicine and Child Neurology* 13:279–303.

Lubchenco, Lula O. 1963. Sequela of Premature Birth. *American Journal of the Disabled Child* 106:101–15.

Lubic, Ruth Watson. 1983. Childbirthing Centers: Delivering More for Less. *American Journal of Nursing* 1053-56.

Luker, Kristin. 1984. *Abortion and the Politics of Motherhood*. Berkeley: University of California Press.

Luria, A.R. 1966. *Higher Cortical Functions in Man*. New York: Basic Books.

Lyons, Jeff. 1985. *Playing God in the Nursery*. New York: Norton.

McCaffery, Margaret. 1984. Breastfeeding: Religious Experience or Hard Work? Editorial. *Canadian Family Physician* 30:1441–42.

MacCormack, Carol P., ed. 1982. *Ethnography of Fertility and Birth*. London: Academic Press.

McCormick, Marie C. 1985. The Contribution of Low Birthweight to Infant Mortality and Childhood Morbidity. *New England Journal of Medicine* 312(2):82–90.

McLain, Carol. 1983a. Perceived Risk and Choice of Childbirth Service. *Social Sciences and Medicine* 17(23):1857–65.

———. 1983b. Home Birth and Social Change. Paper presented at the meeting of the American Anthropological Association, Chicago.

———. 1982. Toward a Comparative Framework for the Study of Childbirth: A Review of the Literature. In *The Anthropology of Human Birth*. M. Kay, ed. Philadelphia: F.A. Davis.

———. 1981a. Women's Perception of Medical Risk and Choice of Childbirth Service. Paper presented at the meeting of the Society for Applied Anthropology, Edinburgh, Scotland.

———. 1981b. Women's Choice of Home or Hospital Birth. *Journal of Family Practice* 12(6):1033–38.

McManus, John. 1979. Ritual and Human Social Cognition. In *The Spectrum of Ritual*. E.G. d'Aquili et al., eds. New York: Columbia University Press.

McNatt, Nona. 1980. A Lesson in Empathy. *Obstetrics and Gynecology* 56(1):131–32.

Magnet, Joseph E., and W. Kluge Eike-Henner. 1985. *Withholding Treatment from Defective Newborns*. Cowansville, Que.: Brown Legal Publications.

Main, T. J. 1983. The Homeless of New York. *The Public Interest* 72:3–28.

Malinowski, Bronislaw. 1954. Magic, Science, and Religion. In *Magic, Science and Religion, and Other Essays*. New York: Doubleday (first published 1925).

Manderino, Mary, and Virginia M. Bzdek. 1984. Effects of Modeling and Information on Reactions to Pain: A Childbirth Preparation Analogue. *Nursing Research* 33(1):9–14.

Manderson, Lenore. 1981. Traditional Food Classifications and Humoral Medical Theory in Peninsular Malaysia. *Ecology of Food and Nutrition* 11:81–93.

Manniello, R., and P. Farrell. 1977. Analysis of the United States Neonatal

Mortality Statistics from 1968 to 1974, with Specific Reference to Changing Trends in Major Casualties. *American Journal of Obstetrics and Gynecology.* 129:667–74.

Margolis, Maxine L. 1984. *Mothers and Such: Views of American Women and Why They Changed.* Berkeley: University of California Press.

Marion, J.P., et al. 1980. Acceptance of Amniocentesis by Low-Income Patients in an Urban Hospital. *American Journal of Obstetrics and Gynecology* 138:11–15.

Marshall, Richard E., and Christine Kasman. 1980. Burnout in the Neonatal Intensive Unit. *Pediatrics* 65:1161–65.

Martinez, Gilbert A., and John P. Nalezienski. 1979. The Recent Trend in Breast-Feeding. *Pediatrics* 64:686–92.

Marut, Joanne S., and R.T. Mercer. 1981. The Cesarean Birth Experience: Implications for Nursing. In *Perinatal Parental Behavior: Nursing Research and Implications for Newborn Health.* R. Lederman et al. New York: Alan R. Liss.

Massenda, Katie. 1984. Comments. *Spokane Week,* October 23: A-3.

Mata, Leonardo. 1978. Breast-feeding: Main Promoter of Infant Health. *American Journal of Clinical Nutrition* 31 (11):2058–65.

Mead, Margaret, and Niles Newton. 1967. Cultural Patterning of Perinatal Behavior. In *Childbearing: Its Social and Psychological Aspects.* S. Richardson and A.F. Guttmacher, eds. Baltimore: Williams and Wilkins.

Mehl, Lewis. 1977. Research on Childbirth Alternatives: What Can It Tell Us About Hospital Practice? In *21st Century Obstetrics Now!* Lee Stewart and David Stewart, eds. Marble Hill, Mo.: NAPSAC.

Melmed, H., and M.I. Evans. 1976. Patterns of Labor in Native and Immigrant Populations in Israel. *Israel Journal of Medical Science* 12:1405–09.

Melzack, Ronald. 1984. The Myth of Painless Childbirth. *Pain* 19:321–37.

Melzack, Ronald, et al. 1981. Labor Is Still Painful after Prepared Childbirth. *Canadian Medical Journal* 125:357–63.

Mercer, Ramona. T. 1981. Factors Impinging on the Maternal Role in the First Year of Motherhood. In *Perinatal Parental Behavior: Nursing Research and Implications for Newborn Health.* R. Lederman et al. New York: Alan R. Liss.

Mercer, Ramona T., Kathryn C. Hackley, and Alan G. Bostrom. 1983. Relationship of Psychosocial and Perinatal Variables to Perception of Childbirth. *Nursing Research* 32(4):202–7.

Merchant, Carolyn. 1983. *The Death of Nature: Women, Ecology, and the Scientific Revolution.* San Francisco: Harper and Row.

Meyer, Herman F. 1968. Breastfeeding in the United States. *Clinical Pediatrics* 7:708–15.

Michigan Department of Public Health. 1984. *Annual Statistics.* Lansing, Mich.

Miller, C. Arden. 1985. Infant Mortality in the U.S. *Scientific American* 253(1):31–37.

Miller, C. Arden, et al. 1985. The World Economic Crisis and the Children: United States Case Study. *International Journal of Health Services* 15(1):95–134.

Minde, K., et al. 1980. Some Determinants of Mother-Infant Interaction in a Premature Nursery. *Journal of the American Academy of Child Psychiatry* 10:1–21.

Montagu, Ashley. 1937. *Coming Into Being among the Australian Aborigines.* London: G. Routledge and Sons.

Moore, Sally Falk, and Barbara Myerhoff, eds. 1977. *Secular Ritual.* Amsterdam, The Netherlands: Van Gorcum.

Morse, Janice M. In press. Cultural Variation in the Behavioral Response to Parturition: Childbirth in Fiji. *Medical Anthropology.*

———. 1984. The Cultural Context of Infant Feeding in Fiji. *Ecology of Food and Nutrition* 14:287–96.

———. 1982. Infant Feeding in the Third World: A Critique of the Literature. *Advances in Nursing Science* 5:77–88.

———. 1981. A Descriptive Analysis of Cultural Coping Mechanisms Utilized for the Reduction of Parturition Pain and Anxiety in Fiji. Ph.D. diss. University of Utah.

Morse, Janice M., M. Harrison, and M. Prowse. 1986 Minimal Breast-feeding. *Journal of Obstetric, Gynecologic, and Neonatal Nursing* 15(4):333–38.

Mulcahy, R.A., and N. Janz. 1973. Effectiveness of Raising Pain Perception Threshold in Males and Females Using a Psychoprophylactic Childbirth Technique During Induced Pain. *Nursing Research* 22:423–27.

Mumma, C., and J. Benoliel. 1984. Care, Cure, and Hospital Dying Trajectories. *Omega* 15(3):275–88.

Mundy, Karen C. 1983. The Medical Control of Female Health Care: An Analysis of a Contemporary Social Issue. Paper presented at the meeting of the Society for the Study of Social Problems.

Munn, Nancy D. 1973. Symbolism in a Ritual Context: Aspects of Symbolic Action. In *Handbook of Social and Cultural Anthropology.* Chapel Hill: Rand-McNally.

Murray, Thomas H. 1985. The Final Anticlimactic Rule on Baby Doe. *The Hastings Center Report* 15(3):5–9.

Murray, Thomas H., and Arthur L. Caplan. 1985. *Which Babies Shall Live?: Medicine, Ethics, and Imperiled Newborns.* Clifton, N.J.: Humana Press.

Nathanson, C.A., and M. Backer. 1985. Client-Provider Relationships and Teen Contraceptive Use. *American Journal of Public Health* 75(1):33–38.

National Center for Health Statistics. 1984a. *Health. United States.* DHHS Pub. No. (PHS) 85-1232. Washington, D.C.: U.S. Government Printing Office.

———. 1984b. *Advance Report of Final Mortality Statistics, 1982.* Monthly Vital Statistics Reports 33(9) Supplement, December 20.

National Institute for Child Health and Human Development. 1980. *Draft Report of the Task Force on Cesarean Childbirth.* Bethsda, Md.: National Institutes of Health.

Navran, L. 1967. Communication and Adjustment in Marriage. *Family Process* 6:173–84

Nelson, Margaret K. 1983. Working-Class Women, Middle-Class Women, and Models of Childbirth. *Social Problems* 30(3):284–91.

Neugarten, B. 1979. Time, Age, and the Life Cycle. *American Journal of Psychiatry* 136:887–94.

New York Times. 1985. Decline Slowing for Death Rate of U.S. Infants. (February 24):1,18.

———. 1984. Unwed Mothers Accounting for Third of New York Births. (August, 13):1,14.

———. 1983. Survey Shows Split on Issue of Treating Deformed Infants. (June 3):A14.

Newland, Kathleen. 1981. Infant Mortality and the Health of Societies. *Worldwatch*, no. 47. Washington, D.C.: Worldwatch Institute.

Newman, Lucile F. 1986. Premature Infant Behavior: An Ethological Study in a Special Care Nursery. *Human Organization* 45(4):327–33.

———.1984. Fitness and Survival: The High Risk-High Risk Spiral. Paper presented at the meeting of the American Anthropological Association, Denver.

———. 1983. Preterm Infants, Their Parents, and the Neonatal Intensive Care Nursery. In *Gynecology and Obstetrics.* J.J. Sciarra, ed. Philadelphia: Harper and Row.

———. 1981. Social and Sensory Environment of Low Birth Weight Infants. *Journal of Nervous and Mental Diseases* 169: 448—55.

———. 1980. Parents' Perception of their Low Birth Weight Infants. *Paediatrician* 9(3-4): 182–90.

Newton, Niles. 1972. Childbearing in Broad Perspective. In *Pregnancy, Birth, and the Newborn Baby.* Boston: Delacorte Press.

Nichter, Mark. 1980. The Layperson's Perception of Medicine as a Perspective into the Utilization of Multiple Therapy Systems in the Indian Context. *Social Science and Medicine* 14B:225–33.

Niswander, Kenneth. 1981. *Obstetrics: Essentials of Clinical Practice.* Boston: Little, Brown.

Niven, Catherine, and Karel Gijsbers. 1984. A Study of Labor Pain Using the McGill Pain Questionnaire. *Social Sciences and Medicine* 19(12):1347–51.

Norris, F., and R. Williams. 1984. Perinatal Outcomes among Medicaid Recipients in California. *American Journal of Public Health* 74(10):1112–17.

Notelovitz, Morris. 1978. The Single-Unit Delivery System—A Safe Alternative to Home Deliveries. *American Journal of Obstetrics and Gynecology* 132:889–94.

———. n.d. *New Understandings of the Physiology and Anatomy of Labor as Applied to Family-Centered Maternity Care.* Continuing Education Module. Spokane, Wash.: The Cybele Society.

Nuckolls, C.H., J. Cassel, and B.H. Kaplan. 1972. Psychosocial Assets, Life Crises, and the Prognosis of Pregnancy. *American Journal of Epidemiology* 95:431–41.

Nunnally, J.C. 1978. *Psychometric Theory.* Second edition. New York: McGraw-Hill.

Oakley, Ann. 1981. *Woman Confined: Sociology of Childbirth.* New York: Schocken.

———. 1980. *Becoming a Mother.* New York: Schocken.

———. 1979. A Case of Maternity: Paradigms of Women as Maternity Cases. *Signs* 4:607–31.

———. 1977. Cross-Cultural Practices. In *Benefits and Hazards of the New*

Obstetrics. T. Chard and M. Richards, eds. Philadelphia: J.B. Lippincott.

Oakley, Ann, A. MacFarland, and I. Chalmers. 1982. Social Class, Stress, and Reproduction. In *Disease and the Environment.* A.R. Rees and H.J. Purcell, eds. Chichester, England: John Wiley.

Obeyesekere, G. 1977. The Theory and Practice of Psychological Medicine in the Ayurvedic Tradition. *Culture, Medicine, and Psychiatry* 1:155–81.

O'Connor, S., et al. 1980. Reduced Incidence of Parenting Inadequacy Following Rooming In. *Pediatrics* 66:176.

Olds, David L. 1983. An Intervention Program for High-Risk Families. In *Minimizing High-Risk Parenting.* R.A. Hoekelman, ed. Johnson and Johnson Pediatric Roundtable 7. Media, Pa.: Harwal Publishing.

Ornstein, R. 1972. *The Psychology of Consciousness.* San Francisco: Freeman Press

Osofsky, Howard J., and Norman Kendall. 1973. Poverty as a Criterion of Risk. *Clinical Obstetrics and Gynecology* 168(1):103–19.

Oxorn, Harry, and William R. Foote. 1975. *Human Labor and Birth.* Third edition. New York: Appleton-Century-Crofts.

Palkovitz, R. 1982. Fathers' Birth Attendance, Early Extended Contact, and Father-Infant Interaction at Five Months Postpartum. *Birth* 9(3):173–77.

Paneth, Nigel, et al. 1982. Social Class Indicators and Mortality in Low Birthweight Infants. *American Journal of Epidemiology* 116(2):3674–75.

Pannabecker, B.J., R.N. Emde, and B.C. Austin. 1982. The Effect of Early Extended Contact on Father Newborn Interaction. *Journal of Genetic Psychology* 141:7–17.

Parfitt, Rebecca. 1977. *The Birth Primer: A Source Book of Traditional and Alternative Methods in Labor and Delivery.* Philadelphia: Running Press.

Parke, R.D., and S.E. O'Leary. 1976. Family Interaction in the Newborn: Some Findings, Some Observations, and Some Unresolved Issues. In *The Developing Individual in a Changing World.* K.F. Reegel and J.A. Meachan, eds. Chicago: Aldine.

Parke, R.D., S.E. O'Leary, and S. West. 1972. Mother-Father-Newborn Interactions: Effects of Maternal Medications, Labor, and Sex of Infant. *Proceedings of the 80th Annual Convention.* American Psychological Association.

Parke, R.D., and D.B. Sawin. 1976. Infant Characteristics and Behaviors and Elicitors of Maternal and Paternal Responsbility in the Newborn Period. Paper presented at the meeting of the Society for Research in Child Development, Denver.

Parmalee, Arthur H., et al. 1983. Social Influences on Infants at Medical Risk for Behavioral Difficulties. In *Frontiers of Infant Psychiatry.* Eleanor Galenson and Robert L. Tyson, eds. New York: Basic Books.

Parsons, Talcott, and Renee Fox. 1952. Therapy and the Modern Urban Family. *Journal of Social Issues* 8:31:44.

Parsons, Talcott, Renee Fox, and Victor M. Lidz. 1972. The Gift of Life and Its Reciprocation. *Social Research.* 39:369–415.

Petchesky, R. 1984. *Abortion and Women's Choice.* New York: Longman.

Peterson, G., and Lewis Mehl. 1984. *Pregnancy as Healing: A Holistic Philosophy for Prenatal Care.* Vols 1, 2. Berkeley: Mindbody Press.

Peterson, G., L. Mehl, and H. Leiderman. 1979. The Role of Some Birth-Related Variables in Father Attachment. *American Journal of Orthopsychiatry* 49(2):330–38.

Poland, Marilyn. 1984. *Unemployment, Stress and Infant Mortality: Detroit.* Monograph. Chapel Hill: University of North Carolina Press.

———. 1976. The Effects of Continuity of Care on the Missed Appointment Rate in a Prenatal Clinic. *Journal of Obstetric and Gynecological Nursing* 5:45–47.

Powledge, Tabitha., and John Fletcher. 1979. Guidelines for the Ethical, Social, and Legal Issues in Prenatal Diagnosis. *New England Journal of Medicine* 300:168–72.

Prenatal Diagnosis Laboratory of New York City. n.d. Counseling protocols, charts, and tables.

President's Commission for the Study of Ethical Problems in Medicine and Biomedical and Behavioral Research. 1983a. *Decisions to Forego Life-Sustaining Treatment: Ethical, Medical, and Legal Issues in Treatment Decisions.* Washington, D.C.: U.S. Government Printing Office.

———, 1983b. *Screening and Counseling for Genetic Conditions.* Washington, D.C.: U.S. Government Printing Office.

Pritchard, Jack A., and Paul C. MacDonals. 1980. *Williams Obstetrics.* 16th edition. New York: Appleton Century Crofts.

Pryor, Karen. 1973. *Nursing Your Baby.* New York: Pocket Books.

Public Health Reports. 1980. *Women and Health: United States 1980.* Supplement to September/October 95(5).

———. 1983. *Pregnancy and Infant Health, Summary of the Problem.* Supplement to September/October 98(5).

Pueschel, Siegfried, ed. 1978. *Down Syndrome: Growing and Learning.* Kansas City: Sheed Andrews and McMeel, Inc.

Quint, Jeanne. 1966. Awareness of Death and the Nurse's Composure. *Nursing Research.* 15: 49-55.

———. 1965. Institutional Practices of Informational Control. *Psychiatry* 18: 119–32.

Radin, R. 1983. Primary Caregiving and Role-Sharing Father. In *Nontraditional Families: Parenting and Child Development.* M.E. Lamb and S. Sagi, eds. Hillsdale, N.J.: Lawrence Erlbaum Associates.

Raphael, Dana. 1973. The Role of Breast-Feeding in a Bottle-Oriented World. *Ecology of Food and Nutrition* 2:121–26.

Rapp, Rayna. 1984. Amniocentesis: The Ethics of Choice. *Ms Magazine,* (April): 97–100.

Rappaport, Roy A., 1971. Ritual Sanctity and Cybernetics. *American Anthropologist* 73(1):59–76.

Redfield, Robert. 1960. The Folk Culture of Yucatan. In *The Anthropology of Folk Religion.* Charles Leslie, ed. New York: Vintage Books.

Reed, Dwayne M., and Fiona J. Stanley, eds. 1977. *The Epidemiology of Prematurity.* Baltimore/Munich: Urban and Schwarzenberg.

Reed, M.L. and J.B. Morris. 1979. Perinatal Care and Cost Effectiveness: Changes in Health Expenditures and Birth Outcome Following the Establishment of a Nurse-Midwife Program. *Medical Care* 17(5).

Rhoden, Nancy K,. and John D. Arras. 1985 Withholding Treatment from Baby Doe: From Discrimination to Child Abuse. *Milbank Memorial Fund Quarterly/Health and Society* 63(1):18–51.

Rich, Adrienne. 1976 *Of Woman Born: Motherhood as Experience and Institution*. New York: Norton.

Richardson, Stephen A., and Alan F. Guttmacher. 1967. *Childbearing: Its Social and Psychological Aspects*. Baltimore: Williams and Wilkens.

Richman, J., and W. Goldthorp. 1978. Fatherhood: The Social Construction of Pregnancy and Birth. In *The Place of Birth*. S. Kitzinger and J. Davis, eds. New York: Oxford.

Richmond, Julius B. 1969. *Currents in American Medicine: A Developmental View of Medical Care and Education*. Cambridge, Mass.: Harvard University Press.

Richmond-Abbot, M. 1983. *Masculine and Feminine: Sex Roles over the Life Cycle*. Reading, Mass.: Addison-Wesley Publishing.

Riordan, Jan. 1983. *A Practical Guide to Breastfeeding*. St. Louis: C.V. Mosby.

Robert Wood Johnson Foundation. 1985. *The Perinatal Program: What Has Been Learned*. Special Report Number 3. Princeton, N.J.: The Robert Wood Johnson Foundation.

Roberts, S. 1969. We Had A Baby. *Good Housekeeping* (May): 102ff.

Robson, Kenneth S. 1967. The Role of Eye-to-Eye Contact in Maternal-Infant Attachment. *Journal of Child Psychology and Psychiatry* 8:13–25.

Rodholm, M., and K. Larsson. 1982. The Behavior of Human Male Adults in Their First Contact with a Newborn Infant. *Behavior and Development* 5:121–30.

Romalis, Shelley, ed. 1981. *Childbirth: Alternatives to Medical Control*. Austin: University of Texas Press.

Rossi, Alice. 1980. Life Span Theories and Women's Lives. *Signs:.*6:4–32.

———. 1968. Transition to Parenthood. *Journal of Marriage and the Family* 30:26–39.

Rothman, Barabara Katz. 1986. *The Tentative Pregnancy*. New York: Viking/Penguin.

———. 1982. *In Labor: Women and Power in the Birthplace*. New York: W.W. Norton. (Reprinted as *Giving Birth: Alternatives in Childbirth*. New York: Penguin, 1985).

———. 1981. Awake and Aware or False Consciousness: The Cooption of Childbirth Reform in America. In *Childbirth: Alternatives to Medical Control*. S. Romalis, ed. Austin: University of Texas Press.

Rousseau, E. H., et al. 1982. Influence of Cultural and Environmental Factors on Breast-Feeding. *Canadian Medical Association Journal*. 127:701–4.

Rubin, Reva. 1963. Maternal Touch. *Nursing Outlook* 11:328–31.

Russell, Christine, and Felicity Barringer. 1983. "Baby Doe" Task Force Hits Snag. *The Washington Post* (May 23): A11.

Russell, G. 1982. Shared-Caregiving Families: An Australian Study. In *Nontraditional Families: Parenting and Child Development*. M.E. Lamb and S. Sagi, eds. Hillsdale, N.J.: Lawrence Erlbaum Associates.

Russell, Louise B. 1975. Intensive Care. In *Technology in Hospitals: Medical Advances and Their Diffusion*. Washington, D.C.: The Brookings Institute.

Sadovnick, A.D., and P. Baird. 1982. A Cost-Benefit Analysis of Prenatal Detection of Down Syndrome and Neural Tube Defects in Older Mothers. *American Journal of Medical Genetics.* 10: 367.

Sagi, A. 1982. Antecedents and Consequences of Various Degrees of Paternal Involvement in Childrearing: The Israeli Project. In *Non-traditional Families: Parenting and Child Development.* Hillsdale, N.J.: M.W. Lamb and S. Sagi, eds. Lawrence Erlbaum Associates.

Salk, Lee. 1970. The Critical Nature of the Postpartum Period in the Human for the Establishment of the Mother-Infant Bond: A Controlled Study. *Diseases of the Nervous System* 331:110–16.

Sargent, Carolyn., John. Marcucci, and Ellen. Eliston. 1983. Tiger Bones, Fire, and Wine: Maternity Care in the Kampuchean Refugee Community. *Medical Anthropology* 7(4):67–79.

Sauls, Henry S. 1979. Potential Effect of Demographic and Other Variables in Studies Comparing Morbidity of Breast-Fed and Bottle-Fed Infants. *Pediatrics* 64: 523–27.

Schafer, R., and R. Braito. 1979. Self-Concept and Role Performance Evaluation Among Marriage Partners. *Journal of Marriage and the Family* 37:263–75.

Scheper-Hughes, Nancy. 1984. Maternal Detachment and Infant Survival in a Brazilian Shantytown. Paper presented at the meeting of the American Anthropological Association, Denver.

Schluderman, S., and E. Schluderman. 1971. Maternal Child Rearing Attitudes in Hutterite Communal Society. *The Journal of Psychology* 79:169–77.

Schramm, W.F. 1985. WIC Prenatal Participation and Its Relationship to Newborn Medicaid Costs in Missouri: A Cost/Benefit Analysis. *American Journal of Public Health* 75(8): 851–57.

Schwartz, W., and P. Poppen. 1982. Measuring the Impact of Community Health Centers on Pregnancy Outcome. Contract #240–81–0041. Submitted to Division of Evaluation and Analysis, Health Resources and Services Administration, U.S. Department of Health and Humand Services.

Scully, Diane, and Pauline Bart. 1980. *Men Who Control Women's Health: The Miseducation of Obstetrician-Gynecologists.* Boston: Houghton-Mifflin.

———. 1973. A Funny Thing Happened on the Way to the Orifice: Women in Gynecological Textbooks. *American Journal of Sociology.* 78(4):1045-50.

Seiden, A. E. 1978. The Sense of Mastery in the Childbirth Experience. In *The Woman Patient.* C.C.. Nadelson and M.T. Notman, eds., New York: Plenum.

Shapiro, Sam, et al 1983. Changes in Infant Morbidity Associated with Decrease in Neonatal Mortality. *Pediatrics.* 72(3):408–15.

———. 1980. Relevance of Correlates of Infant Deaths for Significant Morbidity at 1 Year of Age. *American Journal of Obstetrics and Gynecology* 136:363.

Shapiro, Sam, et al. 1968. *Infant, Perinatal, Maternal ,and Childhood Mortality in the United States.* Cambridge, Mass.: Harvard University Press.

Shaw, Nancy Stoller. 1974. *Forced Labor: Maternity Care in the United States.* New York: Pergamon Press.

Shelp, Earl E. 1986. *Born To Die: Deciding the Fate of Critically Newborns.* New York: Free Press.

Shereshefsky, P., and L. Yarrow. 1973. *Psychological Aspects of a First Pregnancy and Early Postnatal Adaptation.* New York: Raven Press.

Shereshefsky, Pauline, et al. 1973. Maternal Adaptation. In *Aspects of a First Pregnancy and Early Postnatal Adaptation.* P. Shereshefsky and L.J. Yarrow, eds. New York: Raven Press

Sherman, Miriam. 1980. Pyschiatry in the Neonatal Intensive Care Unit. *Clinics in Perinatology* 7:33–46.

Showstack, Jonathan A., Peter Budetti, and Donald Minkler. 1984. Factors Associated with Birthweight: An Exploration of the Roles of Prenatal Care and Length of Gestation. *American Journal of Public Health* 74(9):1003–8.

Sidel, Victor, and Ruth Sidel. 1981. Health and Medical Care in the United States. In *The Sociology of Health and Illiness: Critical Perspectives.* Peter Conrad and Rochelle Kern. New York: St. Martin's Press.

Silverman, William. 1980. *Retrolental Fibroplasia: A Modern Parable.* New York: Grune and Stratton.

Sjolin, S.V., V. Hofvander, and C. Hillervik. 1977. Factors Related to Early Termination of Breastfeeding: A Retrospective Study. *Acta Paediatrica Scandinavica* 66:505–11.

Smilkstein, Gabriel, et al. 1984. Predictions of Pregnancy Complications: An Application of the Biopsychosocial Model. *Social Science and Medicine* 18(4):315–21.

Smith, Jack C., et al. 1984. An Assessment of the Incidence of Maternal Mortality in the United States. *American Journal of Public Health* 74(8):780–83.

Smith, Susan J. 1984. Surgeon General Urges More Moms to Breast-feed Babies. *Times-Union.* Rochester, N.Y. (June 13):58.

Smith-Rosenberg, Carroll. 1975. The Female World of Love and Ritual: Relations between Women in Nineteenth Century America. *Signs* 1:1–29.

Snow, L. F., S. M. Johnson., and H. Mayhew. 1978 The Behavioral Implications of Some Old Wives Tales. *Obstetrics and Gynecology* 51(6):727–32.

Sokal, D.C., et al. 1980. Prenatal Chromosome Analysis, Racial and Geographic Variation for Older Women. *Journal of the American Medical Association* 244:1355–547.

Sokal, R.R. and F.J. Rohlf. 1969. *Biometry.* San Francisco: W.H. Freeman.

Sokol, Robert, et al. 1980. Risk, Antepartum Care, and Outcome: Impact of a Maternity and Infant Care Project. *Obstetrics and Gynecology* 56(2):150–6.

Spanier, G., R. Lewis, and J. Cole. 1975. Marital Adjustment over the Family Life Cycle: The Issue of Curvilinearity. *The Journal of Marriage and the Family.* 37:263–75.

Stack, Carol. 1974. Sex Roles and Survival Strategies in an Urban Black Community. In *Women, Culture and Society.* Michelle Zimbalist Rosaldo and Louise Lamphere, eds. Stanford: Stanford University Press.

Stahlman, Mildred T. 1984. Neonatal Intensive Care: Success or Failure. *Journal of Pediatrics* 105(1):162–67.

Star, R. B.. 1986. *The Healing Power of Birth.* Austin, Texas: Star Publishing.

Starr, Paul. 1982. *The Social Transformation of Medicine.* New York: Basic Books.

Steven, R.J., and F. Heide. 1977. Analgesics Characteristics of Prepared

Childbirth Techniques: Attention Focusing and Systematic Relaxation. *Journal of Psychosomatic Research* 21:429–38.

Stewart, David and Lee Stewart, eds. 1977. *21st Century Obstetrics Now!* Vols. 1, 2. Marble Hill, Mo.: NAPSAC.

Stickle, G., and P. Ma. 1977. Some Social and Medical Correlates of Pregnancy Outcome. *American Journal of Obstetrics and Gynecology* 127:162–66.

Stinson, Peggy, and Robert Stinson. 1983. *The Long Dying of Baby Andrew.* Boston: Little-Brown.

Stone, Christopher I., Deborah A. Demchik-Stone, and John Horan. 1977. Coping with Pain: A Component Analysis of Lamaze and Cognitive-Behavioral Provedures. *Journal of Psychosomatic Research.* 21:451–56.

Sugarman, Muriel. 1979. Toward Really Improving the Outcome of Pregnancy: What You Can Do. *Birth and the Family Journal.* 6:109–18.

Surgeon General's Report on Health Promotion and Disease Prevention. 1979. *Healthy People.* DHEW no. 79-55071. Washington, D.C.: U.S. Department of Health, Education and Welfare.

Swinyard, Chester A. 1978. *Decision Making and the Defective Newborn.* Springfield, Ill: Charles C. Thomas.

Taylor, Jeffrey. 1984. Infant Mortality: Analysis and Recommendations for Action. Testimony presented to Committee of Energy and Commerce. Washington, D.C.

Tew, Marjorie. 1985. The Place of Birth and Perinatal Mortality. *Journal of the Royal College of General Practicioners* 35:390–94.

Thacker, S. B., and H. D. Banta. 1983. Benefits and Risks of Episiotomy. In *Obstetrical Intervention and Technology in the 1980's.* D. Young, ed. New York: The Haworth Press.

Thompson, Sharon. 1983. Felicita Garcia: I Just Came Out Pregnant! In *The Powers of Desire.* Ann Snitow, Christine Stansell, and Sharon Thompson, eds. New York: Monthly Review Press.

Tilden, Virginia P. 1983. The Relation of Life Stress and Social Support to Emotional Disequilibrium During Pregnancy. *Research in Nursing and Health* 6:167–74.

Todd, Alexandra Dundes. 1984. The Prescription of Contraception: Negotiations between Doctors and Patients. *Discourse Processes* 7:171–200.

Toney, Linnie. 1983. The Effects of Holding the Newborn at Delivery on Paternal Bonding. *Nursing Research* 21(1):16–19.

Trevathan, Wenda R. 1981. Maternal Touch at First Contact with the Newborn Infant. *Developmental Psychobiology* 14:549–58.

Turner, R. Jay, and Samuel Noh. 1983. Class and Pyschological Vulnerability among Women: The Significance of Social Support and Personal Control. *Journal of Health and Social Behavior* 24:2–15.

Turner, Victor W. 1979. Betwixt and Between: The Liminal Period in Rites of Passage. In *Reader in Comparative Religion..* W.A. Lessa and E. Vogt, eds. 4th edition. New York: Harper and Row.

———. 1974. *Dramas, Fields, and Metaphors: Symbolic Action in Human Society.* Ithaca: Cornell University Press.

———. 1969. *The Ritual Process: Structure and Anti-Structure.* Chicago: Aldine.

————. 1968. *The Drums of Affliction*. New York: Oxford University Press.

————. 1967. *The Forest of Symbols*. Ithaca: Cornell University Press.

United Nations. 1980. *Demographic Yearbook*. Pub. no. ST/ESA/STAT/SER/R/10. New York: United Nations.

United Nations Children's Fund. 1983. *World Economic Crisis and the Children. United States Case Study*. October 15.

United States Bureau of the Census. 1980. *Census of the Population. General Social and Economic Characteristics, United States* Summary. Washington D.C.: U.S. Department of Commerce.

United States Commission on Civil Rights. 1976. *Puertorriquenos en los Estados Unidos Continentales: Un Futuro Incierto*. Washington, D.C.: U.S. Government Printing Office.

United States Department of Health and Human Services. 1980. *Monthly Vital Statistics Report* 34 (June):4.

Vaillant, G.E. 1977. *Adaptation to Life*. Boston: Little Brown.

van Gennep, Arnold. 1966. *The Rites of Passage*. Chicago: University of Chicago Press. (First published 1908).

Ventura, Stephanie. 1984. Births of Hispanic Parentage, 1981. *Monthly Vital Statistics Reports* 33(8): Supplement.

Veronnen, P., et al. 1980. Promotion of Breast Feeding: Effect on Neonates to Change of Feeding Routine on a Maternity Unit. *Acta Pediatrica Scandinavica* 60: 279-82.

Vogt, Evon Z. 1976. *Tortillas for the Gods: A Symbolic Analysis of Zinacanteco Rituals*. Cambridge, Mass.: Harvard University Press.

Vohr, B.R., and M. Hack. 1982. Developmental Follow-up of Low Birth Weight Infants. *Pediatric Clinics of North America* 19(6):1441-54.

von Baeyer, V. L., M. E. Johnson, and M. J. McMillan. 1984. Consequences of Nonverbal Expression of Pain: Patient Distress and Observer Concern. *Social Sciences and Medicine* 19(12):1319–24.

Vorys, Lucy. 1977. The Age-Old Discrimination Against Midwives. *Mothering* 5: 50–56.

Walker, Bailus. 1983. The Impact of Unemployment on the Health of Mothers and Children in Michigan. Recommendations for the Nation. Hearing before the Committee on Educaiton and Labor. Washington, D.C.

Wallace, Anthony F.C. 1966. *Religion: An Anthropological View*. New York: Random House.

Wallace, Helen M. 1978. Status of Infant and Perinatal Morbidity and Mortality: A Review of the Literature. *Public Health Reports* 93(4): 386-93.

Weil, William, and Martin Benjamin, eds. 1987. *Ethical Issues at the Outset of Life*. Boston: Blackwell Scientific Publications.

Weiner, Carolyn, et al. 1979. Trajectories, Biographies, and the Evolving Medical Technology Scene: Labor and Delivery and the Intensive Care Nursery. *Sociology of Health and Illness* 1(3):261–83.

Weir, Robert. 1984. *Selective Non-Treatment of Handicapped Newborns*. New York: Oxford University Press.

Wellman, B. 1981. Applying Network Analysis to the Study of Support. In *Social Networks and Social Support*. B.H. Gottlieb, ed. Beverly Hills: Sage.

Wente, Arel S., and S.B. Crockenberg. 1976. Transition to Fatherhood, Lamaze Preparaion, Adjustment Difficulty and the Husband-Wife Relationship. *Family Coordinator.* October:351–57.

Wertz, Dorothy, and Richard C. Wertz. 1977. *Lying In: A History of Childbirth in America.* New York: Free Press.

Whichelow, Margaret J. 1982. Factors Associated with the Duration of Breast Feeding in a Privileged Society. *Early Human Development.* 7:273–80.

White, Marjorie, and Carolyn Dawson. 1981. The Impact of the At-Risk Infant on Family Solidarity. In *Perinatal Parental Behavior.* Birth Defects Original Article Series. R. Lederman et al. New York: Alan Liss.

Whiteford, L.M. 1983. Old Dames and New Babies: Gender Roles Among Women Over the Age of Thirty. Paper presented at the meeting of the American Anthropological Association.

Wiles, Leslie S. 1984. The Effect of Prenatal Breastfeeding Information on Breastfeeding Success and Maternal Perception of the Infant. *Journal of Obstetrical, Gynecologic and Neonatal Nursing* 13(4):253–57.

Wilkie, J.R. 1981. The Trend Toward Delayed Parenthood. *Journal of Marriage and the Family.* 43:583–91.

Winsberg, B., and M. Greenlick. 1967. Pain Response in Negro and White Obstetrical Patients. *Journal of Health and Social Behavior* 8:222–27.

Wise, P.H., et al. 1985. Racial and Socioeconomic Disparities in Childhood Mortality in Boston. *The New England Journal of Medicine.* 31(6):360–66.

Worthington, Everett L., Glen A. Martin, and Michael Shumate. 1982. Which Prepared-Childbirth Coping Strategies Are Effective? *Journal of Obstetric, Gynecological, and Neonatal Nursing* 11:45–51.

Yeung, D. 1983. *Infant Nutrition: A Study of Feeding Practices and Growth from Birth to 18 Months.* Ottawa: Canadian Public Health Association.

Zachary, R.B. 1968. Ethical and Social Aspects of Treatment of Spina Bifida. *The Lancet.* 7562 (Aug 3): 274–75.

Zaretsky, Eli. 1973. Capitalism, the Family and Personal Life. *Socialist Revolution.*, Jan-June (reprinted by Harper and Row/Torch, 1976).

Zax, Melvin, Arnold J. Smeroff and Janet E. Farnum. 1975. Childbirth Education, Maternal Attitudes, and Delivery. *American Journal of Obstetrics and Gynecology.* 123(1185–90.

Zborowski, Mark. 1969. *People in Pain.* San Francisco: Jossey-Bass.

———. 1952. Cultural Components in Response to Pain. *Journal of Social Issues.* 8:16–24.

Zemach, Rita. 1984. What the Vital Statistics System Can and Cannot Do. Editorial. *American Journal of Public Health* 74(8):756–58.

Zelizer, Viviana A. 1985. *Pricing the Priceless Child: The Changing Social Value of Children.* New York: Basic Books.

INDEX

Other books of interest

SILENT KNIFE
Cesarean Prevention & Vaginal Birth After Cesarean
NANCY WAINER COHEN & LOIS J. ESTNER
"The bible of cesarean prevention."
—THE WALL STREET JOURNAL
464 Pages   Illustrations

IMMACULATE DECEPTION
A New Look at Women and Childbirth
SUZANNE ARMS
"Essential reading for any woman who plans to have a baby in an American hospital."
—NEW YORK TIMES BOOK REVIEW
416 Pages   Illustrations

TRANSFORMATION THROUGH BIRTH
A Woman's Guide
CLAUDIA PANUTHOS
Foreword by Suzanne Arms
208 Pages   Illustrations

BABIES, BREASTFEEDING & BONDING
INA MAY GASKIN
"A uniquely personal book reflecting the author's extensive breastfeeding experience as both midwife and mother."
—MARIAN TOMPSON, LA LECHE LEAGUE INTERNATIONAL
240 Pages   Illustrations

THE VAGINAL BIRTH AFTER CESAREAN (VBAC) EXPERIENCE
Birth Stories by Parents & Professionals
LYNN BAPTISTI RICHARDS & CONTRIBUTORS
"It is the book for every woman who hopes for VBAC. In fact many first-time cesareans could be avoided if this book were read first. It is thorough, it is compassionate."
—ESTHER ZORN, CESAREAN PREVENTION MOVEMENT
304 Pages   Illustrations

ENDED BEGINNINGS
Healing Childbearing Losses
CLAUDIA PANUTHOS & CATHERINE ROMEO
224 Pages   Illustrations

THE PSYCHOLOGY OF SPIRITUAL GROWTH
Channelled from the Brotherhood by Mary E. Carreiro
160 Pages
A Gentle Wind Book, Volume I

MODERN RELIGON & THE DESTRUCTION OF SPIRITUAL CAPACITY
Channelled from the Brotherhood by Mary E. Carreiro
160 Pages
A Gentle Wind Book, Volume II

THE LAUGHING BABY
Remembering Nursery Rhymes & Reasons
ANNE SCOTT
Illustration by Lura Schwarz Smith
160 Pages   Illustrations/Musical Scores/Rhymes

WOMEN & HEALTH
Cross-Cultural Perspectives
PATRICIA WHELEHAN & CONTRIBUTORS
304 Pages

WOMEN'S WORK
Development & the Division of Labor by Gender
ELEANOR LEACOCK, HELEN I. SAFA & CONTRIBUTORS
320 Pages   Illustrations

WOMEN & COLONIZATION
Anthropological Perspectives
MONA ETIENNE, ELEANOR LEACOCK & CONTRIBUTORS
352 Páges   Illustrations

THE ANTHROPOLOGY OF MEDICINE
From Culture to Method
LOLA ROMANUCCI-ROSS, DANIEL MOERMAN,
LAURENCE R. TRANCREDI, M.D. & CONTRIBUTORS
416 Pages   Illustrations

FAMILIES & CHANGE
Social Needs & Public Policy
ROSALIE GENOVESE
360 Pages

COMING SOON

WOMAN TO MOTHER
A Transformation
VANGIE BERGUM
Foreword by Michel Odent
144 Pages   Illustrations
(June 1988)

HEALTH & DISEASE OF POPULATIONS IN TRANSITION
Epidemiological and Anthropological Perspectives
GEORGE J. ARMELAGOS, ALAN C. SWEDLUND &
CONTRIBUTORS
352 Pages
(September 1988)

IMMUNIZATION
The Reality Behind The Myth
WALENE JAMES
*The up-to-the-minute statement on vaccine damage . . . should
terrify every parent whose child faces immunization."*
—ROBERT S. MENDELSOHN, M.D., FROM THE FOREWORD
240 Pages
(March 1988)

HOME BIRTH, REVISED
ALICE GILGOFF
"[P]rovocative and enlightening . . . ."
                                        —PUBLISHERS WEEKLY

192 Pages   Illustrations
(July 1988)